Magnetic Resonance of the Cardiovascular System

EDITED BY

RICHARD UNDERWOOD

AND

DAVID FIRMIN

National Heart & Lung Institute
and National Heart & Chest Hospitals,
London, UK

OXFORD

BLACKWELL SCIENTIFIC PUBLICATIONS

LONDON EDINBURGH BOSTON

MELBOURNE PARIS BERLIN VIENNA

Editorial Offices:
Osney Mead, Oxford OX2 0EL
25 John Street, London WC1N 2BL
23 Ainslie Place, Edinburgh EH3 6AJ
3 Cambridge Center, Suite 208
Cambridge, Massachusetts 02142, USA
54 University Street, Carlton
Victoria 3053, Australia

Other Editorial Offices:
Arnette SA
2, rue Casimir-Delavigne
75006 Paris
France

Blackwell Wissenschaft
Meinekestrasse 4
D–1000 Berlin 15
West Germany

Blackwell MZV
Feldgasse 13
A–1238 Wien
Austria

First published 1991

Set by Setrite Typesetters, Hong Kong
Printed and bound in Great Britain
By Butler & Tanner Ltd,
Frome and London

DISTRIBUTORS

Marston Book Services Ltd
PO Box 87
Oxford OX2 0DT
(*Orders*: Tel. 0865 791155
Fax: 0865 791927
Telex: 837515)

USA
Mosby-Year Book, Inc.
200 North LaSalle Street
Chicago, Illinois 60601
(*Orders*: Tel: (312) 726–9733)

Canada
Mosby-Year Book, Inc.
5240 Finch Avenue East
Scarborough, Ontario
(*Orders*: Tel: (416) 298–1588)

Australia
Blackwell Scientific Publications
(Australia) Pty Ltd
54 University Street
Carlton, Victoria 3053
(*Orders*: Tel: (03) 347–0300)

British Library
Cataloguing in Publication Data

Magnetic resonance of the cardiovascular system.
1. Man. cardiovascular system. Diagnosis. Diagnosis of cardiovascular system of man.
I. Underwood, Richard II. Firmin, David
616.1207548

ISBN 0–632–02356–2

Contents

List of Contributors

PETER BUSER, MD, *Division of Cardiology, University Hospital, Petersgraben 4, CH–4031 Basel, Switzerland*

GREGORY B. CRANNEY, MB, BS, FRACP, *Assistant Professor of Medicine, Division of Cardiovascular Disease, and Clinical Director, Center for Nuclear Magnetic Resonance Research and Development, The University of Alabama at Birmingham, Birmingham, Alabama 35294, USA*

DAVID N. FIRMIN, PhD, *Senior Lecturer, National Heart & Lung Institute, Magnetic Resonance Unit, 30 Britten St, London SW3 6NN, UK*

CHARLES B. HIGGINS, MD, *Professor of Radiology, and Chief of Magnetic Resonance Imaging, University of California, San Francisco, Box 0628, C309, CA 94143, USA*

DONALD B. LONGMORE, FRCS(Ed), FRCR, *Professor of Magnetic Resonance in Medicine, National Heart & Lung Institute, Magnetic Resonance Unit, 30 Britten St, London SW3 6NN, UK*

CHAIM S. LOTAN, MD, *Research Fellow, Center for Nuclear Magnetic Resonance Research and Development, Division of Cardiovascular Disease, The University of Alabama at Birmingham, Birmingham, Alabama 35294, USA*

RAAD H. MOHIADDIN, MB, ChB, MSc, *Senior Research Fellow, National Heart & Lung Institute, Magnetic Resonance Unit, 30 Britten St, London SW3 6NN, UK*

GERALD M. POHOST, MD, *Director, Division of Cardiovascular Disease, and Director, Center for Nuclear Magnetic Resonance Research and Development, The University of Alabama at Birmingham, Birminghem, Alabama 35294, USA*

BERTIL R.R. PERSSON, DPhil, *Professor of Medical Radiation Physics, Lund University, Lasarettet, S-221 85 Lund, Sweden*

GEORGE K. RADDA, DPhil, FRS, *British Heart Foundation Professor of Molecular Cardiology, University of Oxford, Department of Biochemistry, South Parks Road, Oxford OX1 3QU, UK*

BHEESHMA RAJAGOPALAN, DPhil, FRCP, *Honorary Consultant Physician, Nuffield Department of Medicine, John Radcliffe Hospital, Headington, Oxford OX3 9DU, UK*

SIMON REES, FRCP, FRCR, *Director of Radiology, Royal Brompton & National Heart Hospital, Fulham Road, London SW3 6HP, UK*

UDO SECHTEM, MD, *Oberarzt der Klinik III für Innere Medizin, Universtität zu Köln, Joseph-Stelzmannstraße 9, 5000 Köln 41, Germany*

RICHARD SEMELKA, MD, *Department of Radiology, Magnetic Resonance Section, University of California, San Francisco, CA 94143, USA*

FREDDY R. STÅHLBERG, PhD, *Associate Professor of Radiation Physics, Lund University, Lasarettet, S-221 85 Lund, Sweden*

S. RICHARD UNDERWOOD, MA, MRCP, *Marcus Sieff Senior Lecturer in Cardiac Imaging, National Heart & Lung Institute, Magnetic Resonance Unit, 30 Britten St, London SW3 6NN, UK*

STEFAN WAGNER, MD, *University of Bonn, Department of Radiology, Sigmund Freud Straße 25, 5300 Bonn, Germany*

Preface

As the seasons come and go and hem-lines rise and fall so, to some extent, do fashions in medicine. There is no shortage of enthusiasts to extol the virtues of their own methods of diagnosis or management, and acceptance of new techniques is made the more easy by sophisticated marketing methods against which not even the scientific community is immune. To counter this the medical establishment argues, rightly, that new techniques must be tested against the old and not adopted until their strengths and weaknesses are appreciated and can be applied to best advantage.

Against this background, the growth of magnetic resonance imaging is remarkable. Its immediate acceptance stems from the clarity of the images that it provides, particularly in the central nervous system and other static organs, and it is in these fields that it has been most widely applied. There has been criticism that magnetic resonance has not been adequately compared with established techniques, but the more obvious the advantages, the more difficult it is to impose a rigorous comparison with, for instance, myelography or computed X-ray tomography. No one would deny their patients the benefit of penicillin for a streptococcal infection although we are not aware of a double blind placebo controlled trial proving its efficacy.

The immediate success of magnetic resonance imaging for the neuroradiologist, the orthopaedic surgeon, the rheumatologist, and others has to some extent hindered its application in the cardiovascular system. It is not simply that imaging a moving organ is more difficult. There are practical and financial difficulties in developing a technique using machines that are fully employed with the imaging of other systems. In addition, cardiologists have a tradition of performing their own investigations rather than requesting the help of imaging specialists. This has left many cardiologists ignorant of the capabilities of magnetic resonance and, perhaps more importantly, the resulting lack of demand affects the perception of equipment manufacturers of where their products could be most profitably applied. There are approximately 2000 magnetic resonance scanners worldwide but only a few with expertise in the cardiovascular system, and less than a handful dedicated to the development of cardiovascular magnetic resonance. Contrast this with the fact that disease of the cardiovascular system kills one half of the Western world and disease of the coronary arteries one third.

We are particularly fortunate to work in an institution and with colleagues who have supported our belief that magnetic resonance can play an important role in the management of the cardiac patient. From our own and other centres' work it has been demonstrated that magnetic resonance does have a place in the assessment of cardiac anatomy, function and blood flow, and we believe that with further development, the majority rather than the minority of patients may benefit. No technique can be useful, however, unless it is widely available and widely applied. One is tempted to extend the argument about magnetic field strength—the best field strength is the one that you have—to diagnostic techniques: the best diagnostic technique is the one with which you are familiar.

For these reasons, we wanted to make our own experience available to others. We hope that this book will be valuable to many different groups but we have written and edited it with cardiologists, cardiac and general radiologists, and physicists in mind. We have assumed no knowledge of magnetic resonance but perhaps a little knowledge of clinical cardiology, and we hope that this policy will be suitable not only for those in training but also for workers already in the field. We make no apology for covering the principles of magnetic resonance when some readers may not turn to a specialist book such as this for their initial grounding. We have adopted this approach above all because we hope that clinical cardiologists will be attracted and many of these will be unfamiliar with the physical principles. Another selfish reason is that we both enjoy our daily battles with the many variables that combine to make magnetic resonance such a powerful technique. Some colleagues are confounded by these complexities and it is a pleasure to be able to provide our own view of the subject. Whilst we have not adopted the challenging policy of asking a clinician to cover the physics and vice versa, we hope that our close collaboration has achieved the same effect.

RICHARD UNDERWOOD
DAVID FIRMIN
London

Acknowledgements

No one can be expert in all areas of cardiovascular magnetic resonance and we are indebted to our friends and colleagues who have enriched this book by their contributions. We are most grateful to Professor Donald Longmore who, far sighted as always, saw the power of magnetic resonance in the cardiovascular system before many others. Without his energy and enthusiasm magnetic resonance would probably not be available to us and many of the developments described in this book would have been slow to occur.

Magnetic resonance is a speciality that requires the input of different skills. Many colleagues have contributed directly and indirectly and we should like to acknowledge their contributions. They include Dr Makoto Amanuma, Mr Peter Andrews, Mrs Mary Bailey, Mr Russell Bergman, Dr Charles Bland, Professor Hugo Bogren, Dr David Bryant, Miss Elisabeth Burman, Professor Graham Bydder, Miss Lindsay Carver, Dr Valmai Cook, Dr Brian Dalton, Dr Robert Dickinson, Dr Kim Fox, Mr Alistair Hall, Miss Victoria Harding, Sir Godfrey Hounsfield, Ms Jennifer Keegan, Dr Kok-tee Khaw, Dr Philip Kilner, Dr Richard Klipstein, Dr Eunice Lockey, Mr Karl Lotey, Dr Douglas Lowell, Mr Mark McNeilly, Dr Surya Mohapatra, Dr Raad Mohiaddin, Dr Graham Nayler, Miss Sharmin Obeyesekara, Dr Martin Paley, Mr Kirit Patel, Dr Rami Paz, Dr Dudley Pennell, Miss Jacqueline Pennock, Professor Philip Poole-Wilson, Dr Chris Randall, Dr Simon Rees, Dr Cynthia Sampson, Professor Robert Steiner, Mrs Rosheen Vernon, Dr Samuel Wann, Dr Mikio Watanabe, Miss Marjorie Watson and Dr Ian Young.

As well as people, magnetic resonance research requires funding. We are particularly grateful to the Royal Brompton & National Heart Hospital, CORDA, Picker International Ltd, the League of Friends, the Medical Research Council, Sir Hector Laing and the many firms contributing to his Normal Subjects' Scheme, Marks & Spencer PLC, Sir Robert McAlpine PLC, John Laing PLC, and the trustees of the Wolfson, Viscount Royston, Halley Stewart, and Maurice Laing Trusts.

Chapter 1
The Principles of Magnetic Resonance

DAVID FIRMIN

The physical principles of magnetic resonance are more complex than those underlying other techniques in medicine. A confounding factor is that a full understanding is impossible without resort to quantum mechanics — a topic which those without a grounding in physics find abstract and difficult to grasp. The innocent reader may wonder why he or she should be subjected to these principles in the opening chapter of a book aimed principally at clinicians, but a knowledge of the subject is both rewarding and essential for anybody who works with magnetic resonance. Several excellent and detailed descriptions are available from other sources,[1–7] but this chapter provides a description which is within the grasp of the majority of clinicians, yet includes some of the more difficult concepts.

Two sections follow, the first giving a description based upon quantum mechanics and the second upon classical Newtonian physics. It is fortunate that both of these descriptions are reasonably consistent for the radio wave section of the electromagnetic spectrum, and since the quantum mechanical description is not essential to a basic understanding of magnetic resonance, some readers may wish to jump to the classical description.

The reasons for the similarity between the two descriptions are several. The predictions of quantum theory and classical physics converge as ΔE, the separation of quantised nuclear energy levels, tends towards the mean molecular thermal energy, kT. In addition the quantum mechanical constant, h (Planck's constant), is absent from the principal magnetic resonance equation that relates the angular frequency of nuclear magnetic resonance, ω_0, and the applied magnetic field, B_0:

$$\omega_0 = \gamma B_0 \tag{1.1}$$

where γ is a constant known as the gyromagnetic ratio, which is specific to each nucleus.

1.1 Quantum mechanical description

1.1.1 Nuclear spin and magnetism

Atomic nuclei possess a property referred to as spin, and quantum mechanics dictates that their angular momentum can only have certain discrete values, determined by the nuclear spin quantum number I. The magnitude, p, of the nuclear angular momentum is given by the equation:

$$p = \frac{h}{2\pi} \sqrt{I(I + 1)} \tag{1.2}$$

where h is Planck's constant (6.6×10^{-34} J·s).

The nuclear spin quantum number can only have integral or half integral values, although an explanation of this would involve a venture into the theory of nuclear physics which is beyond the scope of this book. However, the value always conforms to one of three simple rules:

1 Nuclei with even mass have an integral value of I, examples being deuterium-2 and nitrogen-14.

2 Nuclei with even mass and even charge have $I = 0$, examples being carbon-12 and oxygen-16.

3 Nuclei with odd mass have half integral I, examples being hydrogen-1, carbon-13, and phosphorus-31.

Angular momentum is a vector since it has both magnitude and direction. In quantum systems it can only have certain orientations and a further quantum number, m, is used to describe these orientations. For example, the orientation of p with respect to an arbitrary axis z is described by defining the component of p in the z direction which is given by the equation:

$$p_z = m\hbar \tag{1.3}$$

where $\hbar = h/2\pi$.

The quantum number, m, is allowed a total of $2I+1$ values, these being I, $I-1$, $I-2$, ..., $-I$. The hydrogen

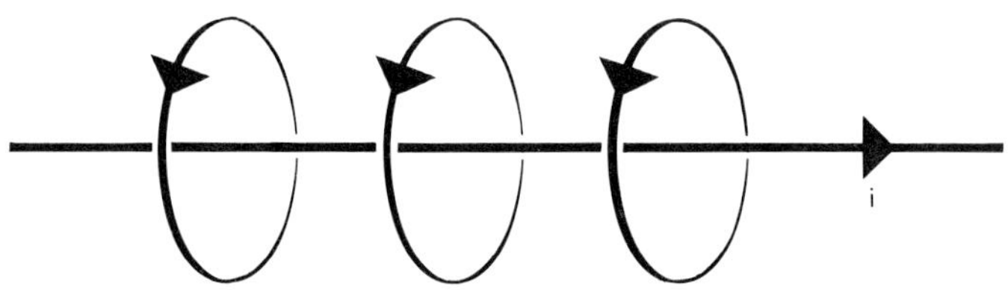

Figure 1.1. A current flowing along a straight conductor creates a circular magnetic field.

nucleus with nuclear spin $I = \frac{1}{2}$ has two orientations with angular momentum:

$$p_z = \pm \tfrac{1}{2}\hbar \qquad (1.4)$$

The combination of charge and spin leads to a magnetic field. We are familiar with this from the circular magnetic field associated with an electrical current flowing along a conductor (figure 1.1). If the conductor is bent into a loop then the magnetic lines accumulate through the centre of the loop to produce a magnetic dipole moment (figure 1.2). Similar effects occur on a nuclear scale. Thus positively charged nuclei with both spin and angular momentum produce a tiny magnetic dipole moment, μ. The magnetic moment and angular momentum of the nucleus are related by a proportionality constant, the gyromagnetic ratio γ.

$$\mu = \gamma p \qquad (1.5)$$

The exact value of the gyromagnetic ratio depends upon the structure of the nucleus and it therefore varies for different nuclei.

1.1.2 Nuclear energy levels in a static magnetic field

Nuclear energy is independent of angular momentum in the absence of an external magnetic field, or in other words the energy levels of nuclei with different angular momentums are degenerate. In the presence of a magnetic field, the nuclear magnetic dipole interacts with the field and the energies of the nuclei are directly related to their angular momentum and to field strength (the energy levels are split by the magnetic field).

$$E = -\gamma p_z B_0 \qquad (1.6)$$

This relationship shows that there are an equal number of allowed energy levels and values of angular momentum. For the simple case of the hydrogen nucleus (1H) which is a single proton, the two energy levels are:

$$E = \pm \tfrac{1}{2}\gamma\hbar B_0 \qquad (1.7)$$

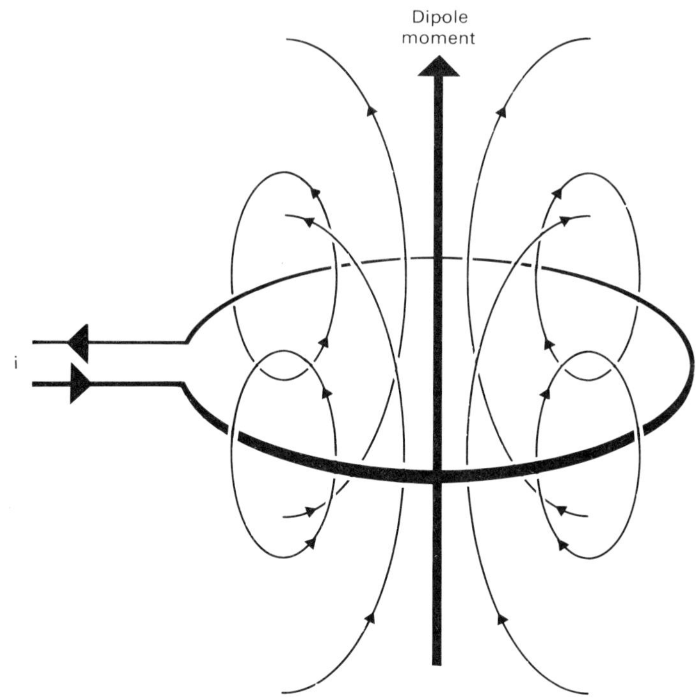

Figure 1.2. When a current flows through a conductor bent into a loop, the lines of magnetic flux accumulate through the centre of the loop to produce a magnetic dipole moment.

and the energy difference between them is:

$$\Delta E = \gamma\hbar B_0 \qquad (1.8)$$

The lower energy nuclei have magnetic moments pointing in the direction of the magnetic field and are said to be in a parallel state, whilst the remainder are said to be anti-parallel. It should be noted though that the terms parallel and antiparallel are borrowed from the classical description. Figure 1.3 shows the relationship between the nuclear magnetic energy levels and the applied magnetic field for hydrogen.

Because we know the magnitude of the angular momentum, p, and the magnitude of its component in the direction of an applied magnetic field, p_z, we also know the angle between the angular momentum vector and the field (figure 1.4). There is, however, no way of determining the components of angular momentum in the x and the y directions. The magnetic dipole of a hydrogen nucleus might therefore be oriented anywhere around the surface of one of two cones, depending upon whether the nucleus is in a parallel or an anti-parallel state (figure 1.5).

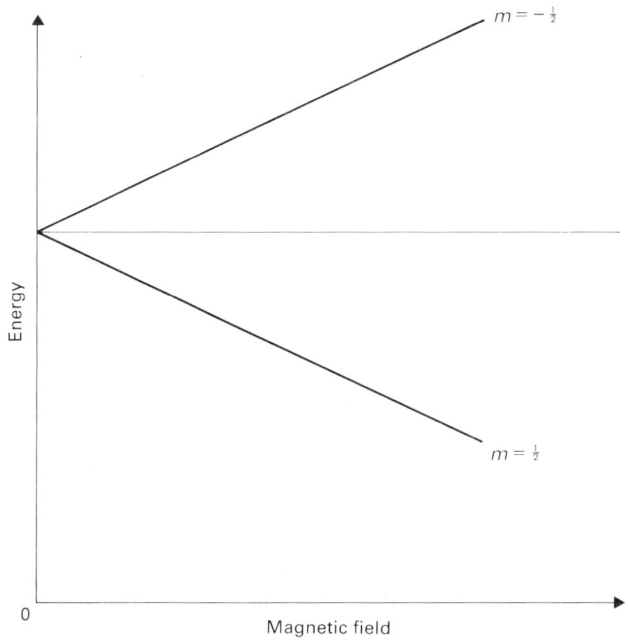

Figure 1.3. The relationship between the nuclear magnetic energy levels and the applied magnetic field for hydrogen.

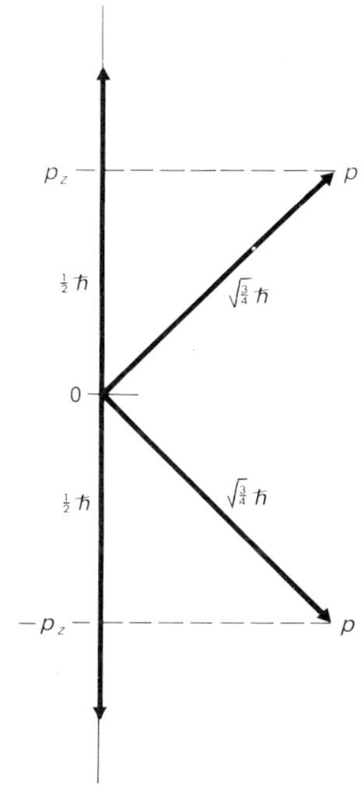

Figure 1.4. The nuclear magnetic dipole moment aligns at a known angle with an applied magnetic field. The angle is derived from the known magnitude of the angular momentum, p, (equation 1.2) and the magnitude of the components in the z direction, p_z (equation 1.3).

1.1.3 Transitions between nuclear energy levels

A nucleus can transfer between energy levels when a quantum of energy exactly equal to the energy difference is supplied or removed from the system. This energy must be in the form of an oscillating magnetic field at a required frequency or, in other words, electromagnetic radiation. The energy of a quantum of electromagnetic radiation is directly proportional to its frequency:

$$E=h\nu \quad (1.9)$$

From equations (1.8) and (1.9) therefore, it can be seen that for a transition to take place the following relationship between the applied field and the frequency of radiation must exist:

$$\nu_0=\gamma B_0 \,/\, 2\pi \quad (1.10)$$

or because the angular velocity ω equals $2\pi\nu$:

$$\omega_0=\gamma B_0 \quad (1.1)$$

We have seen this above as the principal equation of nuclear magnetic resonance describing the resonance condition for magnetic nuclei. The resonant frequency at which transitions will occur is referred to as the Larmor frequency.

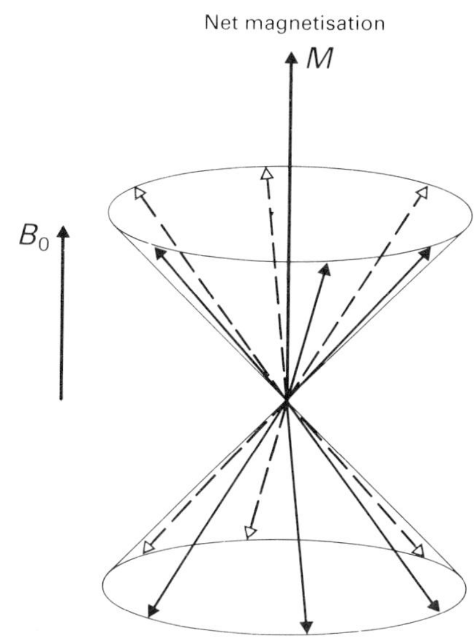

Figure 1.5. The magnetic dipole of the hydrogen nucleus may lie anywhere around the surface of one of two cones, depending on whether the nucleus is in a parallel or an anti-parallel state. In much of the classical description of magnetic resonance, we consider the net effect of a number of nuclei. There is no preferred orientation around the surface of the cone although there are slightly more in the parallel state. The net magnetisation at equilibrium will therefore point in the direction of the applied field, B_0.

1.1.4 The proportion of nuclei in each energy state

The ratio of nuclei in each energy state depends upon the energy separation and thermal energy and is determined by the Boltzman distribution. The greater the separation of energies and the lower the thermal energy, the larger is the proportion in the lower state. For nuclei of spin $I = ½$ the relative number of nuclei in anti-parallel (n_a) and parallel (n_p) states is:

$$\frac{n_a}{n_p} = e^{-\Delta E/kT} \qquad (1.11)$$

where k is the Boltzman constant and T is the absolute temperature. At normal body temperature, $kT = 2.67 \times 10^{-2}$ eV, and in an applied magnetic field of 0.5T, $\Delta E = 10^{-7}$ eV. The proportion of nuclei in the two energy states is therefore very nearly equal, and of one million nuclei only two more are parallel than anti-parallel. This similarity of the energy states means that net signal emission is only seen from a very small proportion of the nuclei during magnetic resonance, and the technique is inherently a low sensitivity technique.

When electromagnetic radiation of the Larmor frequency is applied to an object in a magnetic field, there is an equal chance of inducing transitions from the lower to the upper energy state as in the opposite direction. A transition from lower to upper levels will absorb a quantum of energy and a transition from upper to lower energy will emit energy. Because there are slightly more nuclei in the lower energy state, however, this leads to a net absorption of energy. As energy is absorbed, the proportion of nuclei in the two states will tend to equalise, and when this happens there can be no net energy transfer even though transitions will still occur.

1.2 Magnetic susceptibility

Materials in a magnetic field respond in different ways depending upon the arrangement of nuclei and electrons within the molecular lattice. All materials contain clouds of electrons which will circulate in such a way as to oppose any applied magnetic field. This phenomenon is called diamagnetism and because of this opposition between the diamagnetic and the applied fields a diamagnetic material does not 'like' being in an applied field. A frictionless diamagnetic compass needle would point East–West so that the lines of flux from the earth's magnetic field would pass through it in as short a path as possible.

As well as this bulk effect of the clouds of electrons within the molecular lattice, individual electrons have their own magnetic fields. In many materials the electrons pair up so that these fields cancel, but in materials with unpaired electrons the unopposed magnetic dipoles will line up with an applied field, the effect being considerably stronger than diamagnetism. This phenomenon is called paramagnetism and such materials have an affinity for being in a magnetic field. A frictionless paramagnetic compass needle would point North–South so that the lines of magnetic flux of the earth's magnetic field would pass through with as long a path as possible. The paramagnetic effect of nuclei with net magnetic moments is very much weaker than that of unpaired electrons.

The magnetic susceptibility constant, χ, provides a measure of the affinity of a materials for an applied magnetic field, and it is the proportionality constant between the applied field B_0 and the magnetism M which is induced in the material. Susceptibility is positive in paramagnetic materials, where the induced magnetism is parallel with the applied field, and it is negative in diamagnetic materials.

$$M = \chi B_0 \qquad (1.12)$$

1.3 Classical description

1.3.1 Nuclear spin and magnetism

Atomic nuclei consist of protons and neutrons (together known as nucleons) which can be thought of as spinning particles. The particles are usually paired with opposing spins which produces a net nuclear spin of zero, but nuclei with unpaired nucleons will have a net spin. The combination of net spin and the electrical charge of the nucleus generates a small magnetic field (magnetic dipole moment) which has both direction and magnitude, and is called the nuclear magnetisation vector. The nucleus therefore behaves like a spinning bar magnet.

In an applied magnetic field, the nuclear magnetisation vector will precess about the direction of the field in the same way that the axis of spin of a child's top precesses about a gravitational field (figure 1.6). The frequency of precession (the Larmor or resonant frequency) is directly proportional to the strength of the interaction between the two fields and it therefore depends upon their magnitude. The nuclear magnetic field is constant for any nucleus, but the frequency of

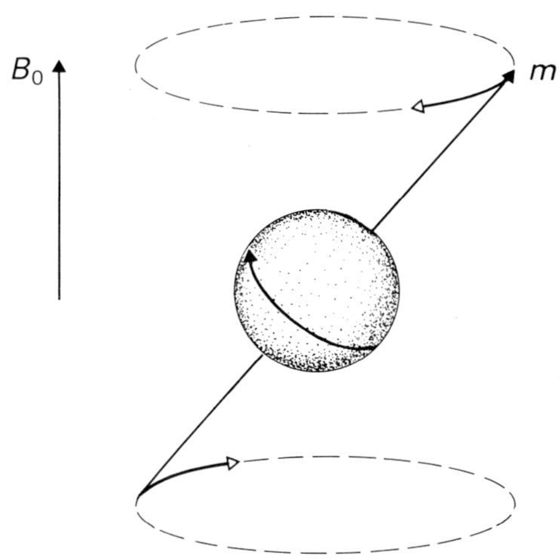

Figure 1.6. The nuclear magnetisation vector precesses around the direction of an applied field in the same way as the axis of spin of a child's top precesses about the gravitational field. The magnetisation vector therefore traces out the surface of a cone.

precession changes with the applied field. The equation relating the angular velocity ω_0 to the applied magnetic field B_0 is:

$$\omega_0=\gamma B_0 \tag{1.1}$$

where γ is the gyromagnetic ratio which is specific to different nuclei and depends upon the structure of the nucleus. Although it is normally positive there are a few exceptions such as nitrogen-15 which precesses in a direction opposite to the more common nuclei such as hydrogen-1. In an applied field of 0.5 T, which is 10 000 times the Earth's magnetic field, the Larmor frequency of the hydrogen nucleus is 21 MHz and that of the phosphorus nucleus is 9 MHz.

When nuclei are placed in a magnetic field they can only adopt certain angles of precession which are dictated by quantum mechanics (see above). The angle of precession is the angle between the nuclear magnetisation vector and the applied field, and the vector therefore traces out the surface of a cone (figure 1.6). Nuclei at different angles posses different energies which are analogous to the different energy states described above. In magnetic resonance, the most common nuclei such as hydrogen have only two allowed states, one with the nuclear magnetisation vector parallel to the applied field and the other anti-parallel. The parallel state is of lower energy than the anti-parallel one, and the difference in energy is proportional to the applied field strength. The proportion of nuclei in each energy state depends upon the energy difference between the states and the temperature. In a magnetic field of 0.5 T at body temperature, in each million hydrogen nuclei there are only two more in the lower energy state than in the higher one.

1.3.2 The net magnetisation vector

In classical physics, magnetic resonance is most easily understood not in terms of the action of individual nuclear magnetisation vectors but in terms of the net effect of many millions of them. Their sum is called the net magnetisation vector (figure 1.5). At equilibrium in an applied field, the net magnetisation vector is parallel to the field because, although the individual magnetisation vectors align at an angle, there is no synchronisation between the individual points on the cone of precession. Their components perpendicular to the applied field therefore cancel leaving only their components in the direction of the field.

Adding energy to the system will disturb the net magnetisation vector from equilibrium so that it takes up an angle to the applied field, which can be anything from 0 to 180° (or beyond) depending upon the amount of energy added. Having disturbed the net vector, like the individual nuclear vectors, it precesses around the field, although it eventually spirals back to equilibrium because of relaxation phenomena which are described below.

1.3.3 The alternating magnetic field

One method of disturbing the net magnetisation vector is to add energy to the system from an alternating electromagnetic field, although it is only the magnetic component of this field that is required. For energy to be transferred, the frequency of alternation must be equal to the Larmor frequency so that there is resonance between the two systems. This frequency is usually radio-frequency, and so the alternating field simply consists of radio waves.

The effect of an alternating magnetic field upon the net magnetisation vector is best understood when considered with respect to a rotating frame of reference, as opposed to the more common static frame of reference. An analogy that may help the understanding of these reference frames would be to imagine the Earth spinning upon its axis and viewed either from a satellite in a geostationary orbit (orbiting with the same angular velocity as the Earth so that it remains fixed over one point on the equator), or from a space craft moving slowly towards the sun. The first is an example of a rotating reference whilst the second is effectively stationary. From the rotating reference frame neither the Earth, nor the nuclear, nor the net magnetisation vectors will appear to spin or precess. This would only occur in the stationary reference frame for the magnetisation vectors if the magnetic field were zero, and this apparent removal of the magnetic field can be likened to the loss of gravity experienced by a man in a lift when the cable breaks.

The coordinates of the rotating reference frame are x', y' and z', (figure 1.7) where x' and y' rotate at the Larmor frequency in the xy plane of the static reference frame, whilst z' and z are equivalent and both point in the direction of the applied magnetic field.

In the rotating reference frame, the applied magnetic field B_0 is effectively removed and the alternating magnetic field (B_1) is in a fixed direction such as the y' direction. Because of the interaction between B_1 and the net magnetisation vector M, M precesses around y', or in other words it precesses in the $x'z'$ plane (figure 1.8). The angular frequency of this secondary precession is given by the equation:

$$\omega_1 = \gamma B_1 \tag{1.13}$$

Usually, the alternating magnetic field B_1 is applied only for a short time so that the net magnetisation vector is rotated through a specific angle such as 90 or 180° (figure 1.9). For a 90° pulse ($\pi/2$ radians), B_1 and the pulse duration t_p, must be such that:

$$\gamma B_1 t_p = \pi/2 \tag{1.14}$$

Viewed from a static reference frame the behaviour of the net magnetisation vector in an alternating mag-

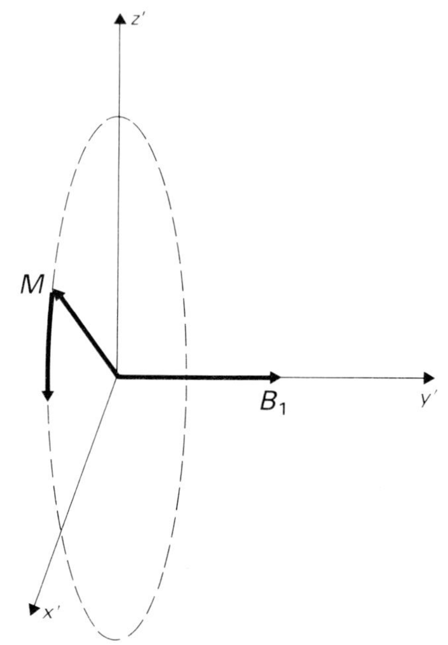

Figure 1.8. In the rotating reference frame, the applied magnetic field B_0 is effectively removed and the alternating magnetic field, B_1, is in a fixed direction such as the y' direction. Because of the interaction with B_1, the net magnetisation vector M precesses around y' or in other words it precesses in the $x'z'$ plane.

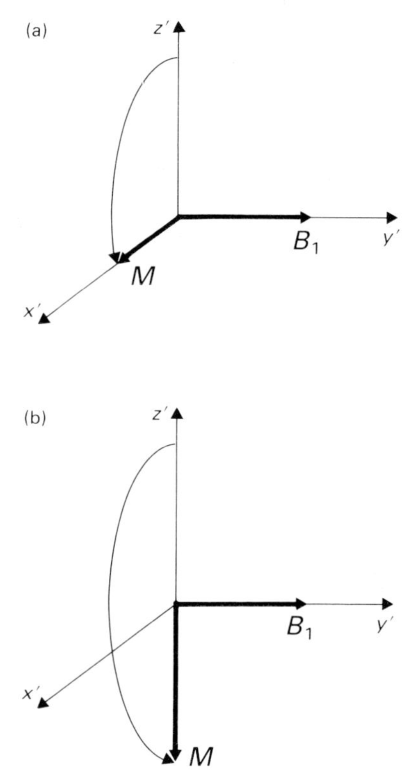

Figure 1.9. The effect of a 90° radio-frequency pulse (a) and a 180° pulse (b) on the net magnetisation vector in the rotating frame of reference.

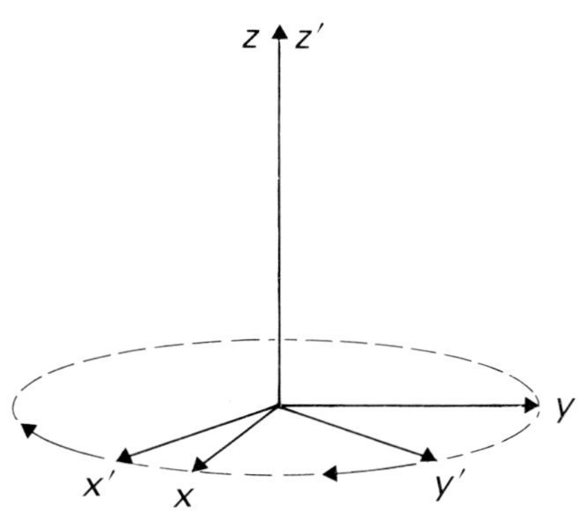

Figure 1.7. In the rotating frame of reference, coordinates x' and y' rotate in the xy plane of the static reference frame whilst z and z' are equivalent and both point in the direction of the applied magnetic field B_0.

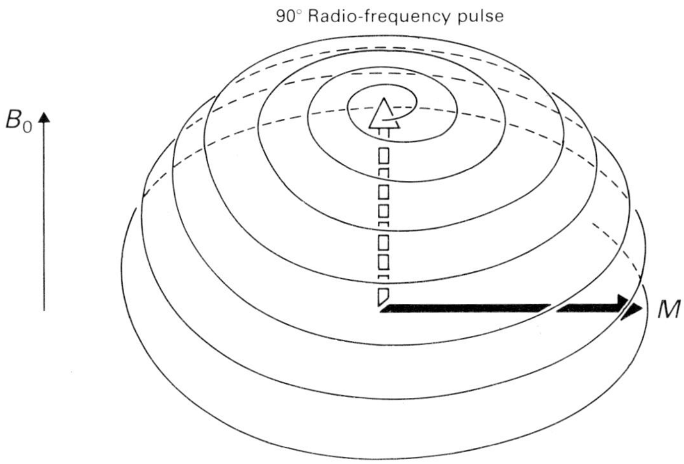

Figure 1.10. The behaviour of the net magnetisation vector in an alternating magnetic field B_1 viewed from the static reference frame is complex. It spirals down with an increasing angle of precession around the static field B_0.

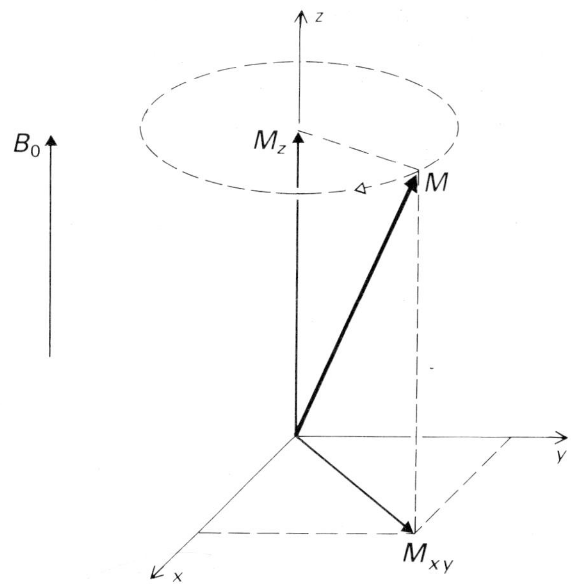

Figure 1.11. When not at equilibrium the behaviour of the net magnetisation vector is best understood by considering two components separately: a longitudinal component in the direction of the static field, M_z, and a transverse component in the plane perpendicular to this, M_{xy}.

netic field B_1 is more complex, and it appears to spiral down with an increasing angle of precession around the static field B_0 (figure 1.10).

Although we have said that it is most helpful to ignore the behaviour of individual nuclei when considering displacement of the net magnetisation vector, some people find it difficult to understand how magnetisation is generated in the xy plane by movement of nuclei from the lower to the upper energy level or vice versa. This is the point where quantum mechanical and classical explanations have difficulty mixing. It is not difficult however to imaging that when nuclei move from the parallel to the anti-parallel state they do so by interaction with the sinusoidal magnetic field B_1 and so they enter the other state in phase with it. The nuclei moved between states are therefore all in phase and they generate a magnetic moment M_{xy} in the xy plane.

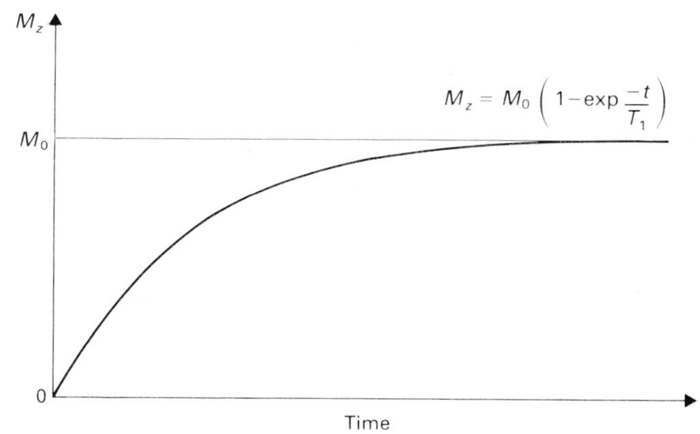

Figure 1.12. Following a 90° pulse, M_z is reduced from its equilibrium value to zero, and it relaxes back at an exponential rate with a time constant T_1.

1.3.4 Relaxation

The behaviour of the net magnetisation vector is best understood by considering two components separately: a longitudinal component in the direction of the static field, M_z, and a transverse component in the plane perpendicular to this, M_{xy} (figure 1.11). After a disturbance, M_z and M_{xy} return to their equilibrium values through processes which are called spin lattice (or longitudinal) relaxation and spin spin (or transverse) relaxàtion respectively.

Following a 90° pulse, M_z is reduced from its equilibrium value to zero, and it relaxes back at an exponential rate with a time constant T_1 (figure 1.12). The relaxation occurs as nuclei that have been displaced into the higher energy anti-parallel state relax back to their equilibrium positions. These changes cannot occur spontaneously and they require an interaction with an alternating magnetic field at the appropriate (Larmor) frequency. Such fields are generated by oscillations of the molecular lattice containing the nuclei, and the spin lattice relaxation is effectively an exchange or equilibration of energy between the nuclei and their surrounding lattice. T_1 tends to be long in solids where oscillations at the appropriate frequency are relatively uncommon (longitudinal relaxation is slow), and short in more mobile liquids (longitudinal relaxation is rapid). In this context, biological tissues are close to liquid because signal is obtained mainly from water in solution, and biological T_1 ranges from hundreds of milliseconds to a few seconds.

At equilibrium in a static field, M_{xy} is zero because the nuclear magnetisation vectors precessing around B_0 are not in phase. A 90° radio-frequency pulse increases M_{xy} by causing transitions between nuclear energy levels that are all in phase, but after the pulse it relaxes back to equilibrium at an exponential rate with a time constant T_2. The nuclear processes which cause this transverse, or spin spin, relaxation are interactions between neighbouring nuclei which alter the local magnetic field for each nucleus and hence the Larmor frequency. The different rates of precession lead to loss of phase so that the individual magnetisation components in the xy plane eventually oppose each other and cancel (figure 1.13). T_2 can never be longer than T_1 because the transitions between nuclear energy levels that cause longitudinal relaxation also lead to loss of phase coherence and so indirectly cause transverse relaxation as well. Transverse relaxation is rapid in solids (T_2 is short) since the positions of nuclei are fixed, and it is slow in liquids where the molecules are in more rapid motion and their magnetic effects are averaged. In biological tissues, T_2 ranges from tens to hundreds of milliseconds.

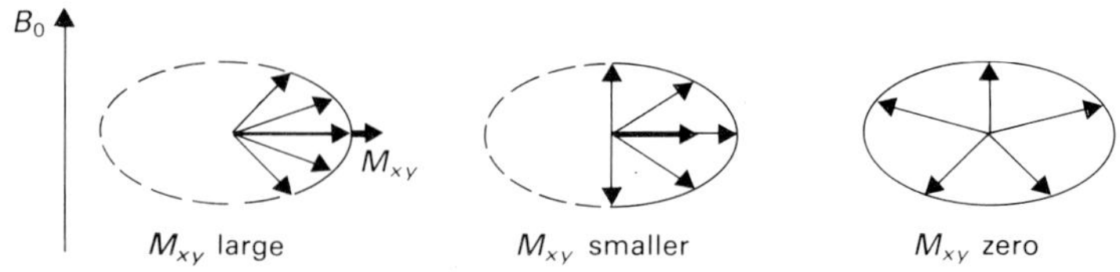

Figure 1.13. Spin spin interactions alter the local field around each nucleus and cause a variation in the Larmor frequency. The different rates of precession lead to loss of phase so that the individual magnetisation components in the plane eventually oppose each other and cancel with a resultant loss of signal.

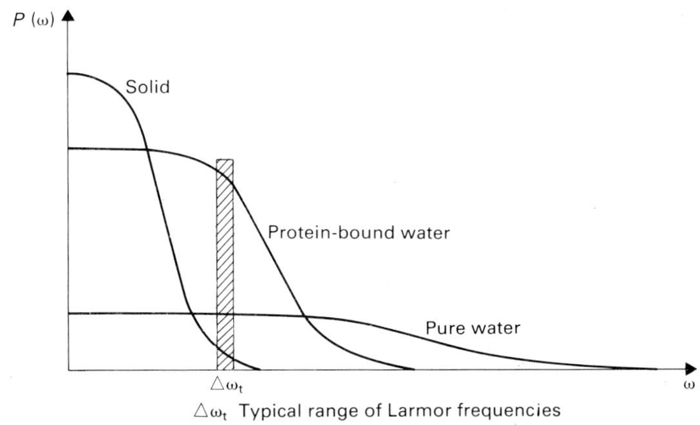

Figure 1.14. Plots showing the ranges of motional frequencies for pure water, protein-bound water and a solid. Long correlation times have a narrow range of frequencies with high amplitude, and short correlation times have a wider range of frequencies with low amplitude. The function $P(\omega)$ tells us the proportion of molecules with a motional frequency ω.

1.4 Molecular mobility

Molecular magnetism is a short range phenomenon and the most important contribution to both spin lattice and spin spin relaxation is thought to be the interaction between nuclear magnetic dipoles within a single molecule. A simple and highly relevant example is the water molecule, where the two protons interact as the molecule tumbles around. Each nucleus will affect the field experienced by the other, but by an amount which depends upon the orientation of the molecule in the field. Rotation of the molecule modulates the effective field at a frequency which depends upon the speed of rotation or motion. Molecular mobility is usually expressed as a correlation time τ_c, which is an inverse measure of the rate at which a molecule moves or rotates in a certain direction. In water where the molecules are small and easily deflected by collisions with others, the correlation time is short (3×10^{-12} s), but for a large enzyme molecule which is much less easily disturbed, it is longer, e.g. 10^{-8} s. In most solids it is longer still, e.g. 10^{-6} s.

A molecule's correlation time does not indicate that it moves or oscillates in a regular fashion with τ_c representing half the period, because the motion is much more random. Analysis of the motion would disclose a range of frequencies from zero to a maximum which depends upon the correlation time. The longer the correlation time, the higher and narrower the range of frequencies, and the shorter the correlation time, the wider the range of frequencies. Figure 1.14

shows a plot of these frequencies for pure water, protein-bound water and a solid, as well as the Larmor frequency for hydrogen. Spin lattice relaxation relies upon a proportion of the molecular motion occurring at the Larmor frequency, but in the solid we can see that the cut-off of frequencies is below the Larmor frequency so that spin lattice relaxation is very slow. For pure water, the cut-off is much higher than the Larmor frequency so that the proportion of motion at this frequency is low and, again, spin lattice relaxation is slow. For protein-bound water, the inverse of the correlation time approximately equals the Larmor frequency and the cut-off of molecular frequencies is only slightly greater so that spin lattice relaxation is fast.

For spin spin relaxation to be effective there should be very little molecular motion because otherwise the effects of the nuclei upon each other are averaged and there is little difference between them. T_2 is shortest therefore when the molecular motion has zero or very low frequency. Figure 1.14 shows that the proportion of molecules with zero frequency increases as the correlation time gets shorter, and therefore solids have the shortest T_2 and pure water the longest.

Figure 1.15 shows a plot of T_1 and T_2 against the correlation time. T_1 has a minimum when τ_c is equal to $1/\omega_0$ (when the molecules oscillate or tumble with a frequency equal to the resonant frequency of the nuclei under study). T_2 increases almost linearly with increasing molecular mobility (as τ_c is reduced) because the magnetic effects of neighbouring spins become more and more averaged. In the body, hydrogen is most commonly found in one of two chemical forms: water (H_2O) or the methylene group of lipid ($-CH_2-$). Because both of these are relatively small we might expect the correlation time to be short. In practice, these small molecules are often bound to much larger ones such as proteins and their correlation times are greatly increased.

Molecular motion and diffusion are very closely linked. The effect of diffusion upon the magnetic resonance signal was noted in very early experiments, and methods of measuring diffusion were soon developed. Diffusion affects the signal in two ways. Because it is closely related to molecular mobility described above, it will have a direct influence on T_1 and T_2. In addition, the movement of nuclear spins in a magnetic field which is not perfectly uniform will cause changes in the resonant frequency and thus phase dispersion leading to loss of signal. The effect of diffusion on the signal from different sequences is described in chapter 2, p. 22.

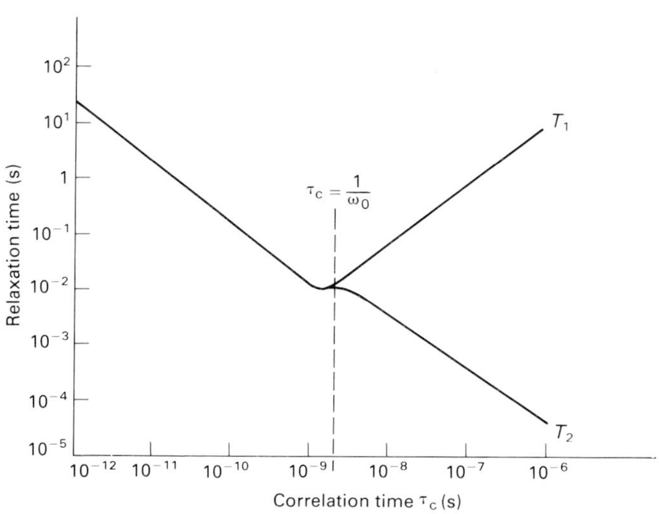

Figure 1.15. The relaxation times of water protons vary with correlation time τ_c. (Reproduced with permission from D.G. Gadian.[3]).

1.5 Free induction decay

If a 90° pulse is applied to a sample, the net magnetisation vector is turned into the xy plane where it precesses. The rotation of M_{xy} gives rise to an oscillating magnetic field or electromagnetic radiation which is usually of radio frequency. This radio signal can be detected by a receiving aerial and it is called the free induction decay (FID) (figure 1.16). It is important to note that it is only the component of the net magnetisation vector in the xy plane that gives rise to the signal. This phenomenon, from the induction of an

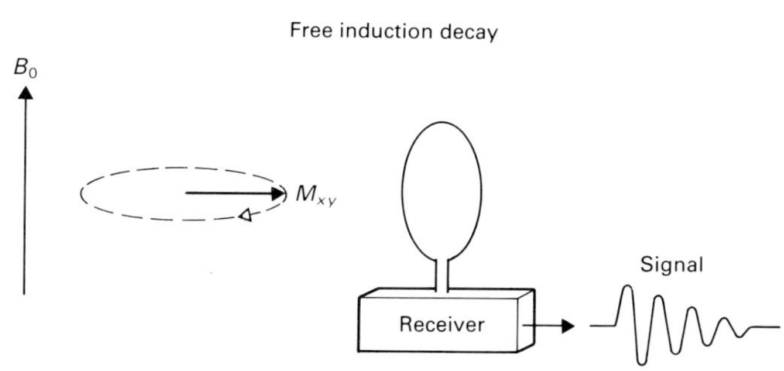

Figure 1.16. The rotation of M_{xy} gives rise to an oscillating magnetic field or electro-magnetic radiation which is usually of radio-frequency. This radio signal can be detected by a receiving aerial and it is called the free induction decay (FID).

electrical potential across the terminals of an alternator when a magnet is rotated within a coil, is well known.

The detected signal decays partly because of transverse relaxation which reduces M_{xy} and also partly because of inhomogeneities in the applied magnetic field, which mean that nuclei in different parts of the sample precess at different rates and fall out of phase even more rapidly.

1.6 Chemical shift and spectroscopy

If a sample is placed in a magnetic field, the electrons surrounding the nuclei circulate in such a way as to produce a small opposing màgnetic field. The nuclei are therefore partially screened from the applied field and the amount of screening depends upon the local electron density. This in turn depends upon molecular structure, and so the same nucleus in different chemical environments will experience different effective magnetic fields and hence precess at different frequencies. These frequency changes are called chemical shifts, and magnetic resonance spectroscopy is a display of the different frequencies of precession of a single nuclear species in the sample. Because chemical shift is proportional to the applied field, spectroscopy is best performed using very strong fields (2 T or greater). The area under each peak is proportional to the number of nuclei contributing to it, and this has not only allowed magnetic resonance spectroscopy to provide a valuable tool in analytical chemistry for many years, but now promises to provide *in vivo* biochemical information.

If all of the chemically equivalent nuclei in the sample precessed at the same frequency, then the spectrum would contain very sharp peaks. However, the same nuclear interactions that lead to spin spin relaxation mean that the nuclei precess at a range of frequencies and each peak has a width that is related to T_2. In addition, inhomogeneities in the applied magnetic field also broaden the peaks, and it is important to tailor the field so that this effect is minimal in comparison with the T_2 effect. Imperfect shimming of the magnetic field during *in vivo* magnetic resonance spectroscopy leads to difficulties in quantifying the peaks accurately and most spectroscopy involves a comparison of peak amplitudes rather than accurate quantification. These principles are discussed in more detail in chapter 12.

References

1 Abragam A. *The Principles of Nuclear Magnetism*. Oxford: Clarendon Press, 1961.

2 Pykett IL, Newhouse JH, Buonanno FS, *et al*. Principles of nuclear magnetic resonance imaging. *Radiology* 1982; **143**: 157–68.

3 Gadian DG. *Nuclear Magnetic Resonance and its Applications to Living Systems*. Oxford: Clarendon Press, 1982.

4 Carrington A, McLachlan AD. *Introduction to Magnetic Resonance*. London: Harper and Row, 1967.

5 Farrar TC, Becker ED. *Pulse and Fourier Transform N.M.R.* New York: Academic Press, 1971.

6 Lyndon-Bell RM, Harris RK. *Nuclear Magnetic Resonance Spectroscopy*. London: Thomas Nelson and Sons, 1969.

7 Slichter CP. *Principles of Magnetic Resonance*. New York: Harper and Row, 1963. (Second edition, Berlin: Springer-Verlag, 1978.)

Chapter 2
Magnetic Resonance Image Formation

DAVID FIRMIN

Magnetic resonance imaging is almost entirely restricted to the hydrogen nucleus, or proton, because of the high concentration of water and fat (and hence protons) in body tissues. An image is a map of the amplitude of the magnetic resonance signal at each point in a thin slice through the patient. Data acquisition consists of an initial exciting pulse or pulses followed by recording of the signal emitted. The amplitude of the signal can be made to depend upon proton density, T_1, T_2, any combination of these or a number of other parameters, and it is this ability to produce maps showing both anatomy (proton density), biochemical (T_1 and T_2) and functional information that makes magnetic resonance such a powerful tool.

The radio signal emitted contains no inherent positional information, and so different methods are used to encode this information in the signal. In conventional imaging, localisation in three dimensions is achieved by a combination of slice selection, frequency encoding and phase encoding. These all rely on a magnetic field gradient superimposed upon the static uniform field and the gradients are produced by passing a current through subsidiary coils within the main bore of the magnet. Gradients in three directions are used to encode the radio signal with spatial information in three dimensions, but the gradients have to be used in different ways because if they were all applied at the same time they would simply summate to create a gradient in an oblique direction.

2.1 Slice selection

If a gradient is superimposed upon the static uniform field then the protons in each slice of the patient will experience different magnetic fields and will precess at different frequencies. A radio-frequency pulse containing a defined band of frequencies will then excite only a selected slice of the patient and the resulting signal, however it is recorded, can come only from that slice (figure 2.1). The imaging slice can be chosen at will by appropriate choice of exciting frequency.

Figure 2.2 shows the radio-frequency pulse and slice selection gradient timings for a simple gradient echo sequence (described later). In order to excite the material within the slice evenly the radio-frequency pulse must be of a certain shape. The shape is that of a sinc function [(sin ωt)/ωt] which is the Fourier transform of a square pulse (see section 2.4 for a description of the Fourier transform). Because the slice is of finite thickness the slice selection gradient, as well as en-

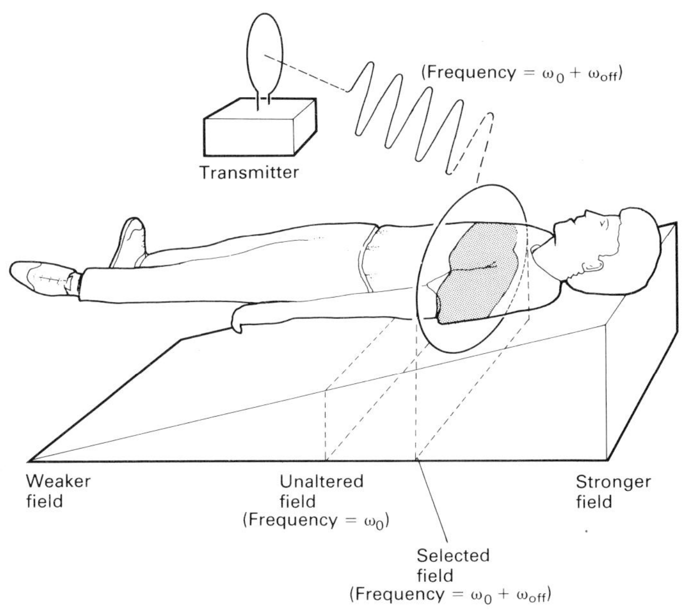

Figure 2.1. Slice selection: a gradient is superimposed upon the static uniform field and the protons in each slice of the patient will experience different magnetic fields and will precess at different frequencies. A radio-frequency pulse containing a defined band of frequencies will excite only a selected slice of the patient and the resulting signal, however it is recorded, can come only from that slice.

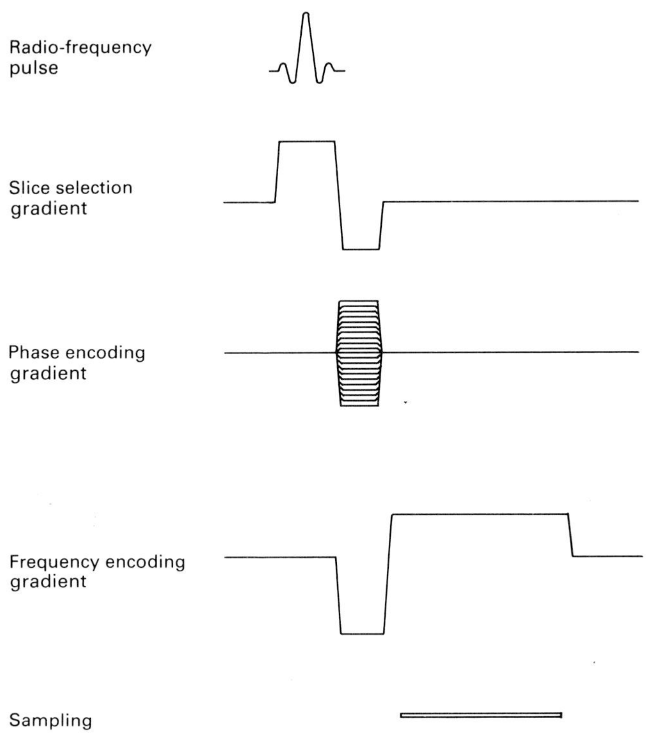

Figure 2.2. Radio-frequency pulse and gradient profiles for a simple gradient echo sequence. The profiles marked slice selection gradient, frequency encoding gradient, and phase encoding gradient indicate the magnitude of the magnetic field gradients applied in these directions. The resulting radio-frequency signal is sampled at the point indicated.

abling the slice to be selected, causes nuclei through the thickness of the slice to be dephased. The negative gradient just after the radio-frequency pulse compensates for this by rephasing the nuclei.

2.2 Frequency encoding

During acquisition of the signal another gradient can be applied, for example in the x direction, and this is called the read gradient (or frequency encoding gradient). Each line in the excited slice is now in a different field and so it emits at an individual frequency. In common parlance, the x direction has been frequency encoded. The signal is a complicated sum of the many frequencies, each with an amplitude proportional to the signal of the corresponding line. Fourier transformation is a mathematical technique that breaks down complex waves into the individual frequencies of which they are composed (see section 2.4). It provides the amplitude of each frequency and a plot of the amplitude against the frequency is equivalent to a projection of the section in a single direction (figure 2.3).

Figure 2.2 shows the timing of the frequency encoding gradient used in a gradient echo sequence. The initial negative gradient causes a dephasing of the nuclear spins which are then rephased by the positive gradient to form an echo at the centre of the frequency encoding gradient.

2.3 Phase encoding

The signal has now been localised in two dimensions, but the third dimension is more complex, and two different techniques can be used. The easiest to understand is similar to the method used in X-ray transmission tomography and gamma-ray emission tomography, and it uses filtered back-projection or what is sometimes referred to as '$r\theta$-reconstruction'. Multiple projections are acquired at angles rotating through 360° using oblique frequency encoding gradients. From these projections, tomographic slices are reconstructed by back-projection. The technique has the virtue of being less sensitive to motion artefact than two-dimensional Fourier transformation (the technique described next), but it is almost never used in commercially available scanners.

In two-dimensional Fourier transformation (sometimes referred to as 'xy-reconstruction'), if the chosen frequency encoding direction is the x direction, then another gradient is applied in the y direction just before (but not during) the read gradient. This is called the phase encoding gradient and it has the effect of altering the phase of the signal by an amount which depends upon the position in the y direction (figure 2.4). The phase encoding gradient can be applied at any time between the slice selection and the frequency encoding gradients (figure 2.2) because the phase alteration is retained until the signal is read. To phase encode only once is insufficient to generate a complete image, and the acquisition has to be repeated a number of times, each time with an increment in the phase encoding gradient. For example, if 128 phase encoding steps are chosen, for the first acquisition a phase encoding gradient of $+n$ is used, for the 64th acquisition the gradient is zero, and for the 128th it is $-n$. The number of phase encoding steps determines the spatial resolution in the phase encoding direction. Typical numbers are 64 for low resolution images but 256 or 512 for high resolution. Clearly, there is a compromise between resolution and imaging time because each phase encoding step means an extra acquisition which for cardiac imaging means an extra cardiac cycle.

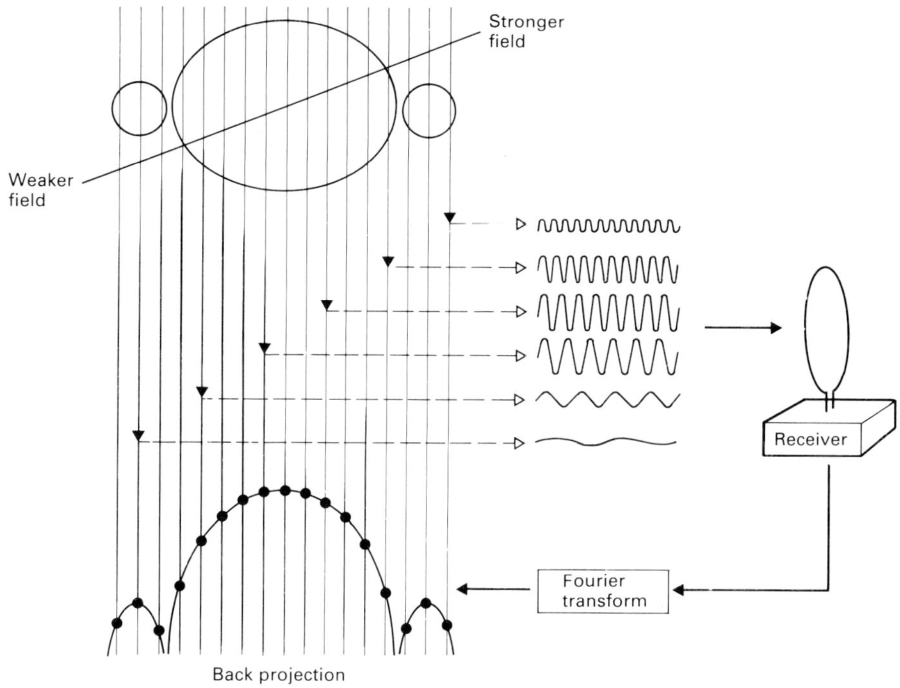

Figure 2.3. Frequency encoding: during acquisition of the signal a magnetic field gradient is applied and each line across the excited slice experiences a different field and emits at a different frequency. The signal is a complicated sum of the many frequencies, each with an amplitude proportional to the signal of the corresponding line. Fourier transformation provides the amplitude of each frequency and a plot of the amplitude against the frequency is equivalent to a projection of the section in a single direction.

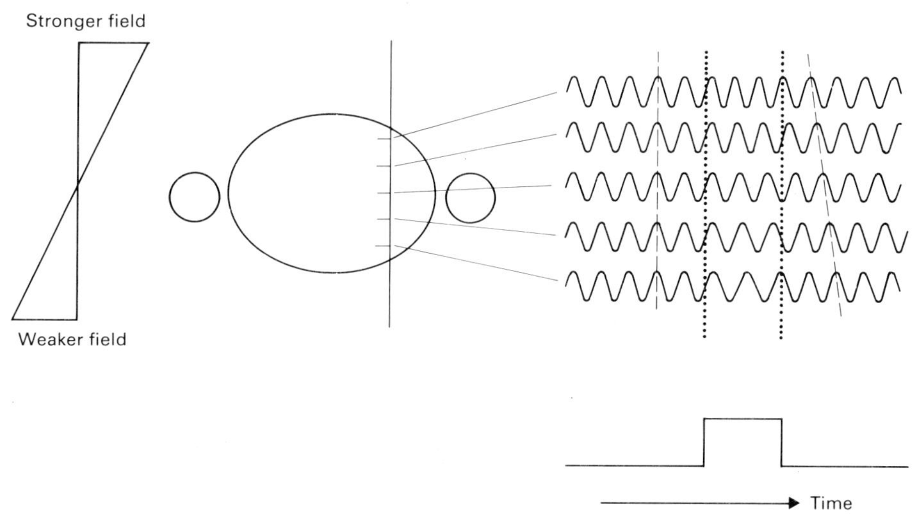

Figure 2.4. The phase encoding gradient has the effect of altering the phase of the emitted signal by an amount which depends on position in the direction of the gradient.

It is difficult to visualise how a set of acquisitions with different phase encoding steps can lead to an image. In order to explain, a case with only eight phase encoding steps will be described. The effect of the phase encoding gradient on signals from a single column in the image (defined by frequency encoding as described above) is first considered. Figure 2.5 shows the upper half of the column and the arrows represent the phase which results from phase encoding. The lower half of the column which is not shown is identical except that the phase is reversed. When the phase shifts for any pixel are viewed consecutively, they generate a frequency of their own. The central pixel that does not experience a change in field strength when the phase encoding gradient is applied has no phase shifts and therefore a frequency of zero. The first pixel above this has a frequency of one cycle per eight phase encoding steps, the second pixel has a frequency of two cycles per eight phase steps, the third pixel has three cycles and the fourth (top) pixel has four cycles.

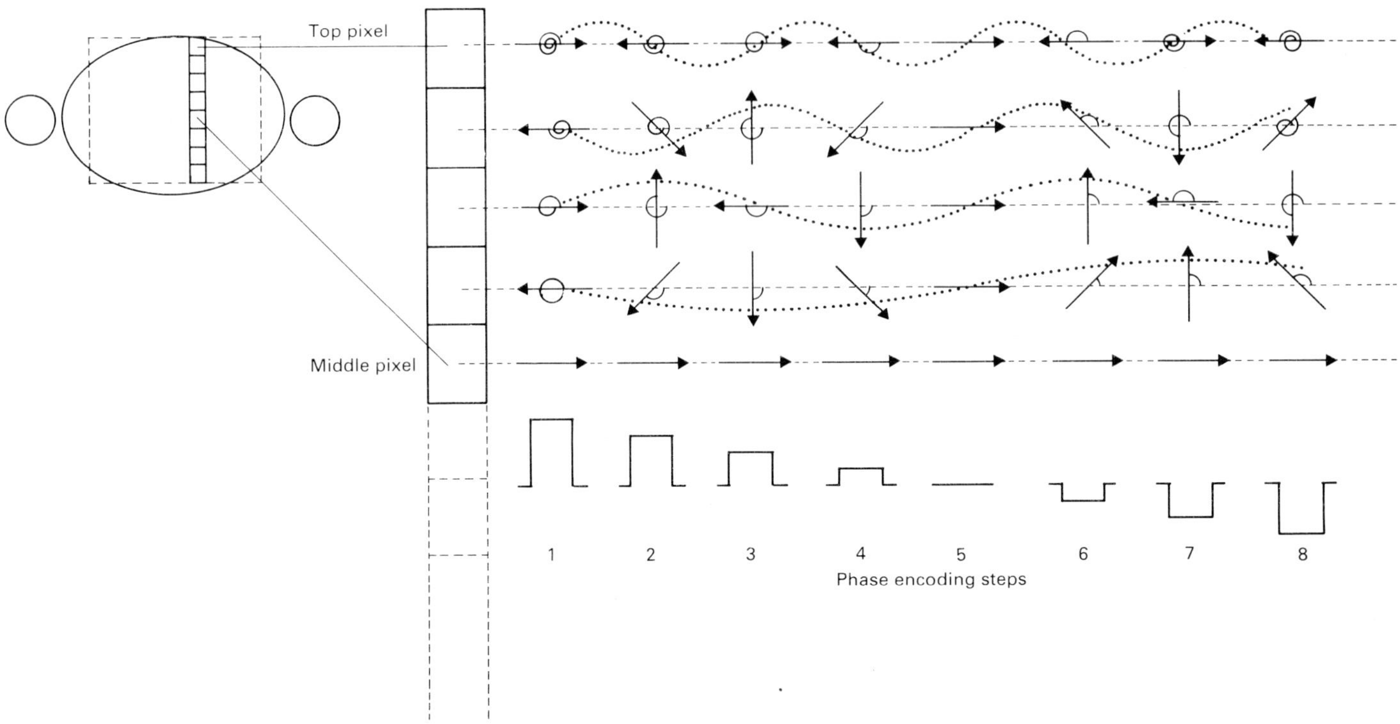

Figure 2.5. The phase encoding effects in a simple case when only eight phase encoding steps are used to define eight points in a single column of an excited slice. The arrows represent the phases of signals after each phase encoding step. When the phase shifts are viewed consecutively, they generate a frequency of their own (dotted lines). The bottom half of the column that is not shown is identical except that the phases are reversed.

Each of the pixels in the chosen column therefore is defined by its own frequency, and the amplitude of this frequency can be extracted by Fourier transformation as described in the frequency encoding section.

The technique can be further illustrated using an eight by eight image matrix to image a pixel sized block of water with frequency encoding in the horizontal direction and phase encoding in the vertical direction (figure 2.6). In (a), the block is positioned in the centre of the image matrix where the application of a gradient in either direction does not affect the signal. In (b), the block is moved sideways by two pixels in the frequency encoding direction. The phase encoding gradient still has no effect and the phase of the signal after each phase encoding step is identical. The signal now has a frequency offset however because of the effect of the frequency encoding gradient. In (c), the block is moved sideways a further two pixels and the frequency doubles although always with the same phase irrespective of phase encoding steps. In (d) and (e), the block is central with respect to the frequency encoding gradient and so the signal after each phase encoding step has zero frequency offset from the Larmor frequency and appears as a straight line. The phase of the signal changes after each phase encoding step, however, and the rate of change of phase generates a frequency which depends upon the offset and is twice as great in (e) as in (d). In (f), the block is offset by two pixels in both directions and the vertical and horizontal signals both have a frequency which is position dependent.

In practice, the signal acquired during each phase encoding step is laid down in successive rows of an image which represents the raw data of the image. A two dimensional Fourier transformation of this raw data image produces the anatomical image. The space in which the raw data image is mapped is called K-space or spatial frequency space and instead of having spatial position along its axes, it has spatial frequency. In order to acquire the data for an anatomical image the whole of K-space must be sampled, and in this conventional imaging method it is sampled as a series of separate lines, each line with its own excitation pulse. This method of sampling is not obligatory how-

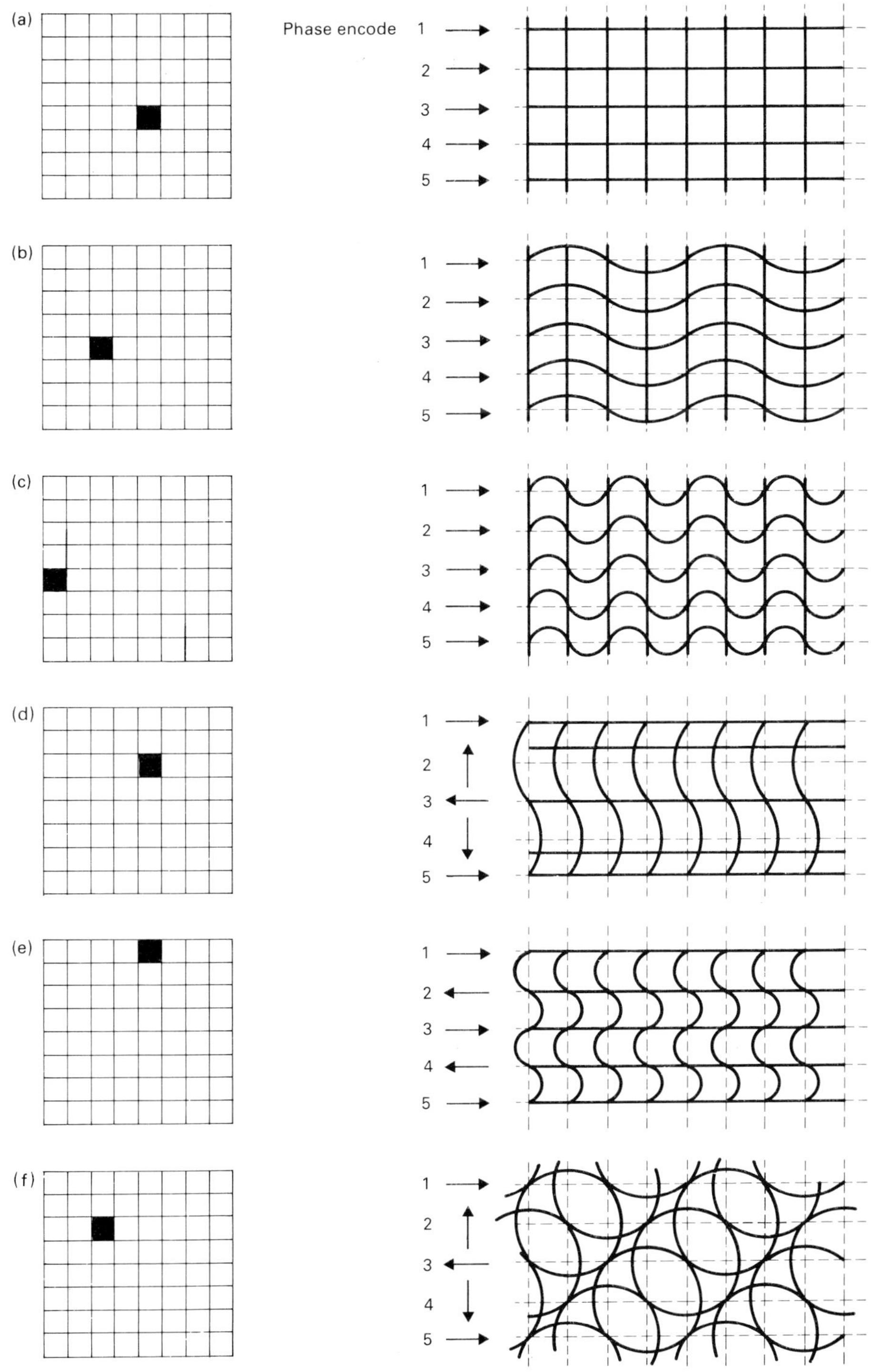

Figure 2.6. An eight by eight matrix is used to image a pixel-sized block of water positioned at various locations. The signals produced after each phase encoding step are shown on the right and the first five phase encoding steps are stacked together. The arrow on the left of each signal represents the memorised phase after encoding and the vertical lines indicate the frequencies that are slowly encoded by the phase encoding gradient.

ever, and in some of the rapid imaging techniques such as echo planar imaging which is described later, the space is covered in a continuous zig-zag line after an initial radio-frequency excitation. Spiral and square-spiral techniques have also been used.

2.4 The Fourier transform

At several points in the description of magnetic resonance a mathematical technique called Fourier analysis is used to transform a plot of signal against time into a plot of signal against frequency or *vice versa*. Although Fourier transformation is a source of mystery to some, it is very simple. In this section we do not consider the basic principles of Fourier transformation but we illustrate the method that is used by imaging computers to perform the calculations.

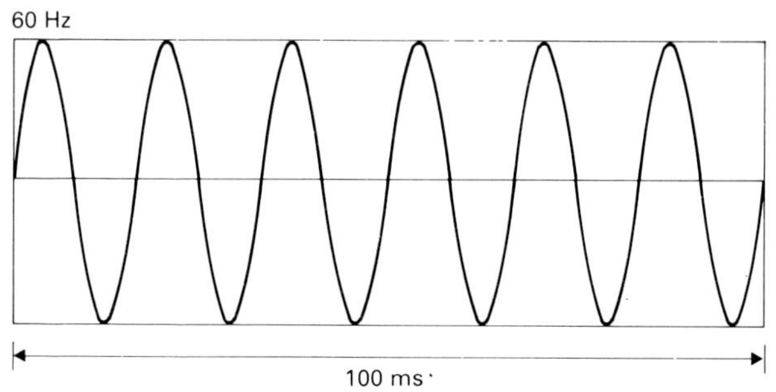

Figure 2.7. A sinusoidal signal with a frequency of 60 Hz sampled for 100 ms.

Consider a sinusoidal signal with a frequency of 60 Hz (cycles per second). If this were sampled for 100 ms the signal would appear as in figure 2.7 and it would contain six complete cycles. The Fourier transform involves a number of repetitive steps to analyse the amount of separate frequencies in the signal. These steps simply involve the multiplication of the signal by a test frequency. Figure 2.8 shows the result of multiplying the 60 Hz signal by test signals between 10 and 90 Hz. For all of the multiplications except 60 Hz, the positive and negative areas under the resultant are equal so that the integral of the resultant is zero. For the multiplication by 60 Hz the resultant is all positive

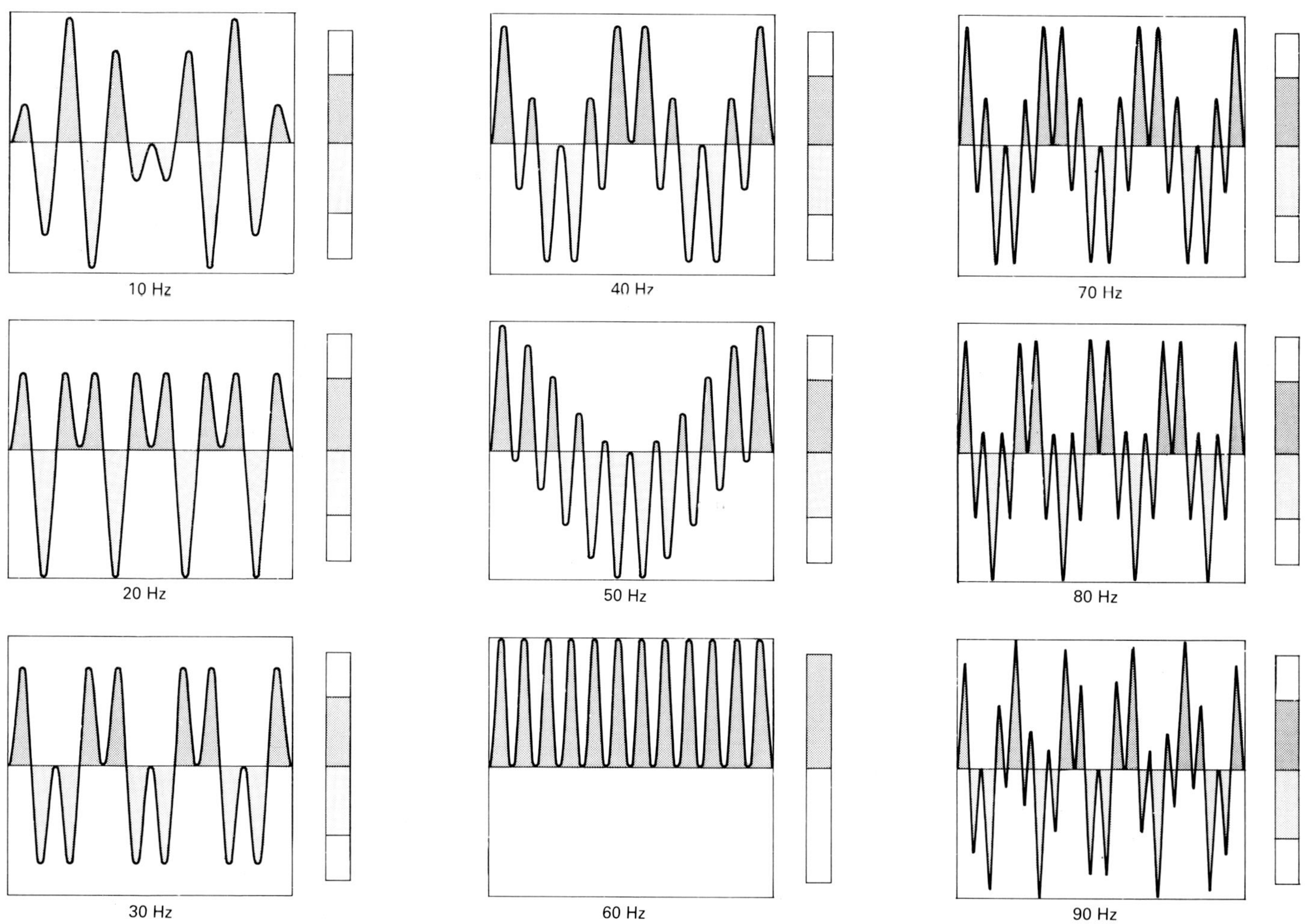

Figure 2.8. The result of multiplying a 60 Hz signal by test signals between 10 and 90 Hz. For all of the multiplications except 60 Hz, the positive and negative areas under the resultant curve are equal and the integral is zero. For the multiplication by 60 Hz the resultant curve is all positive and the integral is proportional to the amplitude of the original signal.

and the integral is proportional to the amplitude of the original signal.

This analysis has detected the frequency and amplitude of the signal, a feat that may seem trivial for such a simple example, but the technique comes into its own when a more complex signal is analysed. Figure 2.9 shows a signal composed of a 30 Hz signal of amplitude 5 mV, a 50 Hz signal (10 mV) and an 80 Hz signal (7 mV). Again these are sampled for only 100 ms. Figure 2.10 shows the analysis and although the results are more complex than before, the multiplications by 30, 50 and 80 Hz are more positive than negative whereas for the other frequencies the resultant integrals are zero.

The method is sensitive to the phase of the signal. If the 60 Hz signal of the first example was shifted by 90° in phase then it would not be detected (figure 2.11). Because two components of the magnetic resonance signal are normally collected, each one being 90° out of phase with the other, analysis of both components allows the phase as well as the amplitude of the signal to be calculated.

The signals of magnetic resonance imaging are even more complex. For a typical image reconstruction with a matrix of 256 × 256 pixels, the Fourier transform analysis requires 256 frequency multiplications and integrations for each of the 256 points in the frequency encoded direction and the same again for the phase encoded direction: in total, 256^4 multiplications and integrations. Mathematical short cuts have been found which reduce the number of steps and so speed up the analysis and this is called the fast Fourier transformation. It is still a major computing task, however, and a dedicated piece of hardware known as an array processor is often employed to speed image reconstruction time to a number of seconds.

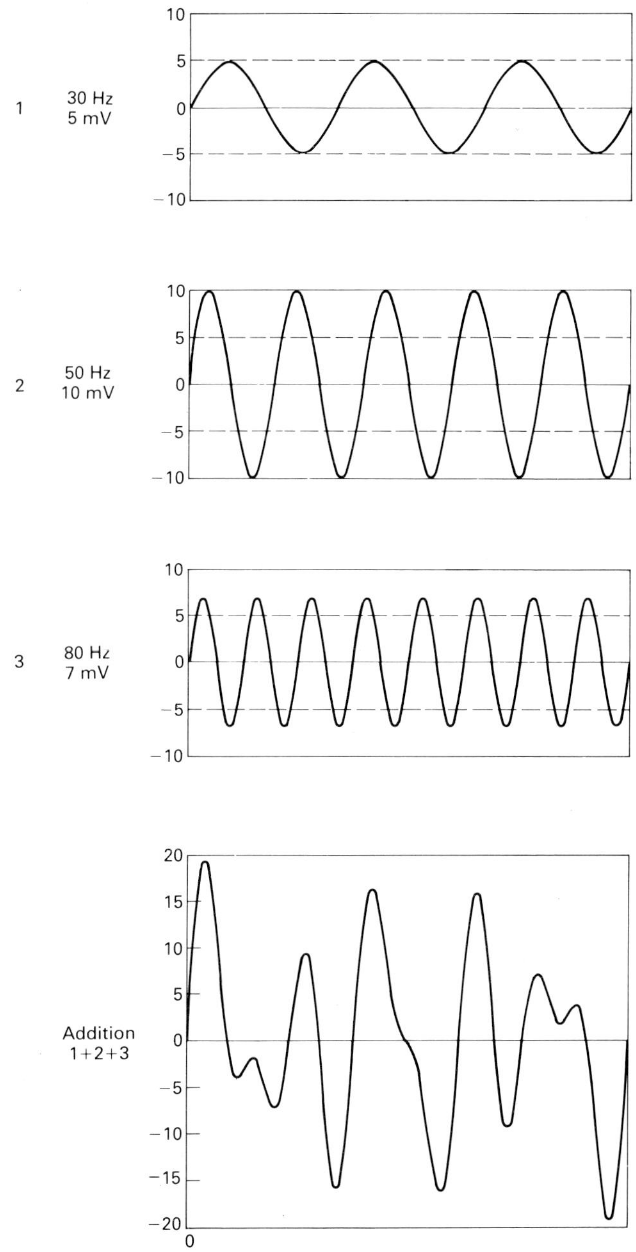

Figure 2.9. A signal composed of a 30 Hz signal of amplitude 5 mV, a 50 Hz signal (10 mV) and an 80 Hz signal (7 mV) sampled for 100 ms.

2.5 Imaging pulse sequences

After a 90° radio-frequency pulse, the free induction decay signal is seen and this could be used to generate an image. For many reasons, including the need to encode the signal spatially, it is not ideal to form an image from this signal and many pulse sequences have been described that allow the signal to be acquired at a stage after the free induction decay signal. A pulse sequence is simply a train of radio-frequency and magnetic field gradient pulses, and we have already been introduced to an important part of the pulse sequence when considering the gradients used to encode spatial information in the image. Some pulse sequences use radio-frequency pulses to produce tissue contrast but in others the timing and amplitudes of applied magnetic field gradients are more important. The common sequences are described below but there are many variations and it is impossible to be comprehensive.

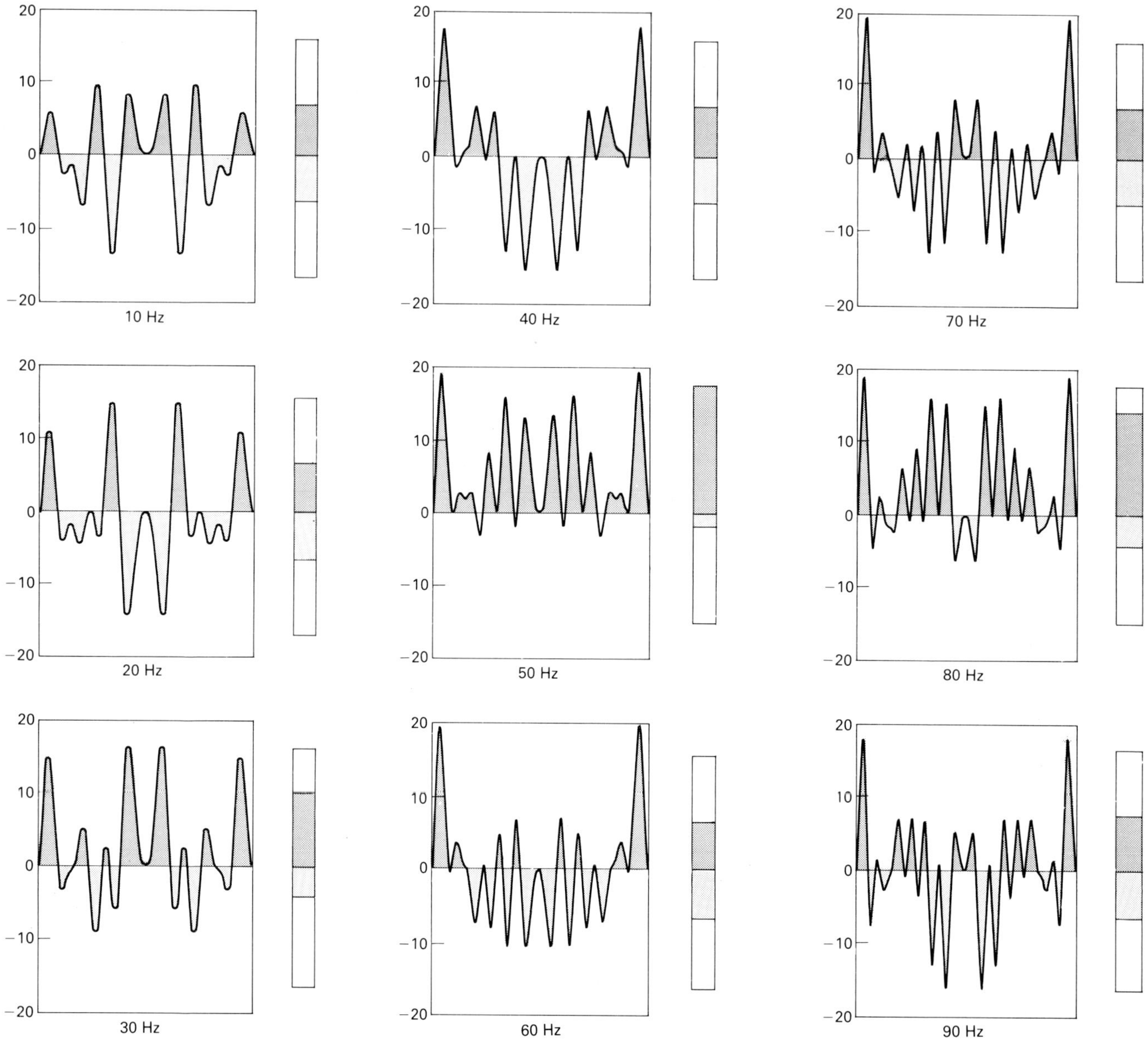

Figure 2.10. The result of multiplying the signal of figure 2.9 by test signals between 10 and 90 Hz. The results are more complex than before but the multiplications by 30, 50 and 80 Hz are more positive than negative, by an amount proportional to the initial amplitude of that frequency, whereas for the other frequencies the resultant integrals are zero.

Unlike computed X-ray tomography where image intensity depends upon only one parameter, the magnetic resonance signal depends upon a large number of parameters including proton density, T_1, T_2, chemical shift, flow effects, diffusion, magnetic susceptibility and more. By using different pulse sequences the signal can be made to depend more or less on each of these parameters in turn. This is one of the greatest strengths of magnetic resonance imaging because of the enormous variety of information available, but it is also a disadvantage because of the complexity of image acquisition and interpretation. Any user of computer software will know that flexibility and user friendliness are sometimes mutually exclusive.

2.5.1 The spin echo sequence

The spin echo effect was initially observed by Hahn in 1950[1] before any imaging methods were developed, but it is now perhaps the most common imaging sequence. It produces images with excellent anatomical resolution and the contrast between tissues with different proton density, T_1 and T_2 can be altered by suitable choice of timing. One disadvantage is that it is a relatively long sequence and so is not ideal for rapid or cine imaging.

After a 90° pulse the induced signal (FID) decays because of field inhomogeneities and also because of spin-spin relaxation (T_2). The combined time constant of these processes is called T_2*. If a 180° pulse is applied at a time τ after the 90° pulse then the individual components of magnetisation remain in the $x'y'$ plane (using the rotating frame of reference) but their phase is inverted so that those precessing at a faster rate now lag behind the slower ones (figure 2.12). After another time τ the faster components will have caught up and all will be in phase again, thus producing a signal called the spin echo. The formation of an echo in this way counteracts only the dephasing caused by field inhomogeneity and at the time of the echo the nuclei are still partly dephased because of the more random effects of transverse relaxation. Figure 2.13 shows a plot of the phase and amplitude of the signal from a number of points within the magnet during a spin echo sequence.

The time at which the signal is obtained can be varied by changing the time between the 90° and 180° pulses (τ), and the time to echo (TE) is always equal to 2τ. Because the effects of transverse relaxation are not reversed by the 180° pulse, the amplitude of the spin echo signal decreases with longer echo times, although the rate of this decrease depends upon T_2. For instance, if transverse relaxation is very rapid (T_2 is short) then very little signal will be obtained with long echo times but if it is slow (T_2 is long) much higher signal will be obtained. Longer echo times therefore impart greater T_2 dependence, and if pathology is sought that is known to have a long T_2 then such sequences will be suitable. On the other hand, T_1 dependence can be imparted by repeating each phase encoding step with

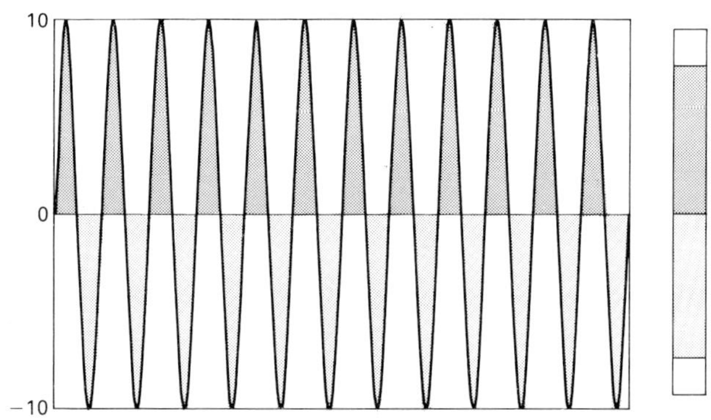

Figure 2.11. The result of multiplying the 60 Hz signal of figure 2.7 with a phase shift of 90° by the 60 Hz test signal. In this case the result is zero because of the lack of phase coherence between the two.

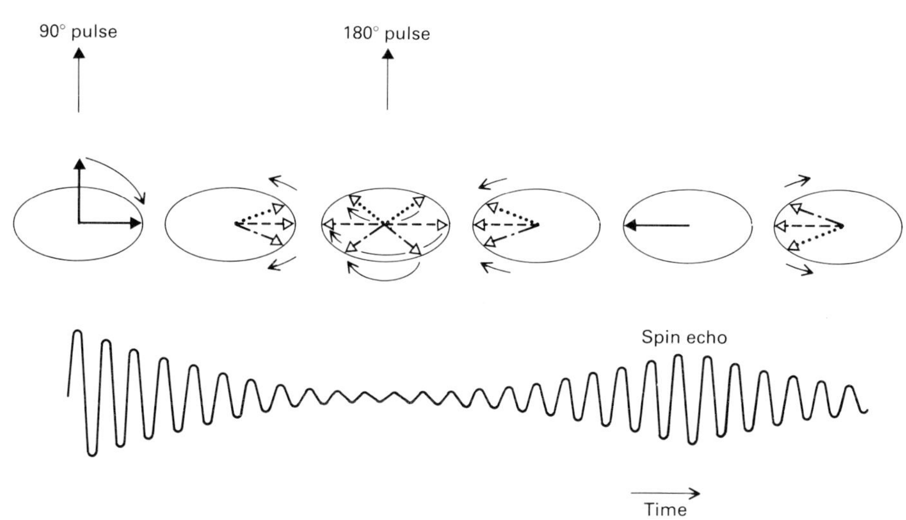

Figure 2.12. The spin echo sequence: After a 90° pulse the induced signal (FID) decays because of field inhomogeneities and also because of spin spin relaxation (T_2). If a 180° pulse is applied at a time τ after the 90° pulse then the phase of each precessing nucleus is inverted and the faster nuclei lag behind the slower ones. After another time τ the nuclei are in phase again, thus producing a signal called the spin echo.

Table 2.1 A summary of the repeat and echo times to weight spin echo images with different parameters. In this context, short and long are with respect to T_1 and T_2

	Repeat time (TR)	Echo time (TE)
Proton density	Long	Short
T_1	Intermediate	Short
T_2	Long	Long

the same repeat time as the T_1 of interest (approximately 500 ms). At this time there will be maximal separation between the longitudinal magnetisation of tissues with different values of T_1 and the signal differences will be greatest. Table 2.1 summarises these effects, but it must be remembered that in cardiac imaging the repeat time is limited to multiples of the cardiac cycle length and so flexibility in choice of the repeat time is limited.

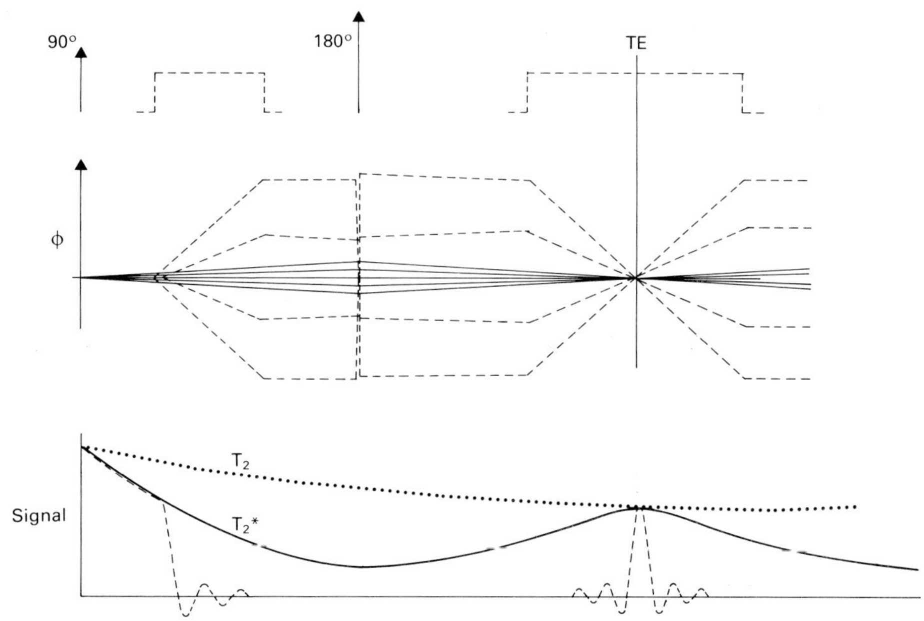

Figure 2.13. The phase and amplitude of the signal from a number of points within the magnet during the application of a spin echo sequence with (dashed) and without (solid) imaging gradients. The theoretical T_2 decay is also shown as a dotted line.

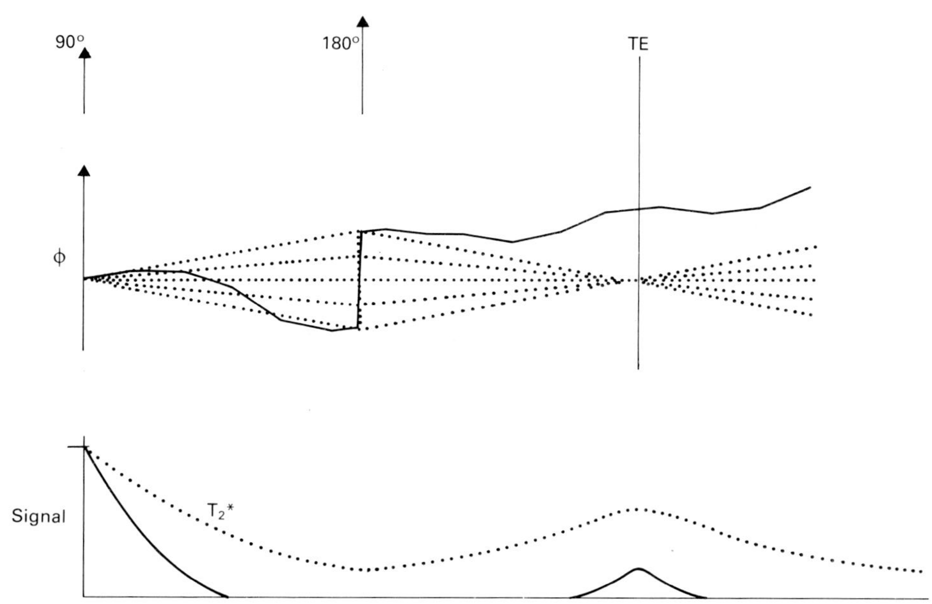

(a)

Figure 2.14. The phases of signals from stationary (dotted line) and diffusing (solid line) material during different spin echo sequences. (a) In the conventional spin echo sequence,[1] nuclei which diffuse through the inhomogeneous field are not perfectly rephased at the time of the spin echo and the signal is reduced.

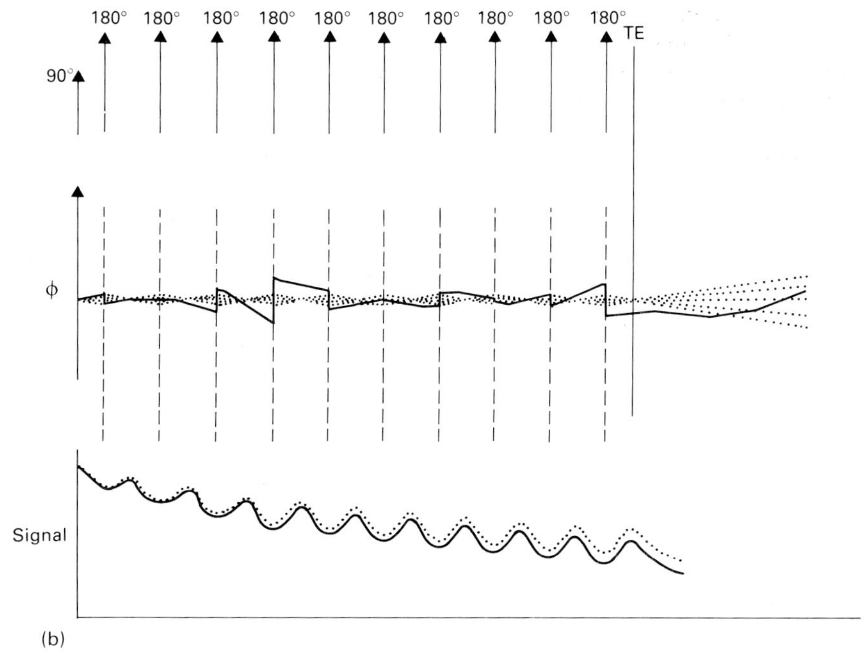

Figure 2.14.(b) The Carr–Purcell multi echo sequence[2] has a short period between 180° pulses and although the echo amplitudes fall off because of transverse relaxation, the phase dispersive effect of diffusion is minimised.

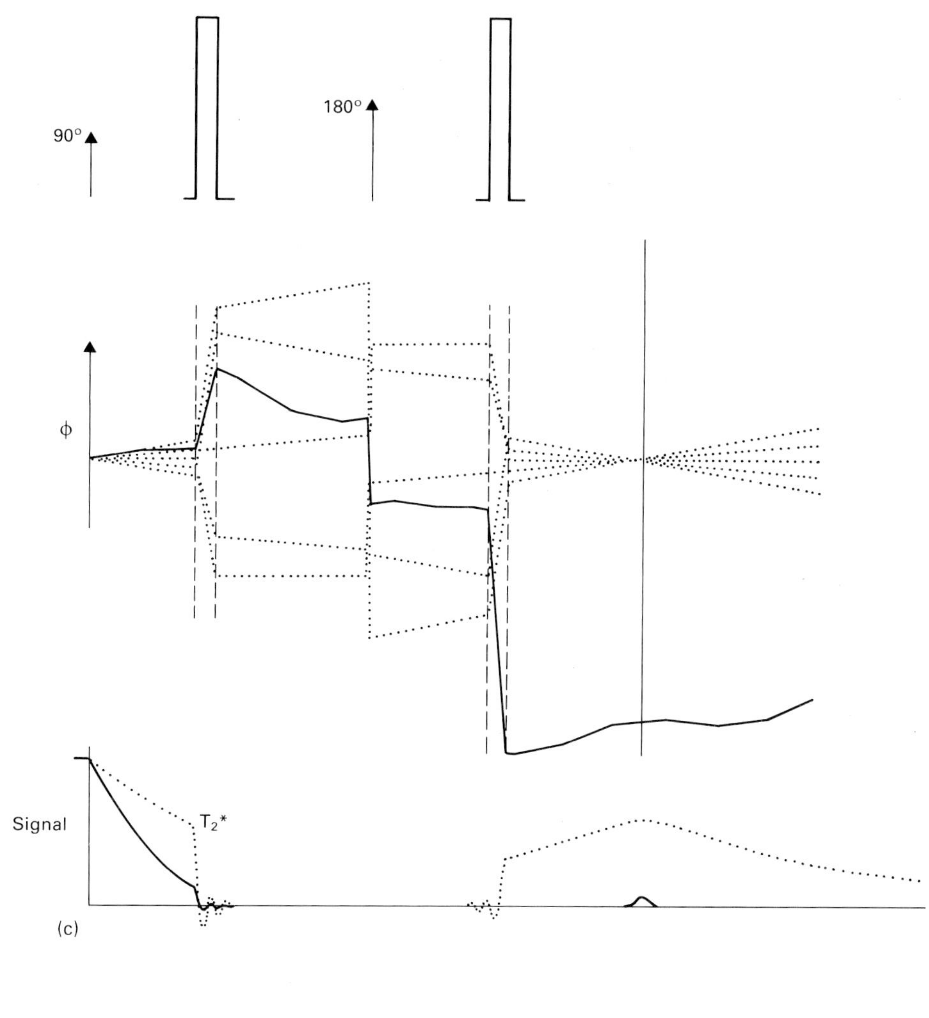

Figure 2.14.(c) In a conventional spin echo sequence with identical field gradients before and after the 180° pulse, the phase dispersion caused by diffusion is maximised.[3] It is assumed for the sake of this diagram that the diffusing spins have a component of motion in the gradient direction.

In addition to the 90° and 180° radio-frequency pulses, slice select, frequency and phase encoding gradients are required in order to form an image. A frequency encoding gradient has been added to figure 2.13. It consists of two parts, the first (sometimes called the dephase gradient) is between the 90° and 180° pulses and it causes rapid dephasing of the nuclei as shown on the plot of phases and also reflected by the sudden decay of the signal amplitude. An equal gradient is applied at the time of data collection and this reverses the dephasing caused by the first lobe as well as frequency encoding the direction in which the gradient is applied. This dephasing and rephasing using a magnetic field gradient is identical to the method of producing an echo described in the next section and is called a gradient echo.

2.5.1.1 *The effect of diffusion*

Figure 2.14(a) shows a plot of the phases of stationary nuclei during a spin echo sequence and also those of nuclei which move randomly by diffusion. Because of inhomogeneities of the static magnetic field, the moving nuclei are not perfectly rephased at the time of the spin echo and this reduces the signal which is obtained. In 1954 Carr and Purcell[2] developed a modification of the spin echo sequence which greatly reduced this effect. They used a rapid series of 180° pulses to produce a series of spin echoes. The amplitude of successive echoes decreases because of transverse relaxation but the phase dispersion of diffusing nuclei is minimised (figure 2.14(b)). If required, the effect of diffusion can be increased by identical field gradients before and after the 180° pulse.[3] Figure 2.14(c) shows that this increases the phase shift of diffusing material and allows accurate measurements of diffusion to be made.

2.5.1.2 *The effect of flow*

Diffusion, which is random in nature, causes random phase shifts leading to phase dispersion and signal loss, especially when gradients such as those used to encode spatial information are used. Flow causes similar phase shifts although, assuming all the material under study is flowing in the same direction and at the same rate, all the phases shifts will be the same and no signal loss will occur. In 1960 Hahn used this global phase shift to develop a technique to measure the flow of sea water.[4] During imaging of the cardiovascular system, much more complicated flow types and flow profiles are experienced and these do normally lead to phase dispersion and signal loss. An advantage of the spin echo sequence for imaging the heart is that flowing blood usually gives no signal and this aids contrast between the different structures of the heart. Methods of imaging blood and measuring blood flow are described in more detail in chapter 10.

2.5.2 The gradient echo sequence

The gradient echo sequence which is also referred to as the field echo or partial saturation sequence, was, despite its simplicity, rather late in its clinical application. It uses a single radio-frequency excitation followed by magnetic field gradients which form an echo at the centre of the data collection period. Figure 2.15 shows the signal amplitude and phase from different positions along the gradient direction during a gradient echo sequence. The initial positive gradient causes rapid phase dispersion and loss of signal which is then reversed by an equal and opposite negative gradient to form an echo. It is not essential that the gradients are of equal and opposite amplitude but the echo forms when the area under the initial positive lobe is equal to that under the negative lobe.

Because this dephasing and rephasing can be achieved very rapidly (echo times shorter than 5 ms can be achieved), the sequence is ideal for rapid repetition and it can be used for cine acquisition (chapter 7). Another property is that the sequence is less susceptible to signal loss caused by flow and blood usually gives a high signal. This is of great benefit for velocity mapping of blood flow (chapter 10).

Because there is no 180° refocusing pulse the magnitude of the signal decays with increasing echo time with the time constant T_2^*, in contrast to the pure T_2 decay of the spin echo signal. This means that signal is lost very rapidly in an inhomogeneous field and this can be recognised in clinical images as a large artefact surrounding metal objects such as sternal sutures or prosthetic heart valves. The absence of a refocusing pulse also makes the image liable to artefacts from chemical shift effects. The protons in lipid and water precess at slightly different rates and the phase relationship between the two signals will vary with echo time. At 0.5 T the two signals are 180° out of phase after about 7 ms and they are in phase again at 14 ms. This has no effect upon the signal from voxels containing pure lipid or pure water, but in voxels that contain

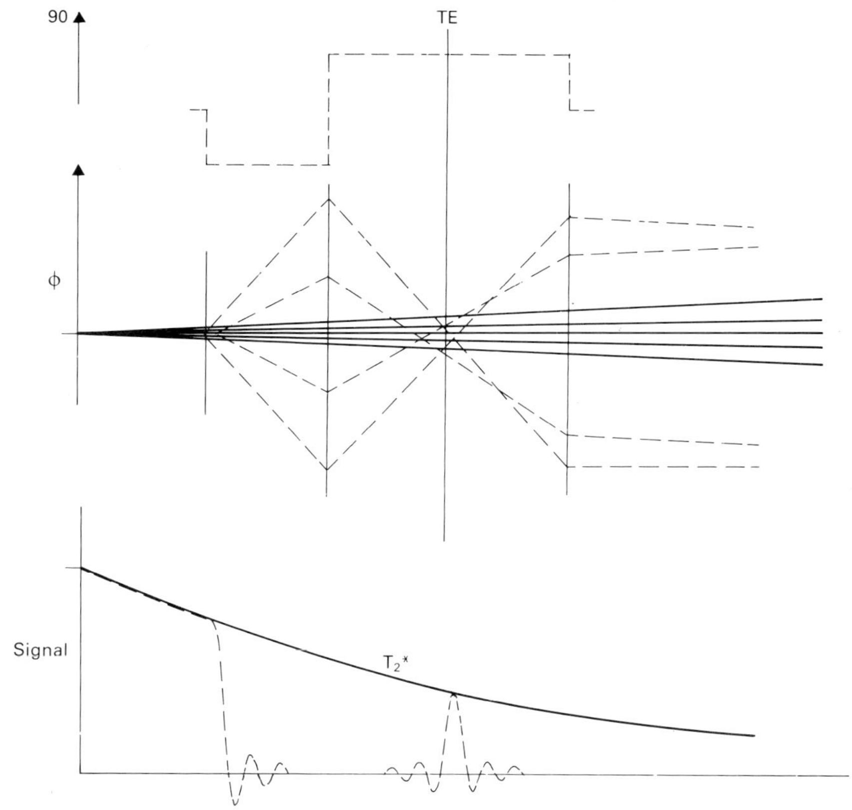

Figure 2.15. The signal amplitude (Signal) and phase (φ) from different positions along the gradient direction during a gradient echo sequence. The solid lines show what would happen without the gradient (slow dispersion and T_2* decay) and the broken lines show the effect of the gradient. The initial negative gradient causes rapid phase dispersion and loss of signal which is then reversed by an equal and opposite positive gradient to form an echo. The magnitude of the echo is reduced because the effect of field inhomogeneity remains.

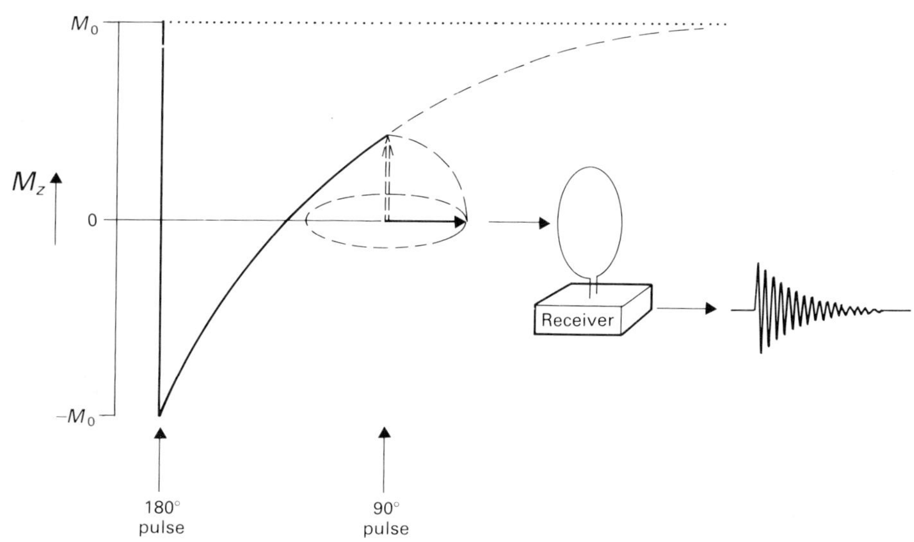

Figure 2.16. Inversion recovery sequence: a 180° pulse inverts the longitudinal magnetisation M_z, which then relaxes back to its equilibrium value exponentially with a time constant T_1. As this relaxation is occurring, a 90° pulse is applied to rotate M_z into the xy plane so that it gives a signal. The amplitude of the signal depends on the size of M_z at the time of the 90° pulse and therefore on T_1.

a mixture of the two, the opposite phases will cancel at echo times of 7 ms (and 21 ms, etc) and cause signal loss. The phenomenon is typically observed as dark lines occurring at boundaries between lipid and water-based tissues and also as low signal from tissues such as the bone marrow.

2.5.3 The inversion recovery sequence

This sequence is longer than the spin echo and gradient echo sequences and so it is less suitable for cardiac imaging. It is very useful for static organs however because the signal can be made to be strongly T_1

dependent. A 180° pulse is first applied to invert the longitudinal magnetisation (M_z becomes $-M_z$), which then relaxes back to its equilibrium value exponentially with a time constant T_1. As this relaxation is occurring, a 90° pulse is applied to rotate M_z into the xy plane so that it gives a signal (figure 2.16). The signal is usually collected in a suitable form for imaging by incorporating a spin echo or a gradient echo sequence after the 90° pulse.

The amplitude of the signal depends upon the size of M_z at the time of the 90° pulse, and so T_1 dependence can be introduced by appropriate choice of timing (figure 2.17). The greatest T_1 dependence is obtained when the time between the radio-frequency pulses (τ) is similar to the T_1 of the tissues being imaged, or between 300 and 600 ms in biological imaging. A variant of the inversion recovery sequence is the short tau inversion recovery (STIR) sequence with an inversion time of the order of 100 ms.[5] At this time, the longitudinal magnetisation of fat is crossing the zero line and no signal is obtained when it is turned into the xy plane by the 90° pulse. This can be particularly helpful when it is required to introduce contrast that depends upon fat content into the image.

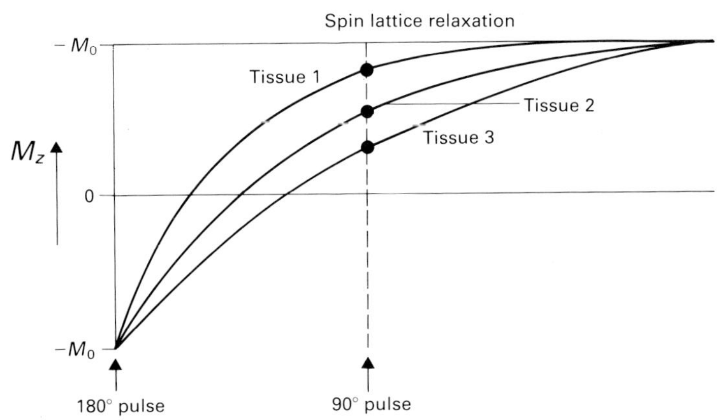

Figure 2.17. Plots showing M_z returning to equilibrium after a 180° pulse for tissues with different T_1 relaxation times. The maximum separation occurs at a time roughly equal to the relaxation times of the tissues.

2.5.4 The echo planar sequence

This sequence was first described by Mansfield in 1977[6] and it allows very rapid imaging with acquisition of a complete image in tens of milliseconds. Because of this speed, cardiac images can be acquired without triggering and it is therefore a very promising technique. In the gradient echo sequence the frequency encoding gradient takes the form of a negative and a positive lobe to form a gradient echo. The sequence is repeated many times with a different phase encoding gradient on each occasion. In echo planar imaging, the frequency encoding gradient is oscillated very rapidly to form a succession of echoes, and phase encoding is achieved by applying a small gradient 'blip' in the phase encoding direction during reversal of the frequency encoding gradient. With suitable hardware it is possible to acquire sufficient information to form a complete image in approximately 30 ms. Figure 2.18 shows the radio-frequency pulses and gradient profiles for a typical echo planar sequence.

Because of the very rapidly switched gradients, the technique is very demanding of imaging hardware, and large gradients have to be used with rapid rise and fall times. Such rapid switching of magnetic field gradients can induce large eddy currents in the main magnet and the object being imaged and it is these eddy currents which complicate application of the technique. At the time of writing, echo planar imaging is just beginning to be implemented on commercially available machines.

An alternative rapid imaging technique is to repeat the gradient echo sequence with a repeat time of only a few milliseconds and in this way an image can be

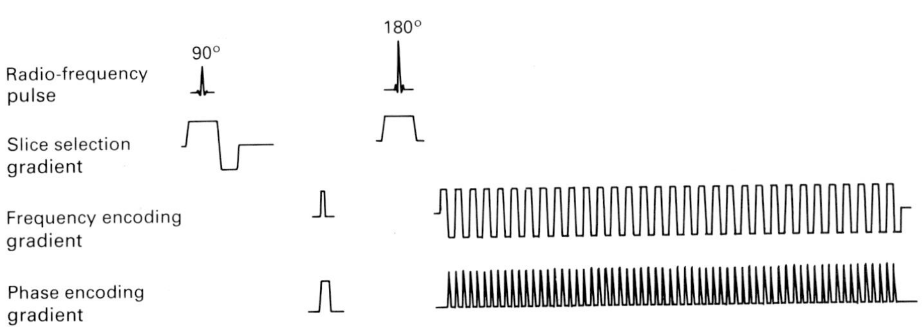

Figure 2.18. The radio-frequency pulse and gradient profiles for a typical echo planar sequence.

acquired in the conventional way in as little as 200 ms.[7] With such a rapid repetition time the method is similar to echo planar imaging except that multiple radio-frequency excitations are used instead of a single one. Because of this, it will never be as fast as echo planar imaging although it does have some advantages in that the hardware requirements are less demanding. Reasonable diastolic images can be acquired since the heart is relatively static in diastole, but systolic images are less good.

References

1 Hahn EL. Spin echoes. *Phys Rev* 1950; **80**: 580–94.

2 Carr HY, Purcell EM. Effects of diffusion on free precession in nuclear magnetic resonance experiments. *Phys Rev* 1954; **94**: 630–8.

3 Stejskal EO, Tanner JE. Spin diffusion measurements: spin echoes in the presence of a time-dependent field gradient. *J Chem Phys* 1965; **42**: 288–92.

4 Hahn EL. Detection of sea-water motion by nuclear precession. *Geophys Res* 1960; **65**: 776–7.

5 Bydder GM, Steiner RE, Blumgart LH, Khenia S, Young IR. MR imaging of the liver using short T_1 inversion recovery sequences. *J Comput Assist Tomogr* 1985; **9**: 1084–9.

6 Mansfield P. Multi-planar image formation using NMR spin echoes. *J Phys C: Solid State Phys* 1977; **10**: 255–8.

7 Haase A, Matthaei D, Norris D. Snapshot-flash NMR imaging. *Procedings of the Eighth Annual Meeting of the Society of Magnetic Resonance in Medicine*. 1989: 364 (Abstract).

Chapter 3 Instrumentation

DAVID FIRMIN

A magnetic resonance scanner has five major components (figures 3.1 and 3.2).

3.1 The magnet

The magnet produces the static magnetic field which is typically between 0.08 and 2 T. Its manufacture is demanding since it is required to produce a field that is homogenous and stable with time, and yet is large enough to contain a human body. Both resistive and superconducting electromagnets are used, and they depend upon a large current circulating in coils to produce the magnetic field. Permanent magnets have also been used although these are usually very heavy and tend only to be used for lower field strengths.

In a resistive magnet the current is driven through the coils at normal temperatures, and one of the major running costs is the power required. The electrical resistance of the coils leads to the generation of a great deal of heat, and water cooling is required. In a superconducting magnet the coils are made of niobium-titanium alloy and they are cooled to 4 K by liquid helium (figure 3.3). At this temperature all electrical resistance is lost, and once the current has started, it will continue to flow without using any power or generating any heat. The main running cost of such a system is the liquid helium although it is possible to condense the helium as it boils off. In addition, the helium can be surrounded by a liquid nitrogen jacket to reduce losses.

The main difference between resistive and superconducting magnets is the stability of the field, and it is very difficult to generate a stable current in a resistive system. On top of this, any slight changes in temperature (either ambient or of the cooling water) can lead to a change in field of a resistive system.

Homogeneity is achieved partly by design of the main coils, partly by a series of subsidiary or shimming coils, and partly by adding magnetic material to correct for distortions in the main field. Variations in field of up to 50 parts per million (ppm) can be tolerated across the imaging volume, although the best magnets are homogenous to nearly 2 ppm. For analytical spectroscopy, homogeneity of 0.1 ppm is needed, and the engineering required to produce such fields is one of

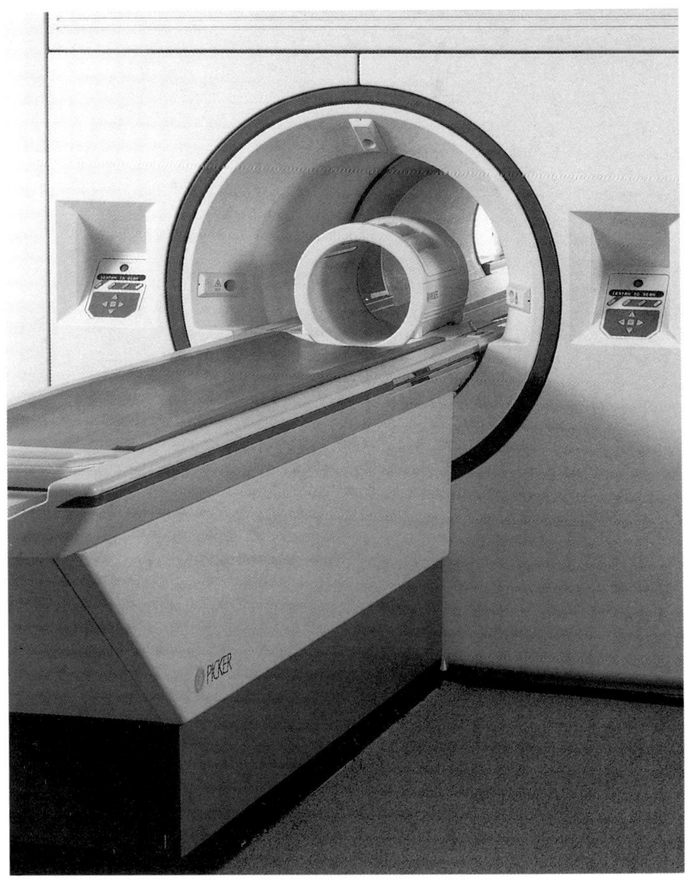

Figure 3.1. A 1.5 T superconducting magnetic resonance scanner.

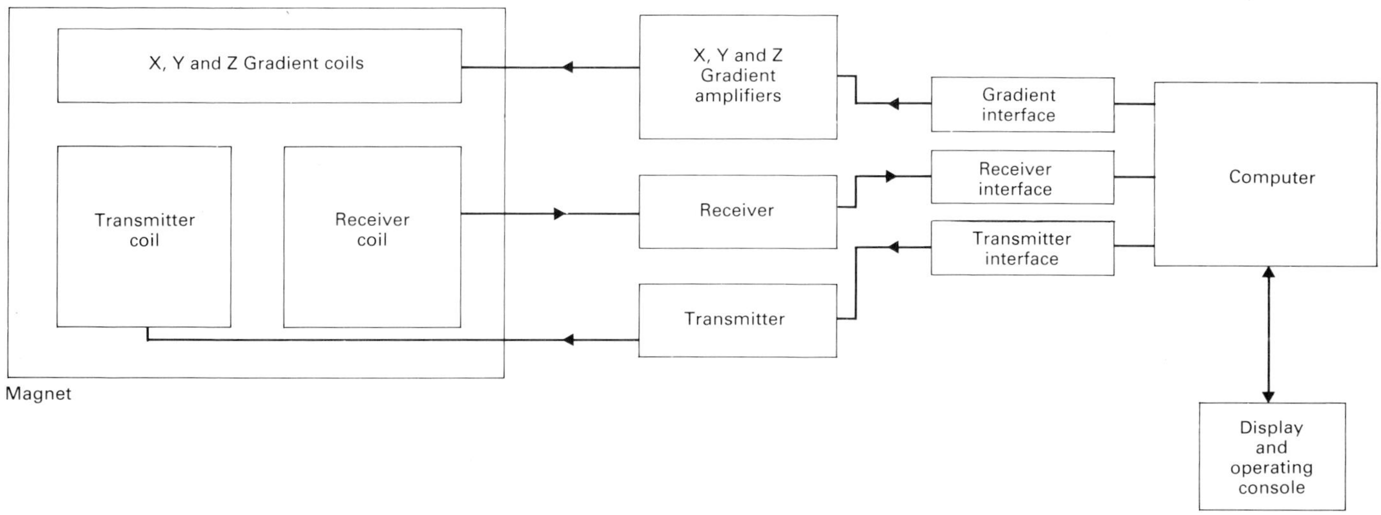

Figure 3.2. Block diagram of a magnetic resonance imaging system.

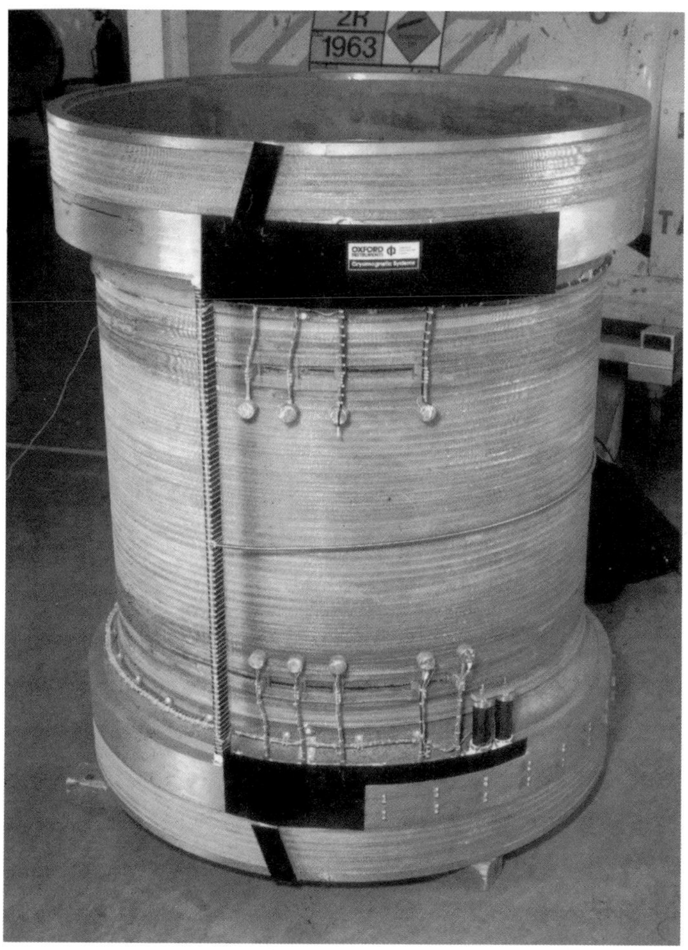

Figure 3.3. The core of a superconducting magnet showing the coils of niobium-titanium wire. This core normally sits inside a cryostat containing liquid helium.

the factors that has determined the rate of development of *in vivo* spectroscopy.

This is not the place to have a detailed discussion of the relative merits of different field strengths, but it is relevant to mention some of the arguments. Many different factors have to be considered and passions tend to run high when the subject is raised. There is no doubt that for imaging of static organs such as the brain and spinal cord, then a high field strength (1.5 T or above) produces higher signal and hence images with higher spatial resolution for an equivalent signal to noise ratio. To set against this, differences in T_1 are reduced at high field and so the contrast to noise ratio is reduced for certain types of pathology. Nonetheless, the neuroradiologist appears to be happiest at high field. For moving organs such as the heart the situation is different because motion artefact increases with field strength and what is gained in signal may be lost in artefact. Electrocardiographic triggering can be more problematical at high field, but good cardiac images can be obtained anywhere from 2 T down to 0.25 T and all of the images presented in this book were acquired between these limits. Below 0.25 T, anatomical information is less good because of the reduced reolution although functional information remains. Another factor is whether spectroscopy is required, although this remains a research tool and the clinical indications for magnetic resonance spectroscopy are still very few. Finally, cost is important and expense increases dramatically with field strength. Until large studies of the cost effectiveness of different field strengths have

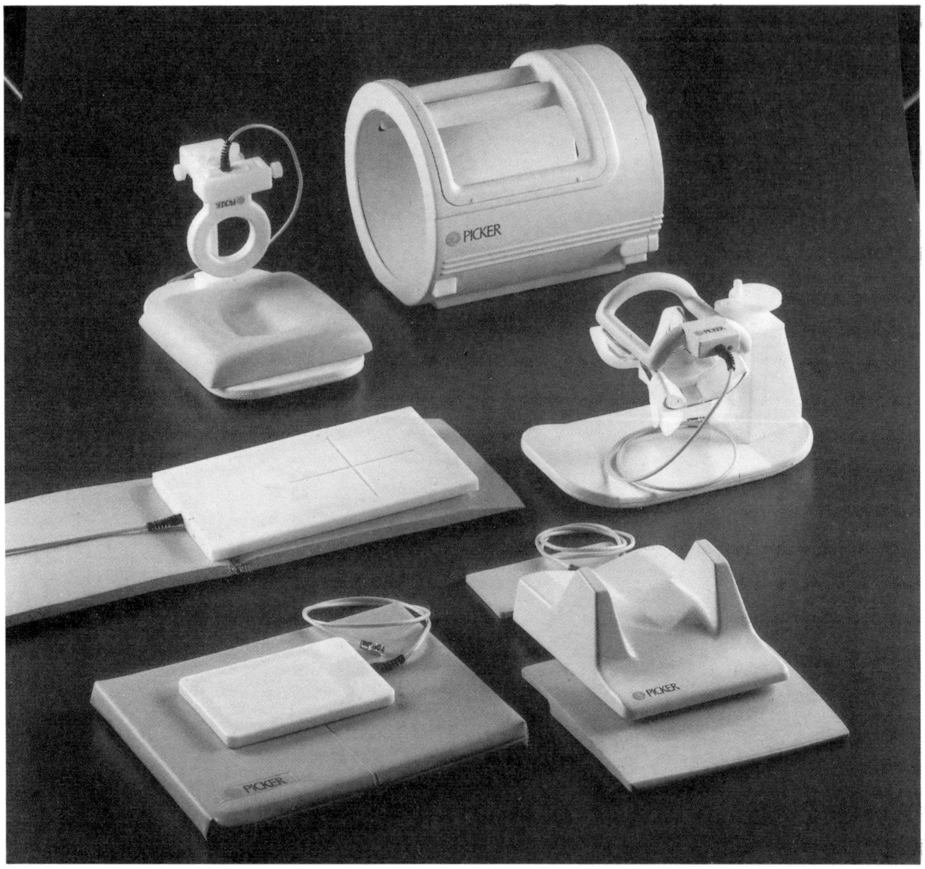

Figure 3.4. Specialised receiver coils for acquisition of the magnetic resonance signal from different regions of the body. Clockwise from the top they are used for the head, the knee, the neck, two for the spine, and the temporomandibular joint.

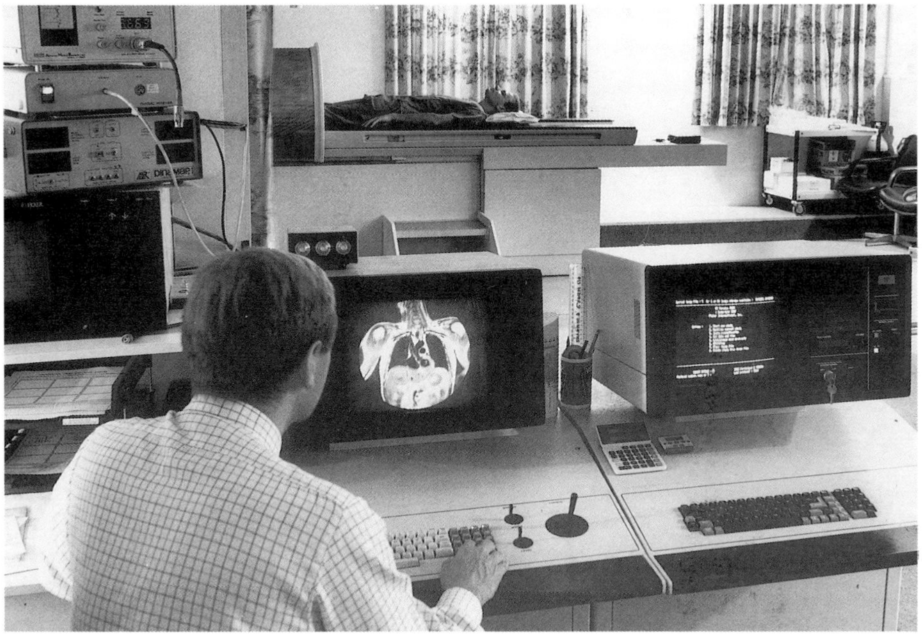

Figure 3.5. The computer console controlling a 0.5 T magnetic resonance scanner. The electrocardiogram triggering unit is seen top left with attached fibreoptic cable link, and remote blood pressure monitoring equipment (used for stress imaging) lies below it. The patient is not positioned for scanning and would be inside the bore of the magnet.

been performed, the idea in some people's minds that low field magnetic resonance is a poor man's tool is unproven.

3.2 The radio-frequency transmitter

The transmitter drives a radio-frequency alternating current through a transmitting coil in order to produce the alternating magnetic field. Its frequency must be equal to the Larmor frequency of the nuclei of interest, and the coil is usually saddle shaped and designed to ensure a constant amplitude throughout the volume of interest.

3.3 The radio-frequency receiver

The receiver coil is a tuned circuit that detects the radio-frequency signal emitted from the body. The signal is amplified by a high quality amplifier, and converted into digital form suitable for storage and manipulation in the computer. The receiver coil is often similar to the transmitter coil although much attention has been paid recently to specialised surface coils that receive signal from localised regions and have a higher signal to noise ratio and hence higher resolution (figure 3.4).

3.4 Magnetic field gradient amplifiers and coils

Magnetic field gradients are superimposed upon the static magnetic field by separate coils and amplifiers which are arranged to produce gradients in the x, y, and z directions. Currents of up to 100 A are required and gradients up to 10 mT/m are required for conventional imaging or 40 mT/m for echo planar imaging. The gradients are small compared with the static field, but they are applied for very short periods and with rapid rise times (200 μs to 10 mT/m). These changing currents give rise to large forces upon the coils carrying them, and the consequent movement produces a sharp noise that may be uncomfortable for the patient. The very rapid field gradients of some sequences, in particular the echo planar sequence, imposes considerable strains upon the coils and special reinforcement may be required.

3.5 The computer

The computer plays a central role since it controls not only the field gradients, but also the radio-frequency pulses. In addition it stores the received signal, and transforms it into the image which it then displays (figure 3.5). An array processor for the rapid handling of data is usual. The latest developments in computers for MR systems incorporate a number of dedicated processors used to interface a main control computer to the various hardware components described above. The demands on the main control computer are thus minimised.

Chapter 4
Practical Aspects of Magnetic Resonance Imaging

RICHARD UNDERWOOD

The major components of commercially available magnetic resonance imagers are very similar and they have been described in chapter 3. Considerable differences exist however in the details of scanning technique and it is important to know the idiosyncrasies of one's own machine in order to apply it well to the cardiovascular system. Unlike other imaging techniques, magnetic resonance has a large number of variables that affect image quality and although predefined protocols are available on most machines, they are often tailored to the imaging of static organs such as the brain and spine. Some 'customisation' may be required but this requires a knowledge of cardiac anatomy and function and also of the many variables that influence the images obtained. This chapter gives a practical guide for those who may find themselves acquiring magnetic resonance tomograms of the heart.

4.1 Patient handling

4.1.1 Comfort

Cardiovascular imaging can take anything from 20 to 90 minutes or more, and if the patient is to stay still for this time it is essential that he or she is comfortable. It is sensible to make sure that he does not want to empty his bladder before the scan. Time spent before the scan explaining what will happen will always be rewarded. In particular the importance of normal breathing and of trying not to cough or swallow should be explained, although in order not to alarm the patient it can also be explained that coughing does not invalidate the whole scan but it introduces artefact into some of the images. The patient can move to become more comfortable between scans but should not move bodily within the scanner otherwise the images will not be acquired in the expected plane. The sound of the sequences can be quite loud, particularly in high field machines and for short echo time cine acquisitions, and it is wise to warn the patient before particularly loud scans. Ear plugs can be used but patients are more likely to tolerate a long scan if they are constantly being told what is happening.

Claustrophobia is not uncommon with the enclosed magnets that are currently available and between 3 and 5% of patients cannot tolerate being in the bore of the magnet. The magnet can be made less forbidding with lighting, fresh air and music but this probably has little effect on true claustrophobia which is an irrational anxiety. Anxiolytics are usually unhelpful. It is difficult to predict in advance which patients will not tolerate scanning and it often arises *de novo* without the patient knowing that he is claustrophobic. Even if the patient does express concern beforehand it is worth trying to perform the scan because many anxious patients can be scanned quite readily.

4.1.2 Positioning

Feet first and supine is the usual orientation. Exact positioning on the couch when outside the magnet depends upon the region to be imaged. Many machines have a system of laser light marking to indicate the point that will be at the centre of the magnet after the patient is moved inside the magnet. It is obviously possible to image planes offset from the centre of the magnet but there is usually a maximum offset (100 mm for instance). This maximum offset is determined by the linearity of the magnetic gradient that can be applied, which is determined in turn by the size of the gradient coils. For an oblique left ventricular volume study a suitable starting position is with the nipple level about 20 mm above the centre of the magnet so that an initial transverse pilot scan with 0 mm offset passes through the body of the ventricle.

The prone position has been used to reduce respiratory chest wall motion but this has the effect of increasing diaphragmatic breathing and is not normally used. In the prone position, the arms may need to be above the head in smaller bore magnets and this is an uncomfortable position if it is required for long periods.

The positioning of the radio-frequency receiver coils varies between manufacturers. In some machines, they are incorporated into the bore of the magnet but in others, local surface coils may need to be worn by the patient.

4.2 Electrocardiographic triggering

Conventional magnetic resonance images are formed from a number of repetitions of a sequence, each with a different phase encoding gradient. For a moving organ such as the heart each sequence must be triggered to occur at the same part of the cardiac cycle. Several different triggering techniques can be used, including finger plethysmography and carotid pulse tracings, but the most widely used is the electrocardiogram because the electrical activity of the heart bears a constant relationship to its mechanical activity and because the most easily recognisable feature, the R wave, preceeds mechanical systole and makes available all other parts of the cycle. The technique is often refered to as cardiac gating, but strictly it is cardiac triggering since a cardiac event is used to trigger the sequence. Gating is used in radionuclide ventriculography, for instance, when the acquisition occurs continuously but the cardiac events are used to assign the information to different frames through the cardiac cycle.

4.2.1 Artefacts in the electrocardiogram

It is not a simple matter to record the electrocardiogram of a patient during imaging. The static magnetic field has a number of effects and the changing fields during imaging introduce additional artefacts. The motion of the blood within the heart and aorta induces potentials that are superimposed upon the electrocardiogram, mainly upon the ST segment and T wave because this is when flow is most rapid. The induced potential is greatest when blood flow is perpendicular to the field, and the direction of the potential is perpendicular to both the field and the flow. The effect is more pronounced in high fields. A well designed gating system will be able to distinguish the R wave from a T wave, even when the T wave is artificially amplified by the flow artefact because it should recognise not only amplitude of deflection but also rate of rise. Some systems however trigger only when a predefined threshold of amplitude is reached and such systems may experience problems with large T waves. Ideally, it should be possible for the user to adjust the sensitivity of the gating system both for amplitude and for rate of rise.

The rapidly switched magnetic field gradients used during imaging sequences also induce potentials in conductors present in the magnetic field, such as the electrocardiographic electrodes and cables. The size of these depends upon the rate of change of magnetic flux through the conductor loop presented to the field and upon the area of the loop. The spike artefacts induced during imaging can be eliminated by clamping the electrocardiogram during the gradient pulses but this makes it difficult to monitor the electrocardiogram during imaging and a better solution is to introduce filters into the circuitry. It is possible to reduce these artefacts by placing the electrodes close together on the patient (although this is partially self-defeating because it also reduces the size of the QRS complex), by minimising the length of cable within the field, and by twisting the leads around each other. Figure 4.1 shows some of the effects of imaging upon the electrocardiogram.

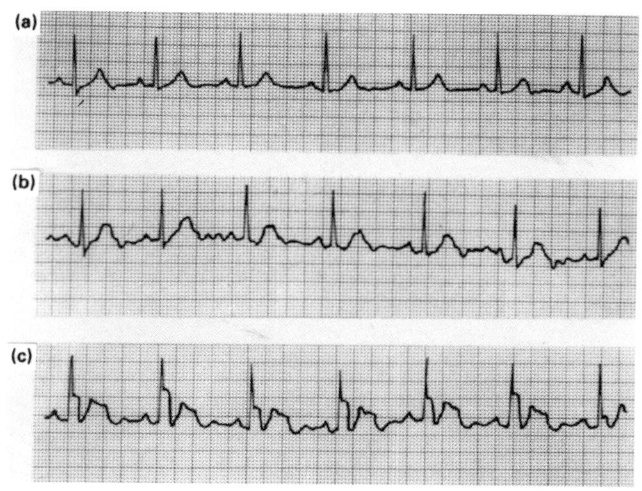

Figure 4.1. Electrocardiogram recorded (a) outside a magnetic field of 0.5 T, (b) inside it and (c) during imaging. The extra potentials seen in (b) are induced by motion of blood within the heart and aorta. In (c) the tracing is clamped briefly at the time of imaging which is on the downstroke of the R wave (end diastole) and close to the end of the T wave (end systole).

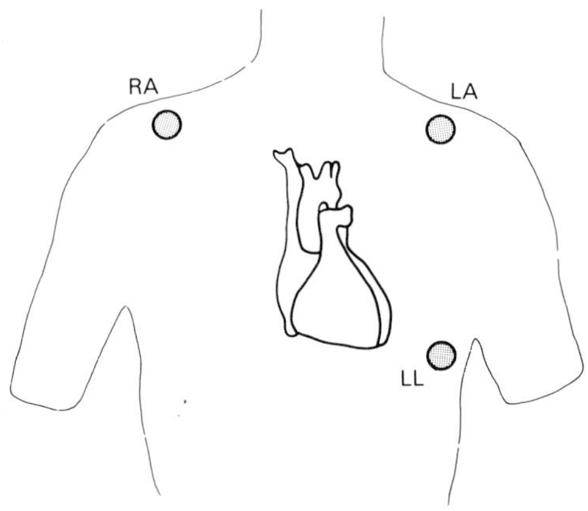

Figure 4.2. Typical positions of the electrodes for recording the electrocardiogram during magnetic resonance imaging. The position of the left leg lead (LL) is slightly modified and bipolar recording between the right arm (RA) and the chest lead (LL) approximates to lead CM5. Reducing the size of the triangle reduces artefacts at the expense of also reducing the size of the QRS complex.

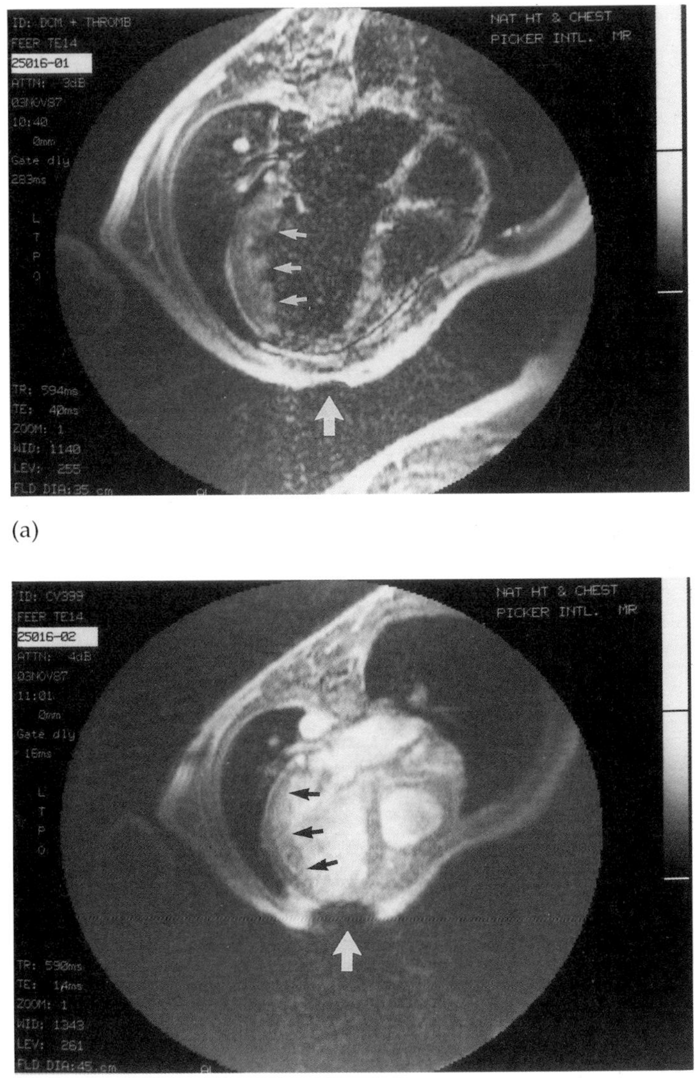

(a)

(b)

Figure 4.3. Artefacts produced by a metallic electrocardiogram electrode placed at the apex (large arrow). On the spin echo image (a) the artefact is very much smaller than on the gradient echo image (b). The images are acquired in the horizontal long axis plane and the patient has a dilated cardiomyopathy with thrombus lining the lateral wall of the left ventricle (small arrows).

4.2.2 Electrode positioning

Dimick and colleagues have shown that the vector of the flow induced potential usually points anteriorly and is slightly depressed from the horizontal.[1] Because the normal QRS vector in the magnetic field is towards the left or posteriorly, a left sided or posterior lead is recommended to maximise the ratio of the QRS complex to the artefact. This can be achieved by placing the electrodes on each shoulder and in the anterior axillary line in the fifth intercostal space, when the bipolar lead recorded between the left chest and the right shoulder approximates to lead CM5 (figure 4.2). Some operators prefer to place the leads in similar positions but on the back.

The material of which the electrodes are made is also relevant. Conventional electrodes are not ferromagnetic but their metallic content induces artefacts on the images by altering the magnetic field locally and by sustaining eddy currents. In spin echo images these artefacts are very superficial and can usually be ignored but field echo images are much more affected by inhomogeneities of magnetic field and larger artefacts are created. It is wise to avoid the region of the apex when using conventional electrodes for cine field echo imaging or to use specialised electrodes containing minimal or no metal. Figure 4.3 shows the artefact produced by metallic electrodes in a spin echo and a field echo image.

Transmission of the electrocardiogram out of the magnet also requires care because wires led into the magnet not only have large potentials induced in them by the imaging sequence but they also introduce radiofrequency noise into the field. To overcome this, the electrocardiogram can either be converted to an optical signal and led out along a fibre-optic cable[2] or it can be transmitted by radiotelemetry at a frequency that does not interfere with imaging (450 MHz).[3]

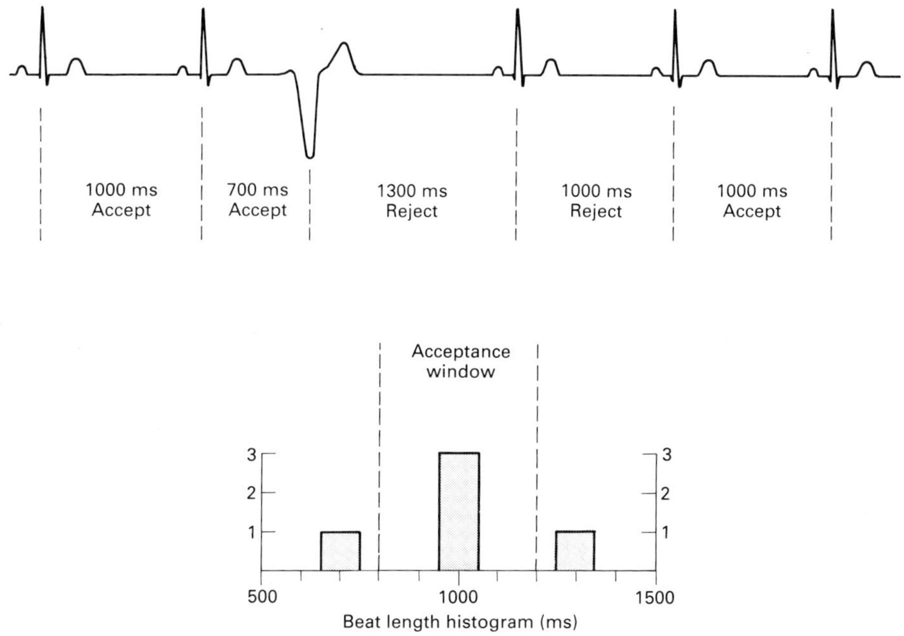

Figure 4.4. Arrhythmia rejection. The user defines a window of beat lengths that will be accepted. The beat following one that falls outside this window is rejected and the effect is to reject the ectopic beat and the following sinus beat. The pulse sequence should continue during every beat but the information from rejected beats is ignored.

4.2.3 Cardiac rhythm

Any irregularity of rhythm invalidates the assumption inherent to cardiac triggering, namely that the cardiac cycles used to construct the image are identical. This produces artefact that is more marked in field echo images than spin echo images. Sinus arrhythmia or infrequent ectopic beats do not seriously interfere with image quality but frequent ectopics and atrial fibrillation may do so. Nevertheless, it is always worth attempting to image because diagnostic information can often be obtained even from patients with marked arrhythmia.

Some systems are able to suspend acquisition for a number of beats after a cycle of abnormal length and this helps to reduced artefact (figure 4.4). A more versatile method is to pulse the imaging sequence continuously and to record the timing of each pulse. The data can be formatted retrospectively according to beat length but this technique is expensive of computer memory and is only available on a few systems.

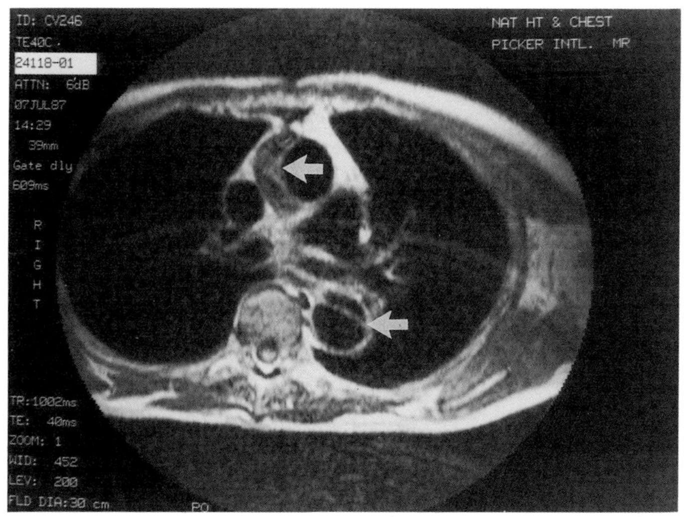

Figure 4.5. The effects of respiratory motion. A shadow of the anterior chest wall is seen overlying the heart. The patient has aortic dissection involving both the ascending and descending aorta (arrows).

4.2.4 Respiratory gating

Respiratory motion is usually ignored and this introduces artefact[4] not only because the heart moves within the chest throughout the respiratory cycle, but also because of the effects of respiration upon cycle length and upon right heart filling. It also means that little information is obtained from the lungs beyond the hila. Figure 4.5 shows the effects of respiratory motion upon the images. Respiratory gating is possible using a number of devices. A pneumograph strapped around the chest monitors chest expansion or a mirror on the chest wall or abdomen can be used to reflect a light beam to record respiratory motion. The respiratory gate can then be used to record information only from cardiac cycles that occur within a predetermined part of the respiratory cycle. This significantly improves image quality but it prolongs acquisition time and for this reason it is not routinely used. For instance, end respiratory gating may prolong a four minute image to 20 minutes.

Other methods of suppressing artefact from respiratory motion have been developed, the most successful of which uses respiratory ordered phase encoding (ROPE).[5] In this technique the phase encoding steps are not acquired sequentially but they are acquired according to the phase of the respiratory cycle in which each beat falls, and acquisition time is only slightly prolonged compared with normal acquisitions. Considerable success has been demonstrated in the abdomen, but there is little experience of cardiac imaging combined with ROPE. Respiratory triggering (as opposed to gating) has also been described[6] but it cannot be combined with cardiac triggering.

4.3 Scanning procedures

This section describes some of the technical factors relevant to static spin echo imaging. Cine imaging and cine velocity mapping are covered in chapters 7 and 10 respectively.

4.3.1 Sequences

A spin echo sequence with an echo time of 24–40 ms is suitable for showing anatomy. Shorter echo times are more likely to have signal from slowly moving blood in the cardiac cavities which may hinder interpretation,[7] but longer echo time images are more likely to suffer from artefact caused by motion during the sequence. On balance, the artefacts caused by signal from moving blood are the worse of the two evils and the longer echo times produce better images. Some centres routinely use multiple echo sequences and display both first and second echo images. The second echo images can be helpful to differentiate blood from myocardium because the phenomenon of even echo rephasing leads to much higher signal from moving structures in all even-echoed images. Images at different echo times may also be used to estimate transverse relaxation times (see chapter 8).

Inversion recovery sequences are more difficult to combine with cardiac triggering because the inversion time, which may be 500 ms, means that only later diastolic images can be acquired. They may be useful for producing different contrast in cardiac tumours but anatomy is not usually so well seen. The short inversion time inversion recovery (STIR) sequence[8] can be more useful for manipulating contrast because of its shorter duration. Using this sequence, the inversion time can be adjusted so that signal from fat is suppressed, and this can be useful for differentiating fat from other structures with high signal on spin echo images. Other sequences that make use of the chemical shift between protons in lipid and those in water can be used to measure the amount of lipid in different tissues such as atheroma and these are discussed in chapter 11.

Sequences that use magnetic field gradients to dephase and rephase the spins after an exciting radiofrequency pulse are very important in cine cardiac imaging and they are discussed in chapter 7.

4.3.2 Field of view

The best field of view depends upon the information required from the image. The small pixels in small fields potentially show fine anatomical detail, but there is a compromise to be made between field of view, signal to noise ratio, and imaging time. The reduced signal from smaller pixels must either be accepted or the imaging time must be increased. Other factors such as motion artefact and artefact caused by irregular rhythms are worse with small fields of view. A 30 cm field of view is usual for transverse images of the heart in adults and 35–45 cm can be used for coronal and sagittal images. Fields of view smaller than 30 cm can present problems with signal to noise ratio and with wrap around in the phase encoding direction if tissue giving signal lies outside the field of view (see next paragraph). Because artefacts are more troublesome with cine field echo sequences, it is better to use a field of view between 40 and 45 cm for cine imaging and velocity mapping.

4.3.3 Phase encoding direction

As explained in chapter 2, localisation of the magnetic resonance signal is achieved by a combination of magnetic field gradients in three dimensions. The slice select gradient defines the plane that is imaged, bt within this plane the frequency and phase encoding directions can be chosen at will. The most important factor governing the direction of phase encoding (vertical or horizontal with respect to the image) is

Table 4.1 Recommended phase encoding direction for each imaging plane

Imaging plane	Phase encoding
Transverse	Vertical
Coronal	Horizontal
Sagittal	Horizontal
Vertical long axis	Horizontal
Horizontal long axis	Vertical
Short axis	Either

whether material that produces a magnetic resonance signal lies outside the field of view. If it lies outside in the direction of phase encoding, then its signal will wrap around back into the image and may confuse interpretation. Other factors being equal, it is therefore best to orientate the phase encoding direction vertically for transverse images and horizontally for coronal and sagittal images. Apart from altering the phase encoding direction, the problem can be avoided by using a larger field of view, receiver coils that are insensitive to tissue outside the field of interest, or one of several other 'anti-aliasing' techniques.

If tissue does not lie outside the field of view then another factor to be considered is motion artefact, which is spread across the image as a band in the phase encoding direction. The band can be orientated to avoid other structures of interest within the image. Moreover, motion in the direction of frequency encoding produces worse artefact than motion in the direction of phase encoding. In the horizontal long axis plane therefore, it is better to have the phase encoding vertically within the image, because blood flow into and out of the heart is mainly in this direction. See Table 4.1 for preferred phase encoding directions.

4.3.4 Pixel size

The ability to resolve small structures in magnetic resonance images is determined by factors such as voxel dimensions, signal to noise ratio, motion artefact and magnet homogeneity. The size of the voxel is entirely operator determined but the other factors such as motion artefact and magnet homogeneity may be outside his or her control. Commonly, the images are anisotropic, i.e. the voxel dimensions differ in each direction. Slice thickness is usually the largest voxel dimension and it can range from 5 to 10 mm although slices as thin as 2 mm can be acquired by most imagers. For adult cardiac imaging 10 mm is usually adequate but 7 or 5 mm may be required for neonates. With slice thicknesses of less than 5 mm the signal to noise ratio is likely to be inadequate unless compensated for by increased imaging time (more averages of each phase encoding step).

Pixel size in the frequency encoding direction is less restricted since it is determined by the rate at which the magnetic resonance signal is sampled. This can be extremely rapid but resolution is usually limited to 256 pixels across the field of view.

Pixel size in the phase encoding direction is determined by the number of phase encoding steps used in the acquisition. Since each phase encoding step requires one cardiac cycle this strongly influences the acquisition time. An adequate number for a pilot scan is 64 phase encoding steps (approximately 1 minute of acquisition if the heart rate is 60 per minute) but 128–256 steps is usual for clinical images. In addition, each step can be acquired more than once and the results averaged; thus an acquisition of 2 averages of 128 phase encoding steps will take 256 cardiac cycles or 3–4 minutes depending upon heart rate.

When reconstructed, the image is displayed with a number of pixels that is often greater than the number acquired and the additional pixels are interpolated between the acquired pixels. A dispay matrix of 512 by 512 pixels is usual.

4.3.5 Delay time

In order to acquire images at any part of the cardiac cycle, a delay between the R wave of the electrocardiogram and the triggering of the sequence is introduced. The timing of the image will be slightly later than the delay time because of the finite duration of the sequence. For instance, using a sequence with an echo time of 40 ms and a delay time of 290 ms, the signal will be acquired 330 ms after the R wave. Thus images can be timed to correspond to end diastole, end systole or any other time in between. The best delay for an end diastolic image is 0 ms and this produces an image approximately 40 ms after the R wave (during isovolumetric contraction) if an echo time of 40 ms is used. Late diastolic images acquired with a delay time slightly shorter than the shortest cycle length are less satisfactory, partly because at this point in the cycle intracavitary blood is often static and gives high signal, and partly because the image will be acquired before atrial contraction and will not represent the end diastolic heart.

End systole is more difficult to define in advance of imaging. A phonocardiogram can be acquired before imaging to locate the second heart sound, but in practice it is usually sufficient to time the image at the end of the T wave of the electrocardiogram or to use the known relationship between the duration of systole and heart rate.[9] Cine imaging is another method of determining true end systole since the time of minimum ventricular volume can be measured.

It is not easy to acquire good images using a long delay time that places the acquisition in the cardiac cycle after the R wave used for triggering, because the variation in cycle length, even in patients in sinus rhythm, is too great. For this reason, images before and after atrial systole are difficult to achieve.

4.3.6 Repeat time

The requirement for cardiac triggering restricts the repeat time of the sequence to the length of the cardiac cycle or multiples thereof. It is usual to specify a minimum repeat time before which the sequence will not be triggered even if an R wave is sensed. In this way premature ectopic beats and artefacts arising from patient motion or from the sequence itself can be prevented from triggering the sequence. The smallest value that can be defined as the minimum repeat time will depend upon the duration of the sequence, and for multislice acquisitions it may be several hundred milliseconds. Although manufacturers differ, some use the minimum repeat time to define the period over which a multislice or a cine acquisition is acquired. In this way, multislice and cine acquisitions can be spread out to cover the entire cardiac cycle, or conversely they can be concentrated into a short period such as systole where spin echo images tend to have higher contrast between soft tissue and moving blood.

4.3.7 Slice offset

This is the perpendicular distance from the centre of the magnet (or other fixed reference point) to the centre of a single slice. For multislice acquisitions, different manufacturers have different conventions but the offset may be to the centre of the group of slices. The direction of positive offset is also a matter of convention but it may either be fixed with respect to the magnet or to the patient. The latter is more convenient since the orientation of the patient within the magnet can be ignored. A typical scheme is for the positive offset to be towards the head for transverse images, towards the anterior chest wall for coronal images, and towards the right of the patient for sagittal images. The problem is more complicated for oblique images, but a simple solution is for the positive offset to be towards the viewer when the image is displayed.

4.3.8 Multislice imaging

Although any individual image is formed from data acquired over a number of cardiac cycles, it is possible to use each R–R interval to acquire several images with different offsets in the same plane. Three dimensional anatomy can therefore be covered very quickly, although the disadvantage of multislice imaging is that each slice is acquired at a different part of the cardiac cycle and it is difficult to control the timing of the slices independently. Because the slice profile of each image is not exactly square, they may overlap slightly and residual magnetisation in neighbouring slices can interfere with data acquisition. In order to overcome this, some manufacturers introduce small gaps between slices but other manufacturers acquire contiguous slices although in an order which minimises interference. Thus the stack of slices may not be acquired in the order 1,2,3,4, . . . but in the order 2,4,6, . . ., 1,3,5, . . .

One method of having more control over the timing of each slice is to perform a multislice acquisition a number of times, rotating the order of acquisition so

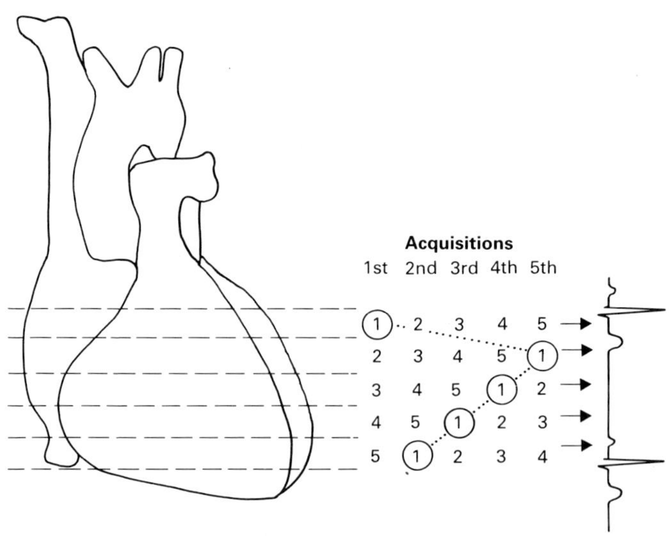

Figure 4.6. In rotating multislice imaging, n slices are acquired n times, each time in a different order. The result is that every slice is acquired at a number of points in the cardiac cycle and can be viewed as a cine display.

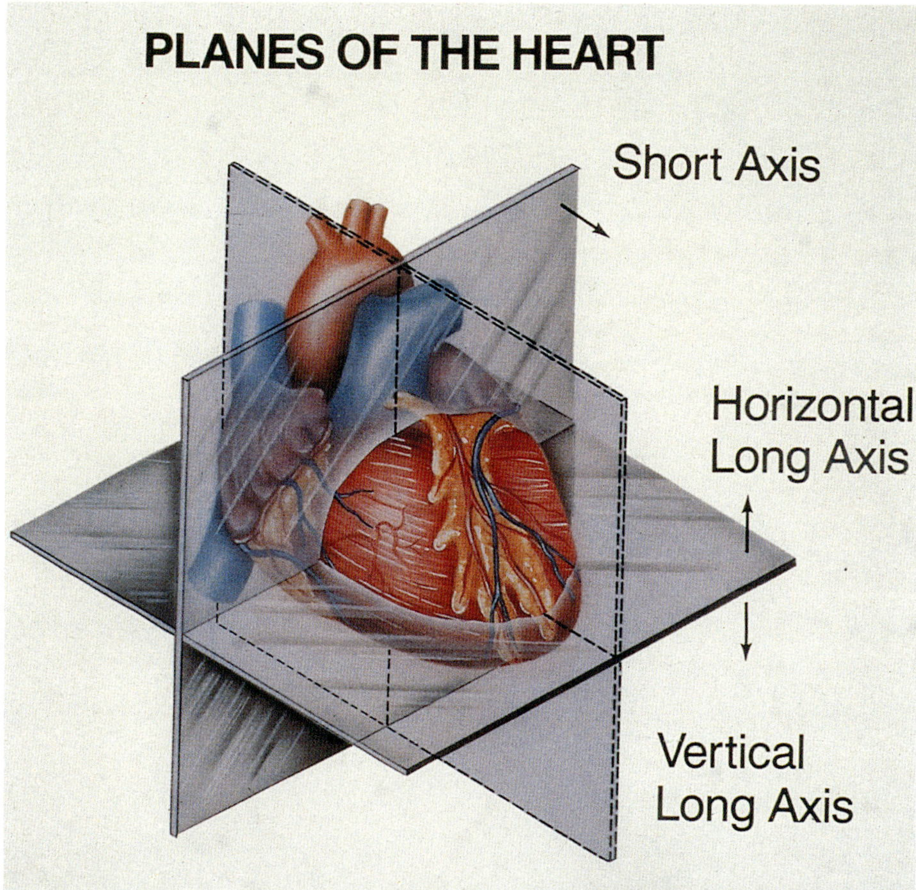

Plate 1. The three planes that are parallel or perpendicular to the long axis of the left ventricle. The vertical long axis plane is equivalent to the right anterior oblique projection except that it is a plane and not a projection, the horizontal long axis plane is equivalent to the apical four chamber view of echocardiography, and the short axis plane is also used in echocardiography.

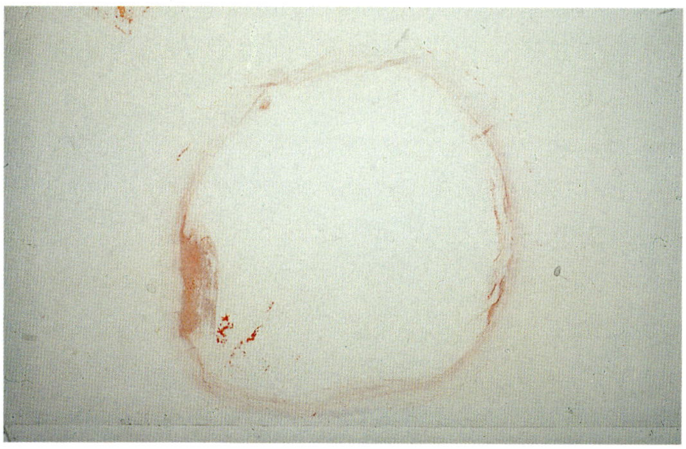

Plate 2. Histology of the plaque seen in figure 11.3, p. 133 (oil red O stain) showing lipid deposition (red) within the intima. (Reproduced with permission from *Br Heart J* 1989; **62:** 81–90.)

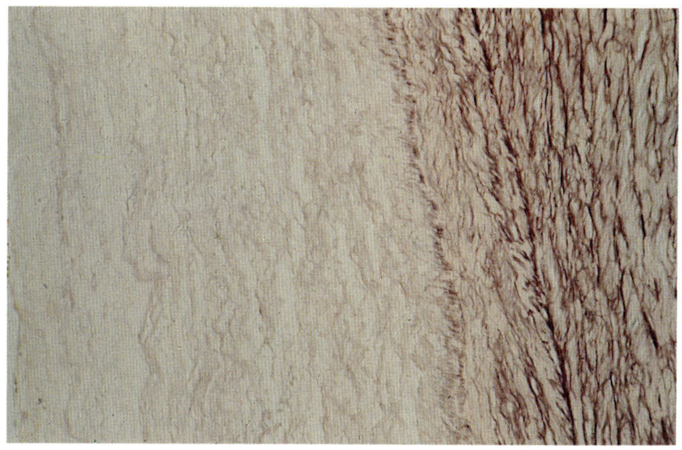

Plate 3. Elastic Van Gieson stain of the plaque seen in figure 11.4, p. 133, which indicates a predominantly smooth muscle and fibrous plaque. Lipid deposition would appear as vacuoles in this alcohol treated stain, but there are none. (Reproduced with permission from *Br Heart J* 1989; **62:** 81–90.)

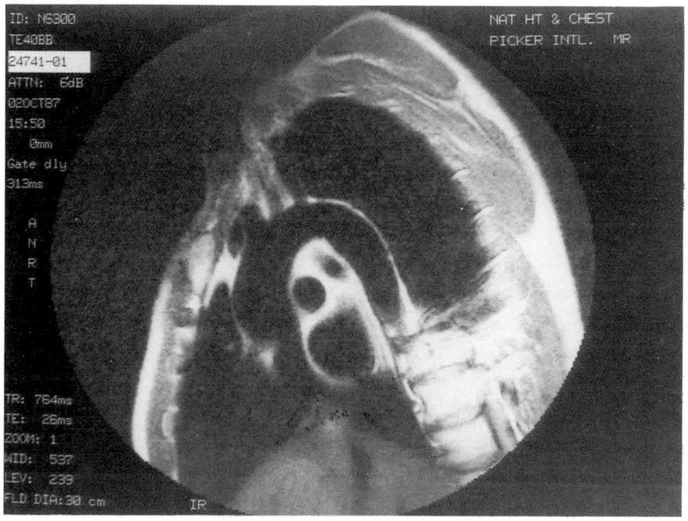

(a)

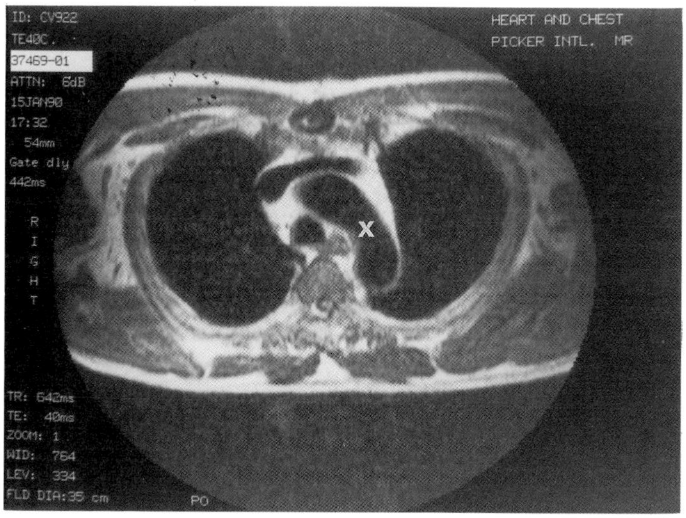

(b)

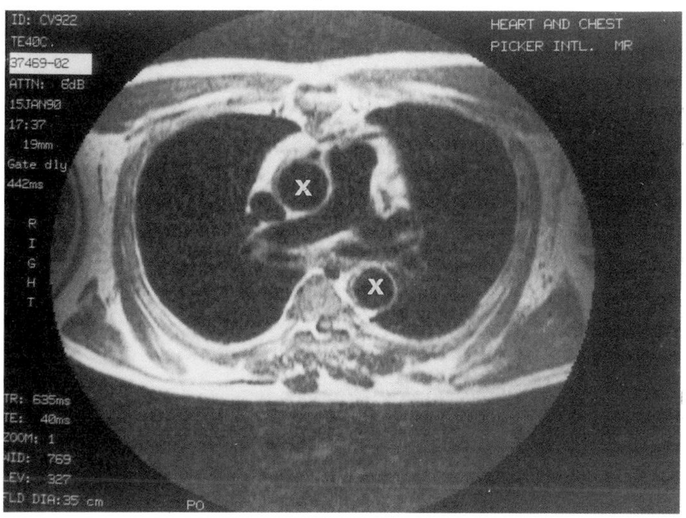

(c)

that every slice is acquired at a number of fixed points in the cardiac cycle (figure 4.6). For instance, five slices can be acquired in the order 1,2,3,4,5, then a second acquisition in the order 2,3,4,5,1, then a third in the order 3,4,5,1,2, etc. After reordering the slices, a five frame cine loop has been acquired at each level. Although this technique was previously common, it is being eclipsed by true cine acquisition using rapidly repeated field echo sequences.

The choice of imaging plane will depend upon the information required but the transverse plane is the best initial plane for anatomy of the ventricles and great vessels, and the coronal plane often provides supplementary information. The sagittal plane is sometimes helpful in patients with congenital heart disease. Oblique imaging is particularly important for the aortic arch and for the left ventricle which is best imaged in planes parallel or perpendicular to its own long axis. The method of acquiring oblique images by using previous images as pilots is described in section 4.3.10, but another method that is particularly helpful for the aortic arch or for the horizontal long axis plane through the ventricles is the three point technique. Three points are chosen anywhere in a stack of images and these points define the oblique plane to be acquired. For the aortic arch, for instance, the top of the arch and points on the ascending and descending aorta could be chosen (figure 4.7).

The maximum number of slices that can be obtained in a single acquisition depends upon the R–R interval and the delay time chosen between the R wave and the beginning of the sequence. Depending upon the heart rate and the echo time of the chosen sequence, between 8 and 16 slices is usual using a 0 ms delay. If this does not cover sufficient ground then the acquisition can be repeated using a different offset. It may be helpful when imaging neonates or small structures such as coronary artery bypass grafts to interleave two sets of 10 mm images offset from each other by 5 mm.

Figure 4.7. To acquire an oblique plane through the aortic arch (a), three points can be defined from a stack of transverse images, for instance the top of the arch [marked with an *X* in (b)], the ascending aorta and the descending aorta (c). Note in image (c) that the patient has had coronary artery bypass grafting, two of which can be seen anterior to the pulmonary artery and one to its left, and also that atheromatous thickening of the aortic wall is seen in both the ascending and the descending aorta.

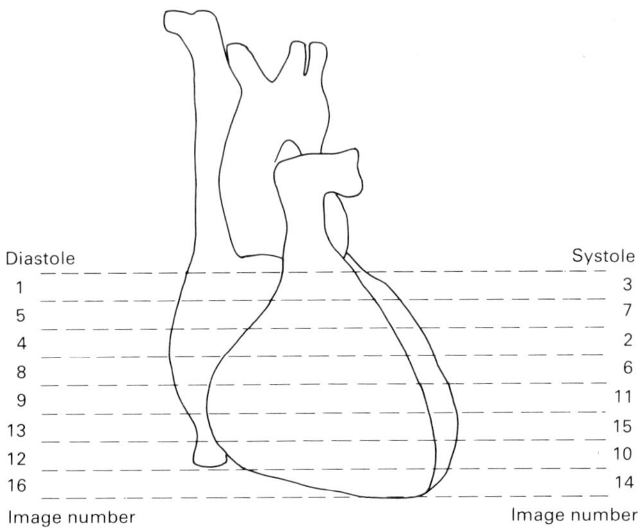

Figure 4.8. A series of two slice acquisitions can be used to calculate ventricular volumes accurately. In each acquisition, one level is acquired at end diastole together with a level 2 cm apart at end systole. A second sequence acquires the first level at end systole and the second level at end diastole, and the two sequences can then be repeated with different offsets to acquire each level at both times in the cardiac cycle. Thus images 1 and 2 are acquired together, then 3 and 4, etc.

4.3.9 Multislice ventricular volume measurement

This is the most accurate method of measuring left ventricular volume and it is the only satisfactory way of measuring right ventricular volume. Contiguous slices are acquired through the heart at end diastole and end systole and the areas of the chambers in each slice are summed. Because each slice must be acquired at the same part of the cardiac cycle a conventional multislice acquisition cannot be used and the slices must either be acquired separately or, to halve the acquisition time, a diastolic and a systolic slice can be acquired at different levels in one acquisition. The technique is illustrated in figure 4.8.

From the end diastolic (ED) and end systolic (ES) volumes, the stroke volume (SV = ED − ES) and the ejection fraction (EF = SV/ED) can be calculated, and the ratio of left and right ventricular stroke volumes allows the regurgitant fraction (RF) to be derived in patients with valvular regurgitation (RF = 1−RVSV/LVSV)[10] and the pulmonary to systemic flow ratio in patients with atrial septal defects (Q_p/Q_s = RVSV/LVSV).[11] With practice, the accuracy of the volume measurements can be better than 5%[12] and the technique is further discussed in chapter 5.

In theory, any plane can be used for volume measurement but the transverse plane or the horizontal long axis plane are the most satisfactory because in other planes, either the position of the atrioventricular valves or the septum can be difficult to judge. Eight levels are usually sufficient for the left ventricle but twelve may be needed for the right ventricle or if the left ventricle is very large. For right ventricular volumes the position of the pulmonary valve should be determined in single sagittal views through the right ventricular outflow tract at end diastole and end systole. If not, a reasonable guess is that the pulmonary valve lies 10 mm below the pulmonary artery bifurcation and is 10 mm lower in systole than in diastole.

The endocardial contours could be assigned by an automatic edge detection program but automatic methods have proved very unreliable on routine images. The boundary between myocardium and blood can be obscured by signal from static blood and in the region of the valves there is no boundary at all to follow. Manual definition is normally required and even this needs considerable experience to become accurate and reproducible. A convention is required on whether to include trabeculae and papillary muscles and we have found it more accurate to include all but the most prominent of papillary muscles in the chamber because they are rarely thick enough to occupy the entire slice.[12] Both extremes of the atrioventricular valve rings can always be identified and it is best to draw a straight line between these to define the valve plane rather than to follow small portions of the valve that may be visible. Another difficult area is in the left ventricular outflow where it may be difficult to distinguish the sinuses of Valsalva from the left ventricle. It is also sometimes necessary to extrapolate the position of the endocardium if it is hidden by signal from static blood, and the most common areas for this are under the anterior cusp of the tricuspid valve and in the left ventricular apex in bad ventricles.

4.3.10 Area-length volume measurement

Multislice volume measurements are accurate but relatively lengthy. An alternative technique for measuring the left ventricular volume is to measure the area (A) and length (L) of the ventricle in an image containing its long axis and to assume that the ventricle is an ellipsoid of revolution about the long axis. Its volume can then be calculated using the technique applied by Sandler and Dodge to X-ray contrast ventriculography:[13]

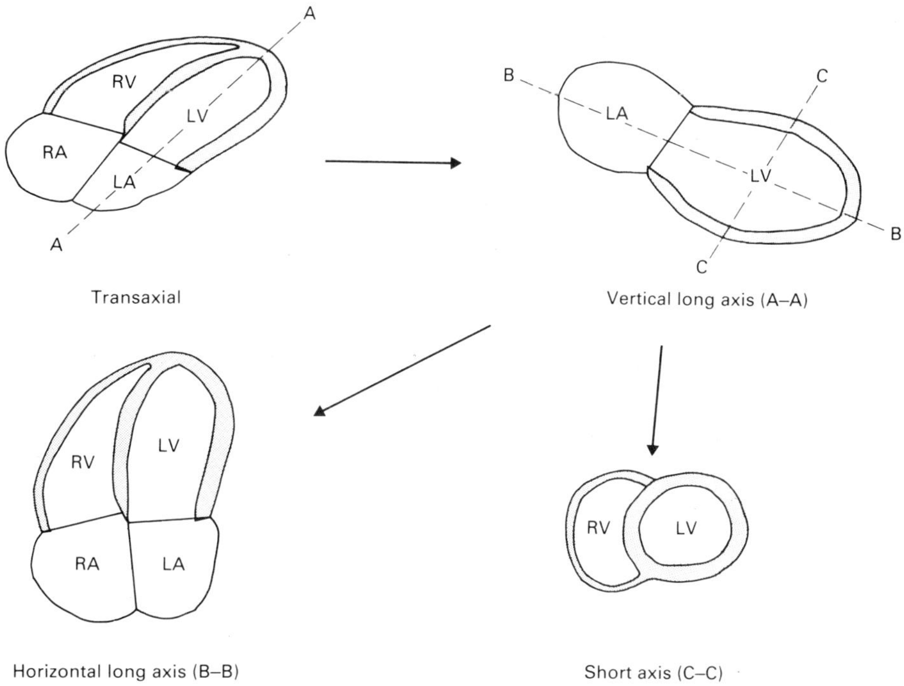

Figure 4.9. Oblique images of the left ventricle are acquired by using the transverse image as an initial pilot and then the vertical and horizontal long axis and the short axis images in turn.

$V = 8/3\pi \times A^2/L$ for single plane measurements

or

$V = 8/3\pi \times A_v \times A_h/L_{min}$ for biplane measurements

where A_v and A_h are the areas in vertical and horizontal long axis planes, and L_{min} is the lesser of the two long axes.

This is only appropriate for the left ventricle since the geometry of the right ventricle is more complex. Single plane measurements are adequate in normal ventricles but the biplane technique is more accurate in patients with previous infarction.[14]

The oblique planes that are used for the left ventricle are the vertical and horizontal long axis planes and the short axis plane (Plate 1, facing p. 36). These can be determined from pilot scans and a simple method is to acquire an initial transverse image through the body of the left ventricle (figure 4.9). From this the rotation of the ventricle towards the left can be seen and the vertical long axis image acquired to contain the long axis. From the vertical long axis image the depression of the long axis from the horizontal is seen and the horizontal long axis image acquired. The short axis image can be acquired using either of the long axis images as a pilot. After acquisition it should be possible to check where each image cuts the others to ensure that the true long axis has been obtained.

References

1 Dimick RN, Hedlund LW, Herfkens RJ, Fram EK, Utz J. Optimizing electrocardiograph electrode placement for cardiac-gated magnetic resonance imaging. *Invest Radiol* 1987; **22**: 17–22.

2 Lanzer P, Botvinick E, Schiller NB, *et al*. Cardiac imaging using gated magnetic resonance. *Radiology* 1984; **150**: 121–7.

3 Wendt RE, Rokey R, Vick GW, Johnston DL. Electrocardiographic gating and monitoring in NMR imaging. *Magnetic Resonance Imaging* 1988; **6**: 89–95.

4 Axel L, Summers RM, Kressel HY, Charles C. Respiratory effects in two-dimensional Fourier transform MR imaging. *Radiology* 1986; **160**: 795–801.

5 Bailes DR, Gilderdale DJ, Bydder GM, Collins AG, Firmin DN. Respiratory ordered phase encoding (ROPE): a method for reducing respiratory motion artefacts in MR imaging. *J Comput Assist Tomogr* 1985; **9**: 835–8.

6 Lewis CE, Prato FS, Drost DJ, Nicholson RL. Comparison of respiratory triggering and gating techniques for the removal of respiratory artifacts in MR imaging. *Radiology* 1986; **160**: 803–10.

7 Edelstein WA, Hutchinson JMS, Johnson G, *et al*. Gated MR imaging of the heart: intracardiac signals in patients and healthy subjects. *Radiology* 1985; **156**: 125–32.

8 Bydder GM, Steiner RE, Blumgart LH, Khenia S, Young IR. MR imaging of the liver using short T_1 inversion recovery sequences. *J Comput Assist Tomogr* 1985; **9**: 1084–9.

9 Boudoulas H, Geleris P, Lewis RP, Rittgers SE. Linear relationship between electrical systole, mechanical systole, and heart rate. *Chest* 1981; **80**: 613–7.

10 Underwood SR, Klipstein RH, Firmin DN, *et al*. Magnetic resonance assessment of aortic and mitral regurgitation. *Br Heart J* 1986; **56**: 455–62.

11 Underwood SR, Klipstein RH, Firmin DN, *et al*. Magnetic resonance assessment of the accuracy of radionuclide methods for the quantification of valvular regurgitation and atrial shunting. In: Hoefer R, Bergman H (eds). *Radioactive Isotopes in Medicine and Research*. Vienna: Verlag H Egerman 1986; **17**: 299–305.

12 Longmore DB, Klipstein RH, Underwood SR, *et al*. Dimensional accuracy of magnetic resonance in studies of the heart. *Lancet* 1985; **i**: 1360–2.

13 Dodge HT, Sandler H, Ballew DW, Lord JT Jr. The use of biplane angiocardiography for measurement of left ventricular volume in man. *Am Heart J* 1960; **60**: 762–76.

14 Underwood SR, Gill CRW, Firmin DN, *et al*. Left ventricular volume measured rapidly by oblique magnetic resonance imaging. *Br Heart J* 1988; **60**: 188–95.

Chapter 5
Imaging of Acquired Heart Disease

RICHARD UNDERWOOD

5.1 Normal appearances

It is important to have an appreciation of normal appearances when interpreting patient scans. Three dimensional anatomy is seen from a multislice acquisition in any plane, but in practice the transverse plane is the most commonly used, sometimes supplemented by the coronal and sagittal planes and also by oblique planes for specialised purposes such as the left ventricle or aortic arch. The demonstration of anatomy depends upon the high contrast between moving blood, which gives no signal in spin echo sequences, and other soft tissues. Signal is very low from lung, cortical bone, and fibrous tissue such as the pericardium, because of the low concentration of water and hence mobile protons. It is intermediate from myocardium, skeletal muscle and other soft tissues because of the much higher concentration of water (approximately 80 mol/l) and variations between the different soft tissues arise mainly from differences in T_1 and T_2. High signal is obtained from fat, static blood and thrombus, particularly in longer spin echo sequences, because of their long T_2 values.

Figures 5.1, 5.2, and 5.3 show normal appearances in the transverse, coronal and sagittal planes respectively. Figure 5.4 shows normal appearances in oblique planes through the left ventricle.

5.2 The great vessels

Because of the absence of signal from rapidly moving blood, the aorta and other major thoracic arteries are seen very clearly and it is in this area, together with congenital heart disease, that magnetic resonance imaging has been applied most successfully and has been able to avoid invasive investigation in selected patients. The suitability of the aorta for magnetic resonance imaging is illustrated by the large literature that has arisen (table 5.1).

Aortic dissection is readily detected and its extent can be seen including the involvement of the arch and other vessels (figure 5.5). The ability to demonstrate aortic regurgitation and rupture into the pericardial space are important additional features when assessing these patients. Because the intimal flap is thin it may not be seen easily in spin echo images unless static blood in the false lumen leads to natural contrast with the true lumen. If there is any doubt, then the flap will be more easily seen using a field echo sequence, and velocity mapping will confirm the diagnosis by demonstrating the differential flow velocities in each lumen (figure 5.6).[17] There are few large comparisons of magnetic resonance with other imaging techniques for the detection of dissection but Goldman *et al.* have compared echocardiography, magnetic resonance and X-ray computed tomography[12] and although computed tomography was not performed in all patients it appears that magnetic resonance has at least equivalent sensitivity or that it is superior. The advantages of magnetic resonance are its ability to image in oblique planes and the fact that it does not require contrast injection, but it is undoubtedly more difficult to image sick patients in the current generation of scanners. In most cases, the investigation performed will depend upon practical problems such as local expertise and availability of equipment.

An important question is whether magnetic resonance can avoid the need for invasive aortography. One consideration is whether it is possible to demonstrate the entry and exit points because surgical strategy is sometimes aimed at sealing the tear. Although the tear is not always seen in spin echo images, cine imaging and velocity mapping can be helpful. A further consideration is the coronary arteries but, because most surgeons believe that it is meddlesome to perform coronary arteriography in patients with dissections involving the ascending aorta, this is rarely a reason for

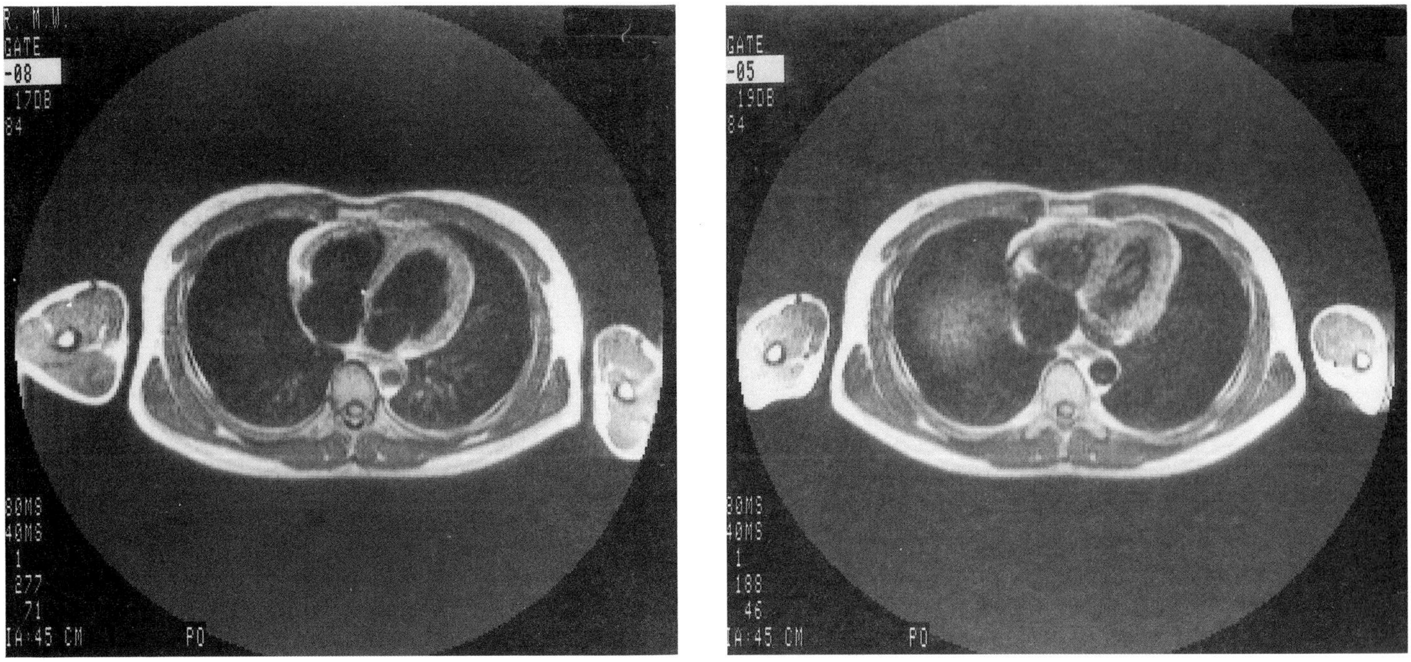

(a) (b)

Figure 5.1 Normal transverse spin echo images at different levels through the heart. (a) All four chambers are seen with some detail of the mitral valve cusps which are open in diastole. (b) At a more caudal level, the coronary sinus is seen draining into the right atrium.

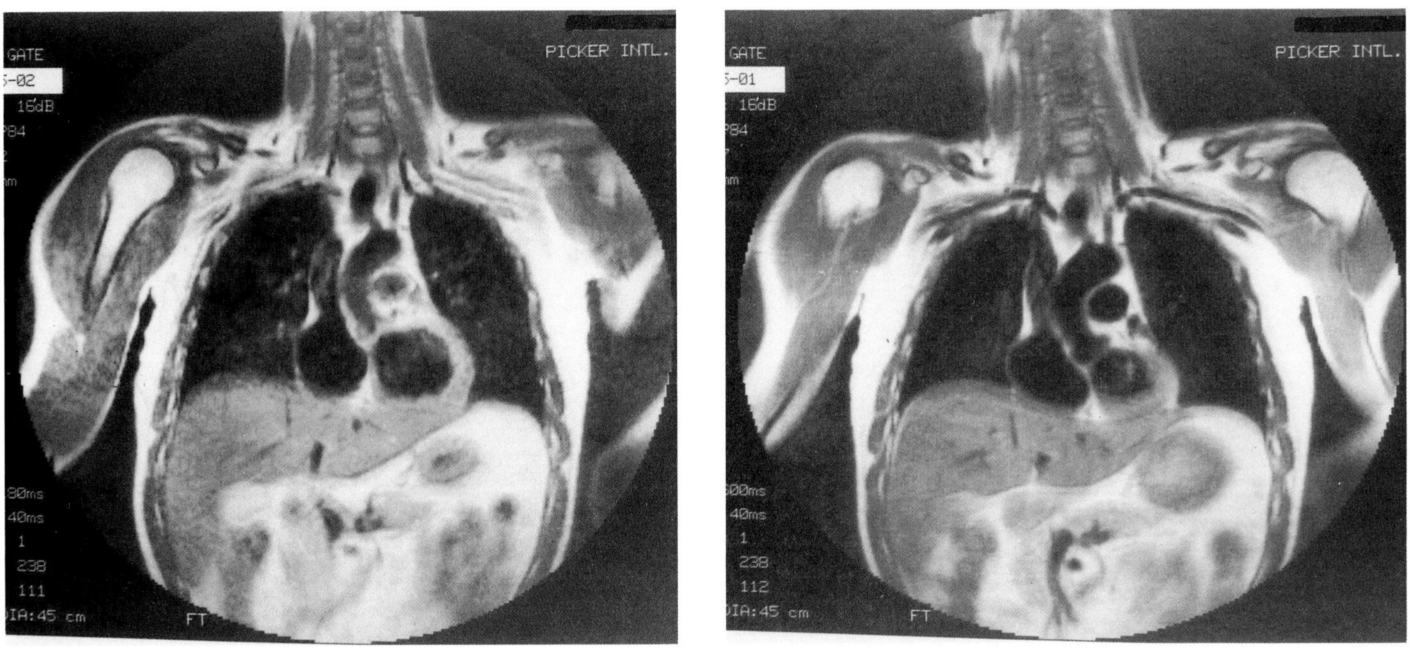

(a) (b)

Figure 5.2. Normal coronal spin echo images through the aortic valve in diastole (a) and systole (b). Some signal from static blood is seen in the aorta and pulmonary artery in the diastolic image.

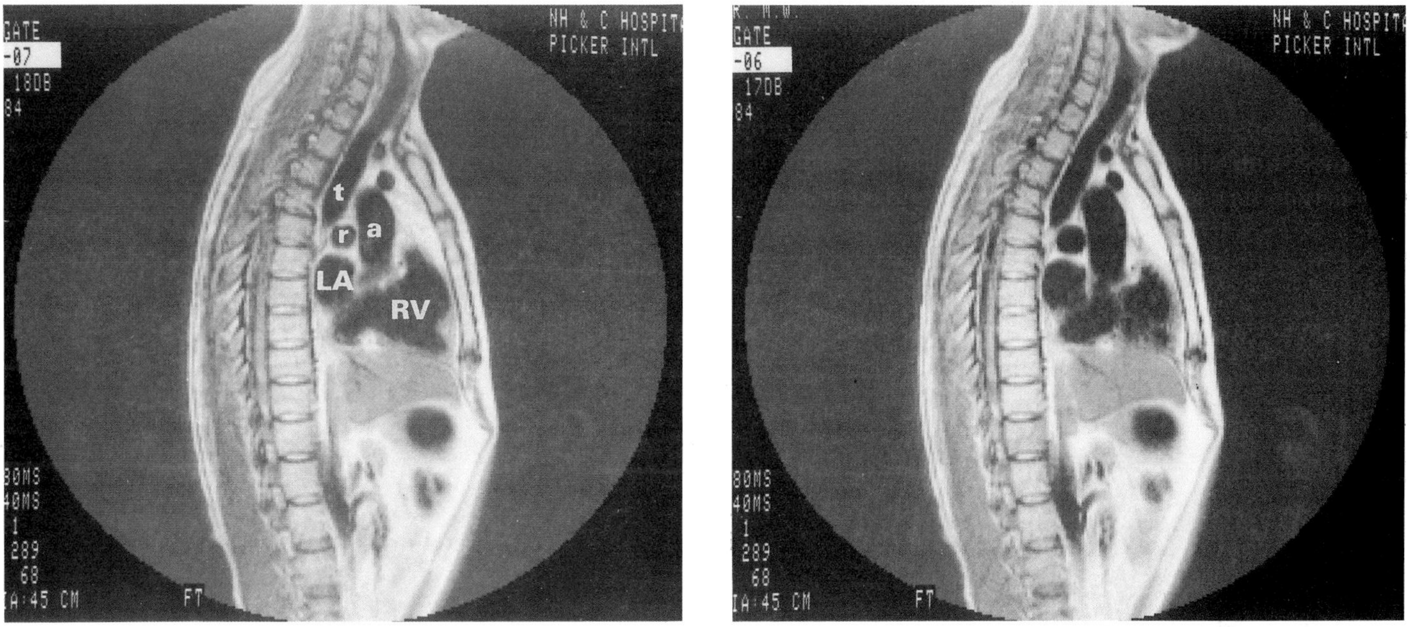

(a) (b)

Figure 5.3. Normal sagittal spin echo images at end diastole (a), and end systole (b). RV, right ventricle; LA, left atrium; a, aorta; r, right pulmonary artery; t, trachea.

cardiac catheterisation. Every case must be assessed individually, but there is no doubt that aortography can be avoided in selected cases using a combination of echocardiography and magnetic resonance.

Other aortic abnormalities that are well seen by magnetic resonance are aneurysms, stenoses including coarctation, and other congenital abnormalities which are more fully discussed in chapter 6. It is an ideal method for the long-term follow-up of patients following coarctation repair and patients with Marfan's syndrome (figure 5.7). A further application is in suspected abscess in the heart or around the aortic root in post-operative patients with infection which is difficult to control. Echocardiography is often equivocal in such patients and magnetic resonance will usually produce a definitive answer.

Takayasu's arteritis has also been studied by magnetic resonance (figure 5.8). It is an arteritis of unknown aetiology affecting the aorta and its major branches, principally the arch vessels although it may also involve the pulmonary and renal arteries. Initial experience using spin echo imaging was that magnetic resonance was sensitive for demonstrating involvement of the largest vessels but was less sensitive for the smaller branches.[45] Improvements in technique and the development of magnetic resonance angiography may lead to more reliable results.

The pulmonary artery is seen equally well and this is most useful in patients with congenital heart disease, as discussed in chapter 6. Of acquired diseases of the pulmonary circulation, there has been some interest in the detection of venous thrombosis[46–48] and pulmonary emboli[49–53] but it appears unlikely that magnetic resonance will prove to be sensitive in the detection of pulmonary emboli because it is only possible to see large emboli that are impacted within the central pulmonary arteries. More peripheral arteries are not well seen without respiratory gating.

5.3 Tumours and thrombus

The ability of magnetic resonance to demonstrate anatomy has given it a small but important role in the investigation of cardiac and paracardiac masses, and a more common reason for referral is to adjudicate upon the presence of possible intracardiac thrombus seen by echocardiography. As with the aorta, a large literature has evolved, ranging from individual case reports[54–62]

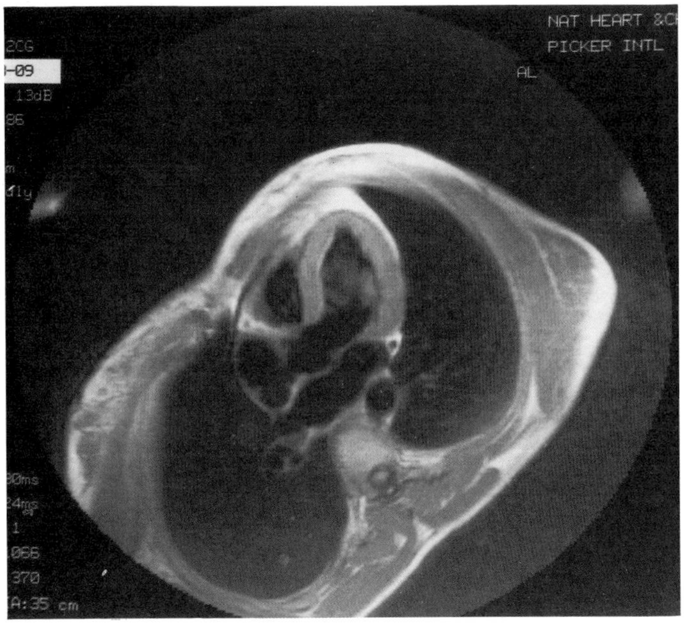

(a)

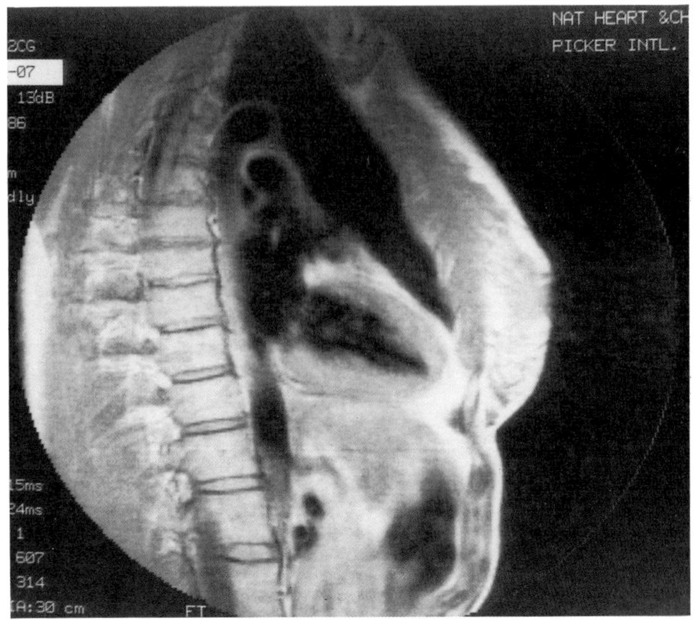

(b)

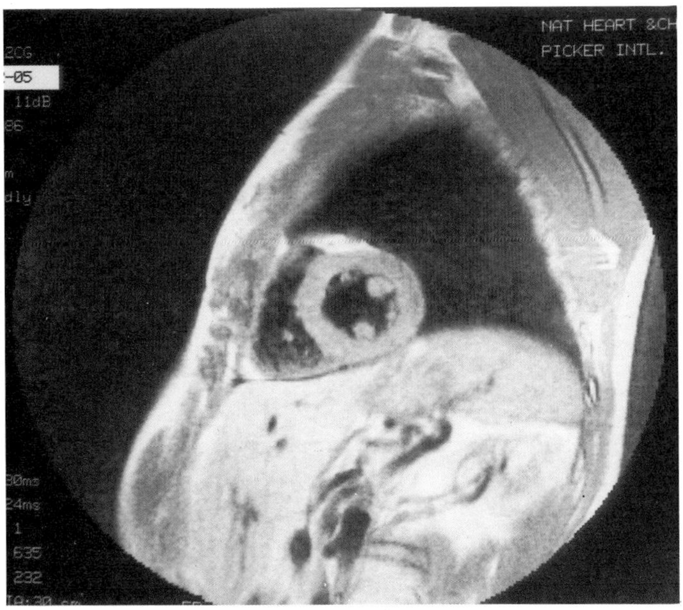

(c)

Figure 5.4. Normal spin echo images in the horizontal long axis plane (a), the vertical long axis plane (b) and the short axis plane (c).

to reviews of larger numbers of tumours[63–71] and thrombi.[72] Magnetic resonance imaging is unlikely to displace echocardiography as the initial investigation in such patients, but it often provides a superior three-dimensional view of the tumour, and shows the extent and attachments better than echocardiography. Figure 5.9 shows a lobulated tumour which echocardiography clearly demonstrated within the right atrium and the most likely diagnosis was thought to be an atrial myxoma. The magnetic resonance images however showed that the tumour extended into the inferior vena cava and the differential diagnosis was revised to thrombus or hypernephroma. In fact, it was an haemangiopericytoma arising from the inferior caval vein.

The difficulty of providing a specific tissue diagnosis arises from the overlap in relaxation times of many

Table 5.1. Recent literature on magnetic resonance imaging of the aorta

Subject	Reference	First author	Year
Aorta	1	Amparo	1984
	2	Glazer	1985
	3	Dooms	1986
	4	Mossard	1986
	5	Auffermann	1987
	6	Lois	1987
	7	Garbagnati	1988
Dissection	8	Amparo	1985
	9	Geisinger	1985
	10	Dinsmore	1986
	11	Goldman	1986
	12	Goldman	1986
	13	Akins	1987
	14	Barentsz	1987
	15	Pernes	1987
	16	Kersting-Sommerhoff	1988
	17	Bogren	1988
	18	Mitchell	1988
	19	Yamada	1988
Aneurysms	20	Moore	1984
	21	Dinsmore	1986
	22	Globits	1989
	23	Spielmann	1989
Coarctation	24	Amparo	1984
	25	Boxer	1986
	26	von Schulthess	1986
	27	Bank	1987
	28	Simpson	1988
	29	Pucillo	1989
Congenital	30	Boxer	1986
	31	Coscina	1986
	32	Guit	1986
	33	Bisset	1987
	34	Brown	1987
	35	Gomes	1987
	36	Bernard	1988
Marfan's sydrome	37	Boxer	1986
	38	Kersting-Sommerhoff	1987
	39	Schaefer	1987
	40	Soulen	1987
Infection	41	Winkler	1986
	42	Miller	1987
Abdominal aorta	43	Amparo	1985
	44	Flak	1985

common tumours. Figure 5.10 illustrates a pericardial cyst and a chondrosarcoma that were impossible to distinguish using relaxation times alone. An observation that may be helpful however is that fat has a

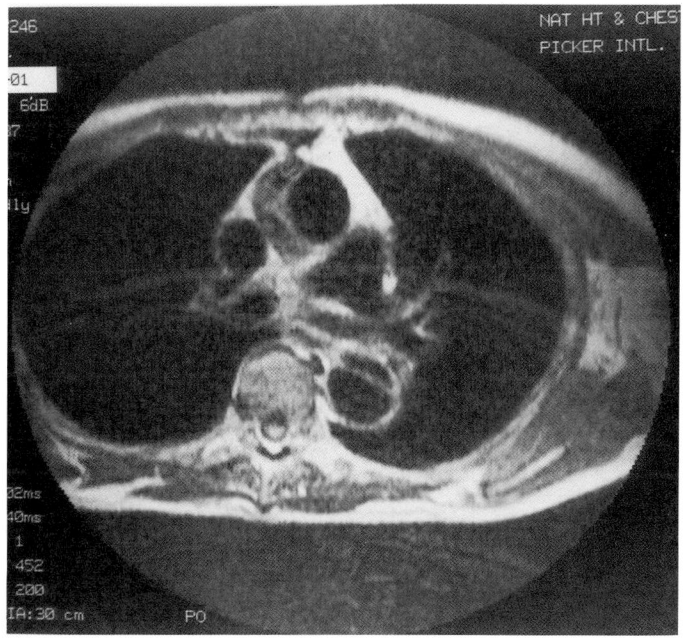

(a)

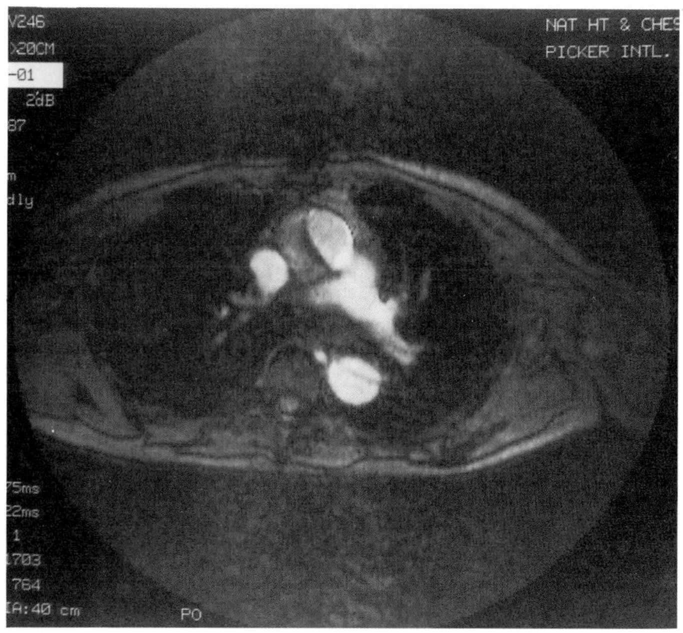

(b)

Figure 5.5. (a) Transverse spin echo image showing aortic dissection involving both the ascending and the descending aorta. The false lumen in the ascending aorta contains signal and it is not possible to be confident whether this is thrombus or static blood. The field echo image (b) confirms that it is thrombus from the characteristic lower signal. Both lumens in the descending aorta are patent.

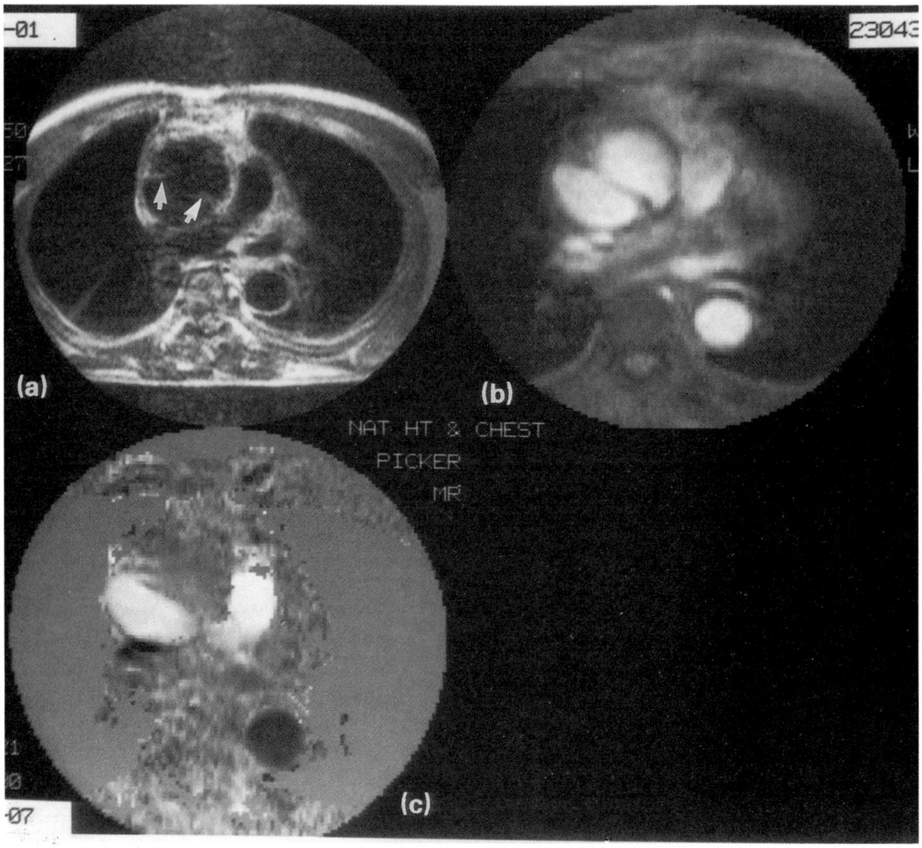

Figure 5.6. (a) Spin echo image showing a dilated ascending aorta divided by an intimal flap (arrows). (b) In the field echo image the dissection is more obvious. (c) Velocity mapping through the plane of the image clearly shows rapid velocity in the true lumen (posteriorly in white) and zero velocity in the false lumen (anteriorly in grey). For a full description of velocity mapping, see chapter 10.

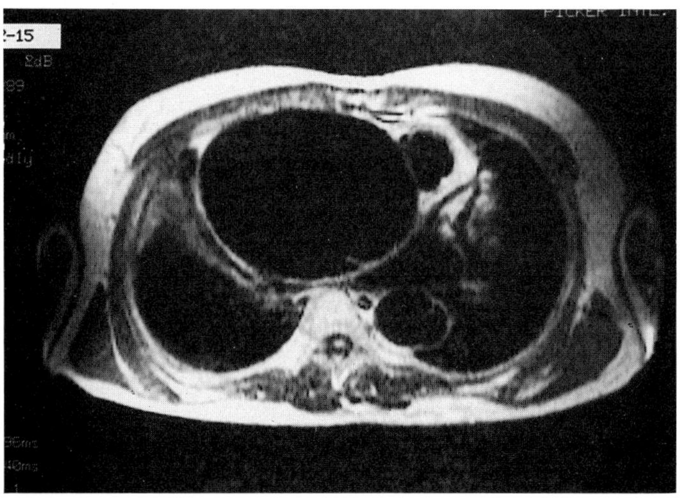

Figure 5.7. The ascending aorta is massively dilated in a patient with Marfan's syndrome and there is a small intimal flap on the posterior wall. Coronary vessels are particularly well seen behind the pulmonary artery. Surgery is recommended when the diameter exceeds 5 cm and regular scans can be performed to monitor the size of the aneurysm.

long T_2 and so it appears with high signal in spin echo images: lipomata are not difficult to characterise.[73] Conversely, acellular or collagenous material has a short T_2 and appears with much lower signal:[74] fibromas may have areas of low signal although this is by no means a general rule since the cellularity of fibromas is very variable (figure 5.11). Calcification within a tumour will also lead to areas of absent signal (figure 5.12).

Intracavitary thrombus is readily seen using a spin echo sequence but a potential pitfall is that slowly moving blood can give signal and be mistaken for thrombus. There are a number of strategies that can be used to overcome the problem including the use of second echo images and phase or velocity mapping which can highlight moving material, but the simplest method is to use cine field echo imaging. Thrombus appears with reduced signal compared with blood in cine images and the constancy of the filling defect throughout the cycle confirms the diagnosis (figure 5.13).

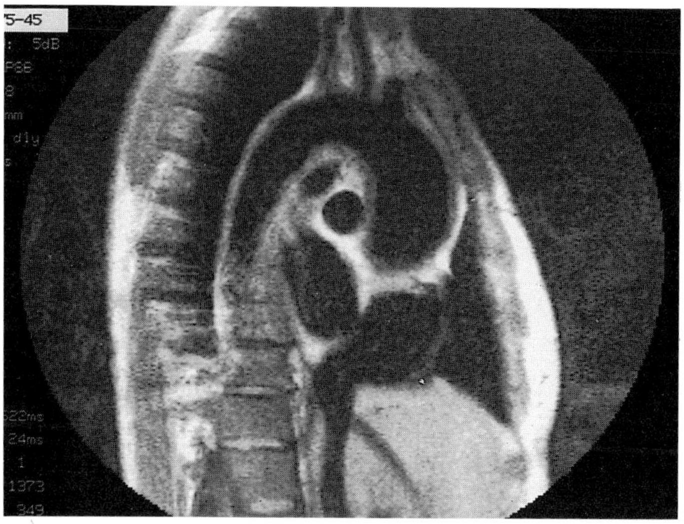

(a)

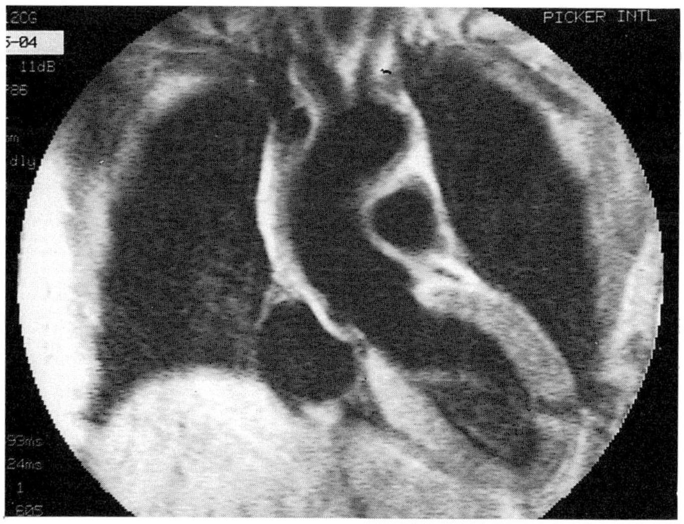

(b)

Figure 5.8. (a) Oblique view of the aortic arch of a woman with Takayasu's arteritis. There is thickening of the aortic wall, the left subclavian artery is almost occluded, the left carotid artery is stenosed but the innominate artery is patent. (b) In the coronal plane the pulmonary artery is seen to be involved in addition to the aorta.

5.4 The myocardium

5.4.1 Global ventricular function

A starting point in the assessment of global ventricular function is the measurement of volume, particularly at end diastole and end systole. The most accurate method, which makes no assumptions about ventricular geometry, is to sum the areas of the chambers in multiple contiguous slices and the technique has been discussed in chapter 4. Although the accuracy of such an approach can be demonstrated in phantom experiments and by comparison with other techniques (figure 5.14),[75–78] the best *in vivo* validation is to compare left and right ventricular stroke volumes in normal subjects, since these should be equal over the period of image acquisition.[79] Figure 5.15 illustrates this approach and it can be calculated from these data that individual volume measurements are accurate to within 5%. Table 5.2 shows the mean values for right and left ventricular volumes in a group of 20 normal subjects.

Although the multislice technique is accurate and is applicable to both the right and left ventricles, it is relatively time consuming. Eight slices are usually needed for the left ventricle and up to twelve for the right. A more rapid method for the left ventricle alone is to assume that it is an ellipsoid of revolution about its long axis and to use the same formula that has been used successfully in X-ray contrast ventriculography and in echocardiography for many years (see chapter 4 and figure 5.16).[80–84] Left ventricular volume can then be measured from a single image although biplane measurements are more accurate.[85] The assumption that the ventricle approximates to an ellipsoid of revolution is reasonable for normal ventricles but significant errors can be made in patients with previous infarction (figures 5.18 and 5.19).

The ability to measure right ventricular volumes accurately allows the regurgitant fraction in patients with regurgitation of a single valve to be measured and such measurements of regurgitation are now the standard against which other techniques should be compared (figure 5.20).[86] Figure 5.21 shows that conventional grading of mitral and aortic regurgitation using X-ray contrast ventriculography gives an estimate of the regurgitant fraction as measured by magnetic resonance, but patients with grade IV (severe) regurgitation by angiography, have a wide range of regurgitant fractions that are better assessed by magnetic resonance. Figure 5.22 shows that the ratio of left and right ventricular stroke volumes measured by radionuclide ventriculography is over estimated when compared with magnetic resonance, the inaccuracy of radionuclide ventriculography arising because of the overlap between the right atrium and ventricle in the left anterior oblique projection.[87] If more than one valve is leaking then the situation is more complicated

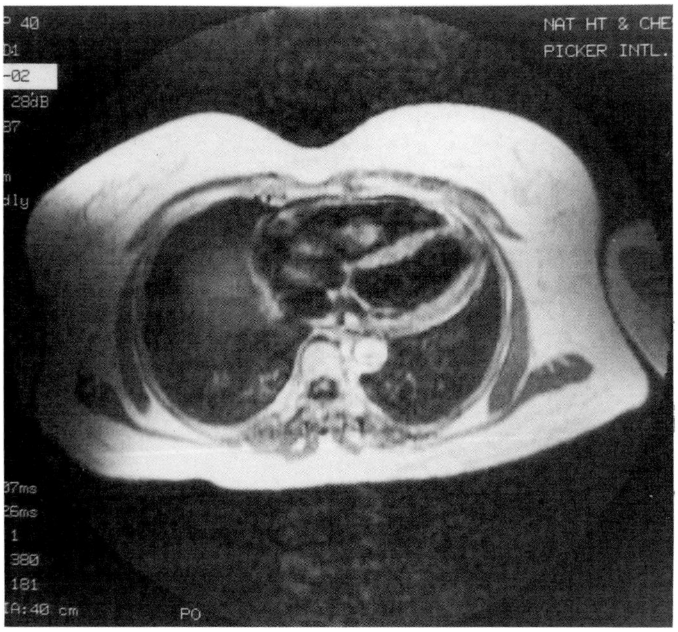

(a)

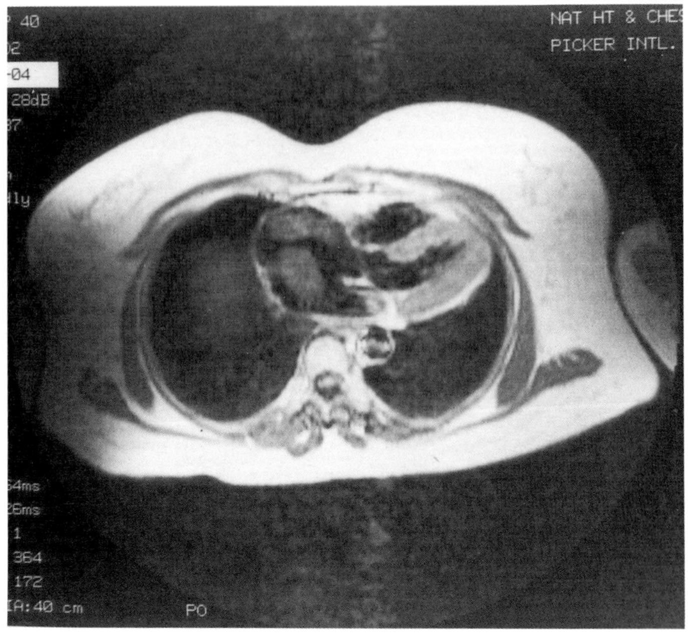

(b)

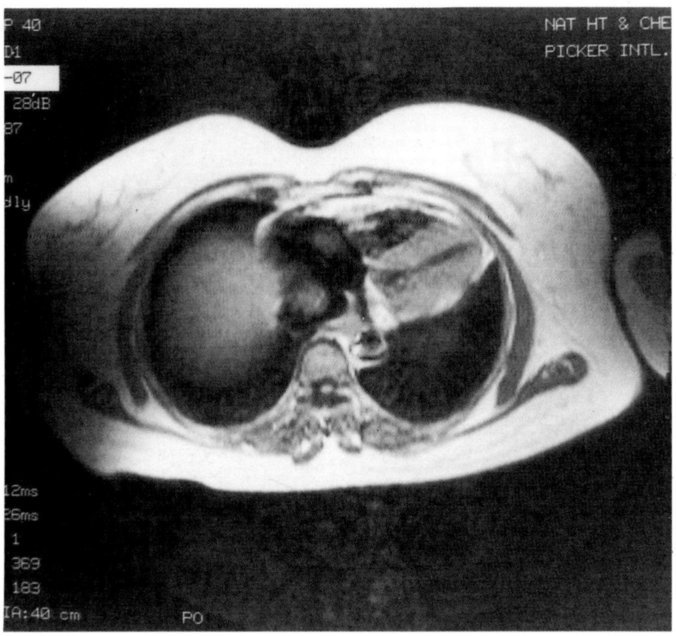

(c)

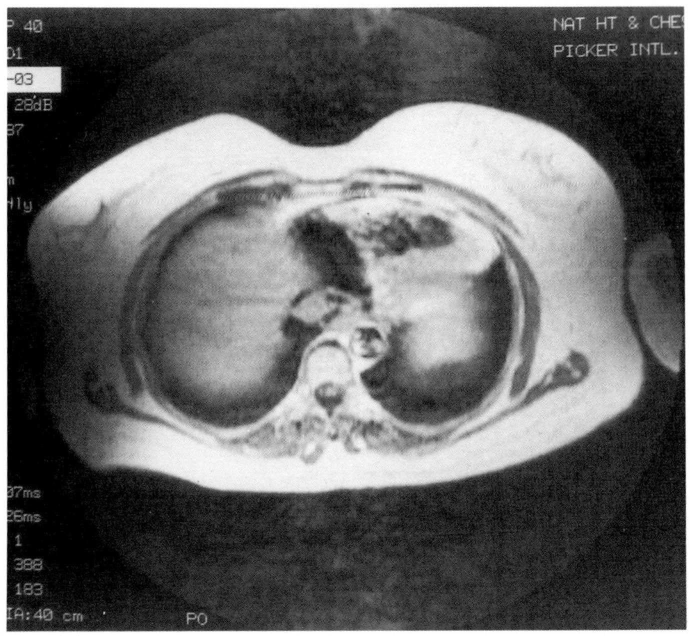

(d)

Figure 5.9. (a) Diastolic and (b) systolic images showing a lobulated tumour in the right atrium, prolapsing into the right ventricle in systole. (c) and (d) show that the tumour extends into the inferior vena cava and histology showed it to be a haemangiopericytoma.

and the ratio of stroke volumes gives the net regurgitant fraction with right sided lesions counterbalancing left sided lesions. Cine imaging can help to apportion the severity of individual lesions from the size of the regurgitant jet and this is further discussed in chapter 7.

The ratio of stroke volumes can also be helpful in measuring shunting through congenital defects because

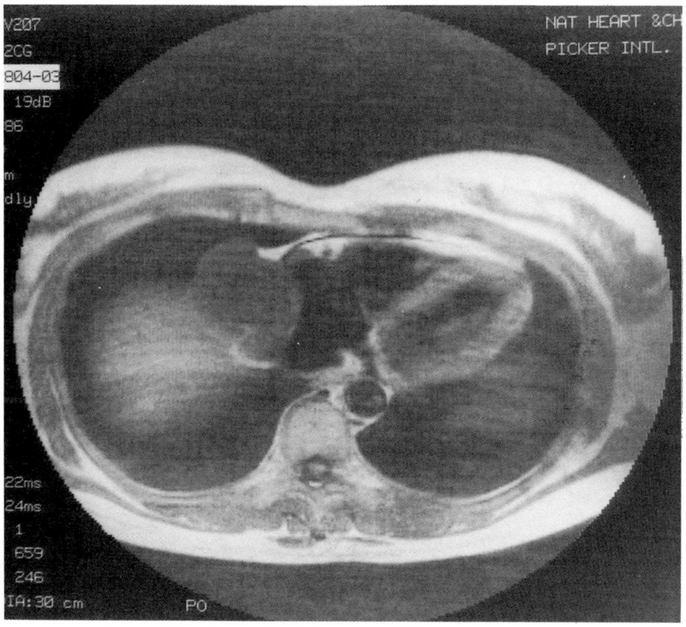

(a)

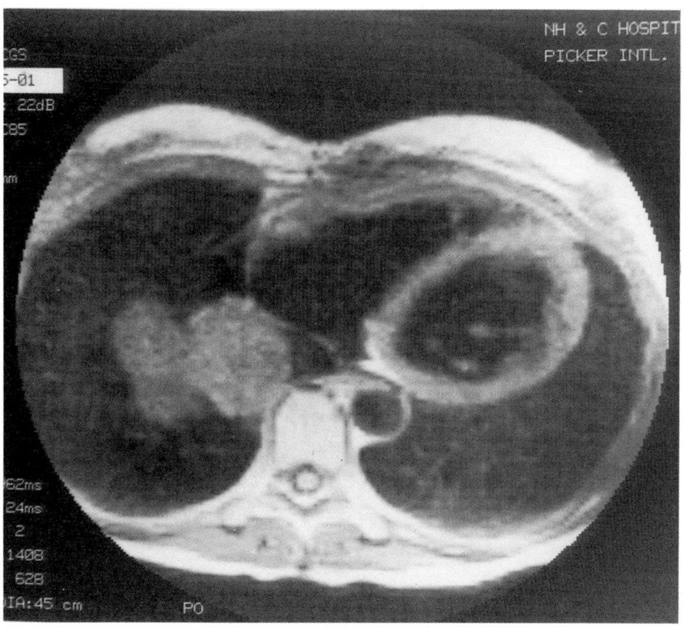

(b)

Figure 5.10. A pericardial cyst (a) and a recurrent chondrosarcoma invading through the diaphragm (b) were impossible to distinguish using relaxation times alone. The cyst however is homogeneous with a capsule in parts and the sarcoma is irregular and inhomogeneous.

left to right shunting at atrial level leads to an increase in right ventricular stroke volume (figure 5.23), and shunting through a patent ductus arteriosus increases

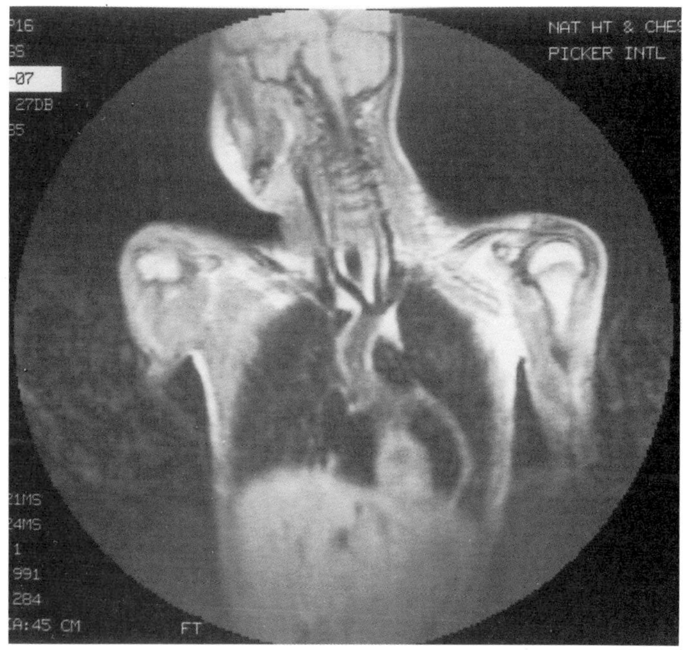

Figure 5.11. Fibroma sitting in the septum of an 8-year-old boy (spin echo sequence, echo time 24 ms, repeat time 820 ms). There is a central area of low signal compatible with reduced cellularity but there are also areas of higher signal within the tumour.

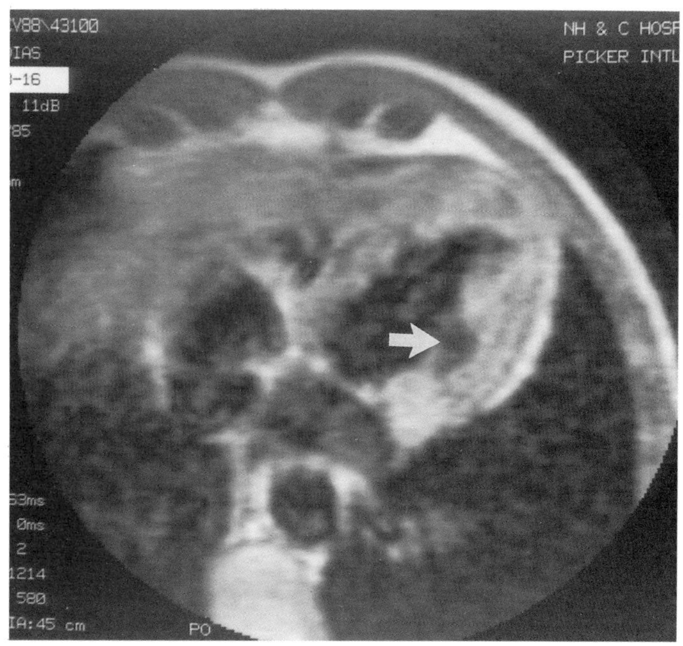

Figure 5.12. Calcification within a myocardial tumour is seen as loss of signal. The histology of the tumour was unknown (it was benign and was not biopsied) but it is likely to be a fibroma because of the calcification.

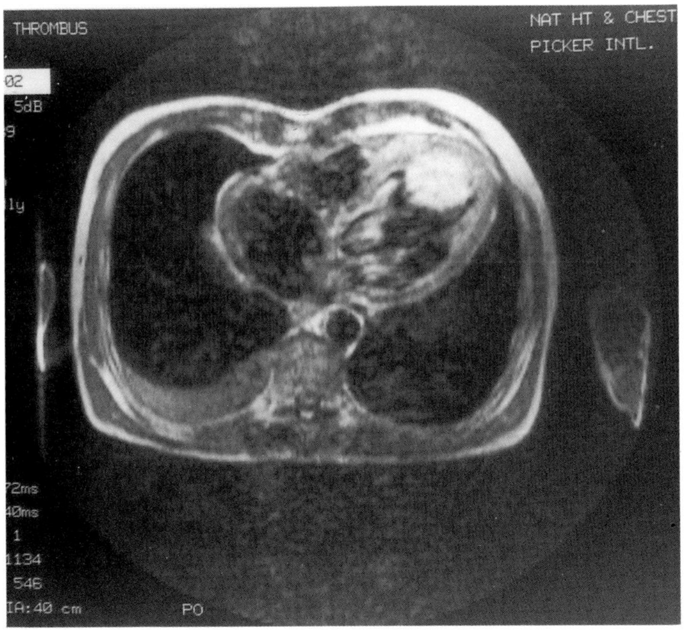

(a)

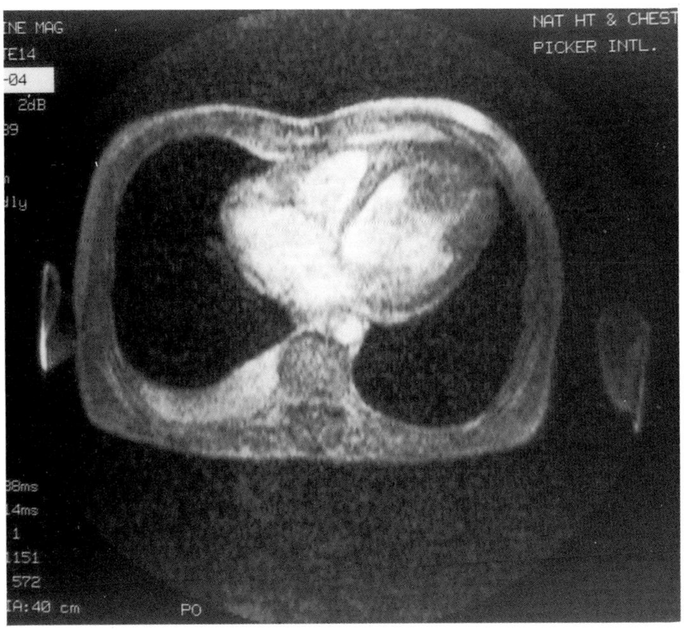

(b)

Figure 5.13. (a) Spin echo image of a patient with coronary artery disease and congestive heart failure. There is a large thrombus at the apex of the left ventricle extending around the lateral wall. There is also some signal from slowly moving blood within the left ventricular cavity. (b) The equivalent field echo image shows the distinction between the high signal of blood and the intermediate signal of thrombus.

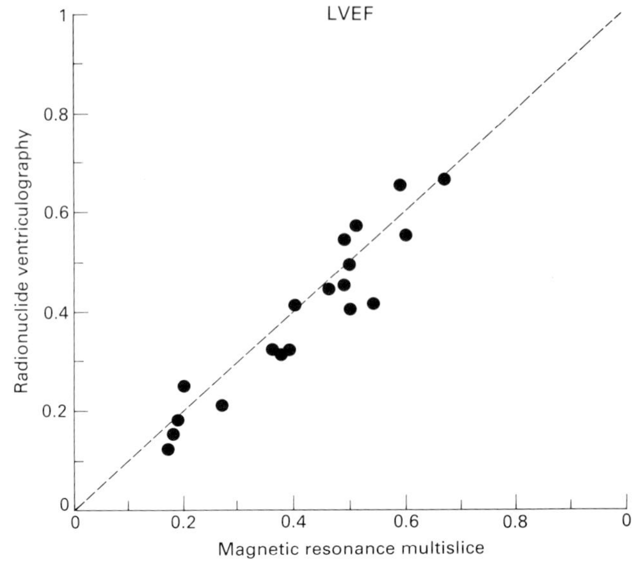

Figure 5.14. A comparison of left ventricular ejection fraction measured by radionuclide ventriculography and by the multiple slice magnetic resonance technique in a series of patients with previous infarction. There is good agreement over a wide range of values (the line of identity is indicated).

Table 5.2 Mean and standard deviation (SD) of left (LV) and right ventricular (RV) end diastolic volume (EDV), stroke volume (SV) and ejection fraction (EF) in 20 normal volunteers. From these figures, normal ranges can be established

	Mean	SD
LVEDV (ml)	132	14.7
LVSV (ml)	81	16.2
LVEF (%)	61	7.2
RVEDV (ml)	152	20.9
RVSV (ml)	80	16.4
RVEF (%)	53	7.4
LVSV/RVSV	1.01	0.067

the left ventricular stroke volume. Shunting through ventricular septal defects is more involved because although the right ventricle acts as a conduit for the shunted volume in systole and the volume is only reflected in the left ventricular stroke volume, diastolic shunting can complicate the matter.

5.4.2 Regional ventricular function

The measurement of regional ventricular function is a complex subject and many different parameters can be investigated including myocardial thickness, thickening

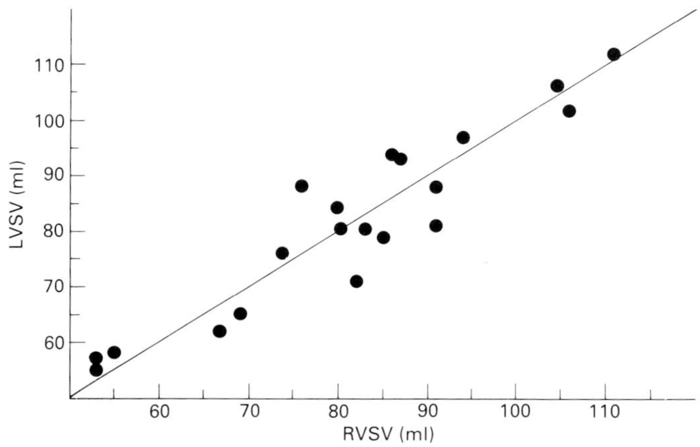

Figure 5.15. The comparison of left (LVSV) and right ventricular stroke volumes (RVSV) in normal subjects illustrates the accuracy of the multislice technique for measuring ventricular volumes. From the spread of points around the line of identity it can be estimated that individual volume measurements are accurate to within 5%.

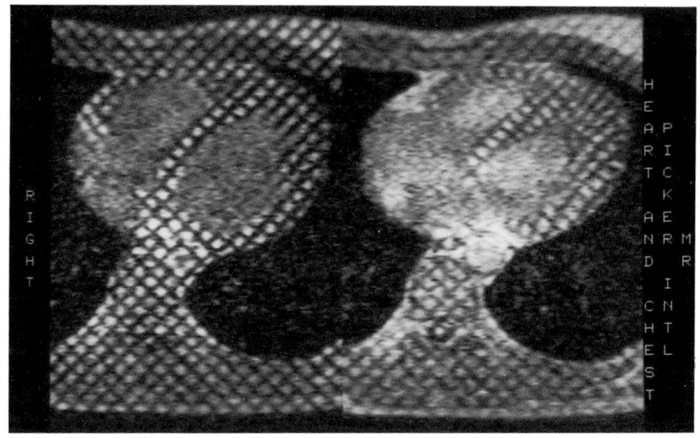

Figure 5.16. Diastolic (left) and systolic (right) transverse images from a cine gradient echo acquisition using spatial modulation of magnetisation to impose a grid of magnetically tagged material. The distortion of the grid caused by contraction is best appreciated in the lateral wall and apex.

between diastole and systole and both the extent and timing of endocardial motion.[88–90] Because of the ability of magnetic resonance to show regional myocardial thickness at any chosen point of the cardiac cycle, magnetic resonance could, in theory, be used to investigate any of these parameters. In practice, it is very time consuming to acquire and to analyse images at all parts of the cardiac cycle, and studies of regional function have usually concentrated on changes between end diastole and end systole. The advent of cine imaging makes more sophisticated analyses possible, and some of these are discussed in chapter 7. Muscle thinning is readily recognised, and previous infarction can be detected and quantified by the presence and extent of thinning and wall motion abnormality (figure 5.24).[91–95]

Methods of assessing regional contraction that involve magnetic tagging of the myocardium have recently been developed. They provide for the first time a method of studying true myocardial motion non-invasively. The importance of this is that motion of an endocardial boundary may differ from that of any individual segment of myocardium. Two different methods have been described, both of which are applicable to spin echo and to cine gradient echo imaging. The first method involves radio-frequency excitation using a slice selective 90° pulse in a plane perpendicular to the imaged plane in order to produce a stripe of saturated material.[96] Imaging at different times after the excitation shows how the stripe moves subsequently. A number of planes can be tagged in this way and an ideal method for studying myocardial motion and torsion is to arrange them as radial lines from the centre of a short axis image. A disadvantage is that each plane is tagged sequentially and recovery of signal may occur in the planes that are tagged first. The technique has successfully shown normal myocardial torsion in the short axis and has demonstrated abnormalities in patients with hypertrophic cardiomyopathy.

An alternative method of spatial modulation of magnetisation has subsequently been described involving two 45° radio-frequency pulses separated by a magnetic field gradient.[97] The field gradient alters the phase of the magnetisation produced by the first pulse and regions of similar phase occur in stripes across the plane. Depending upon this phase, the second pulse will either add or subtract from the effect of the first and so stripes of saturation will appear in the final image. By applying stripes in perpendicular directions a grid can be made to appear, and motion of the intersecting points of the grid can be tracked. An advantage of this method is that all the stripes are applied at the same time but recovery of magnetisation

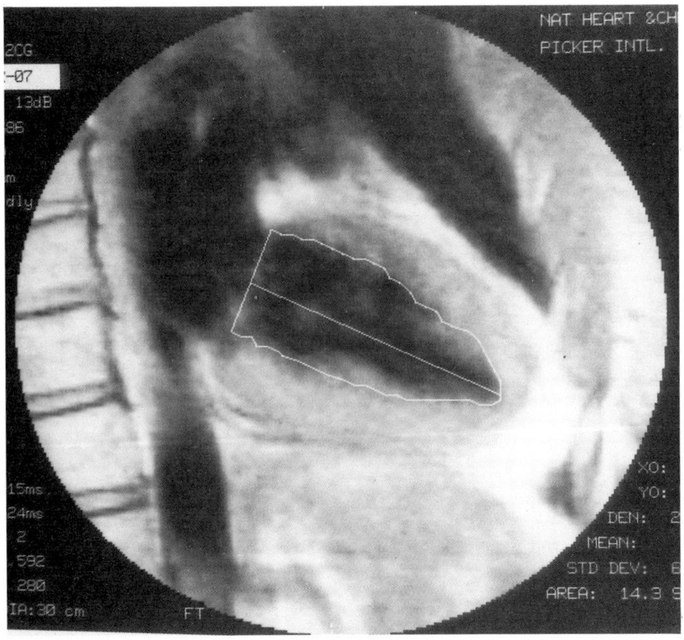

Figure 5.17. (a) Vertical long axis image through left ventricle.

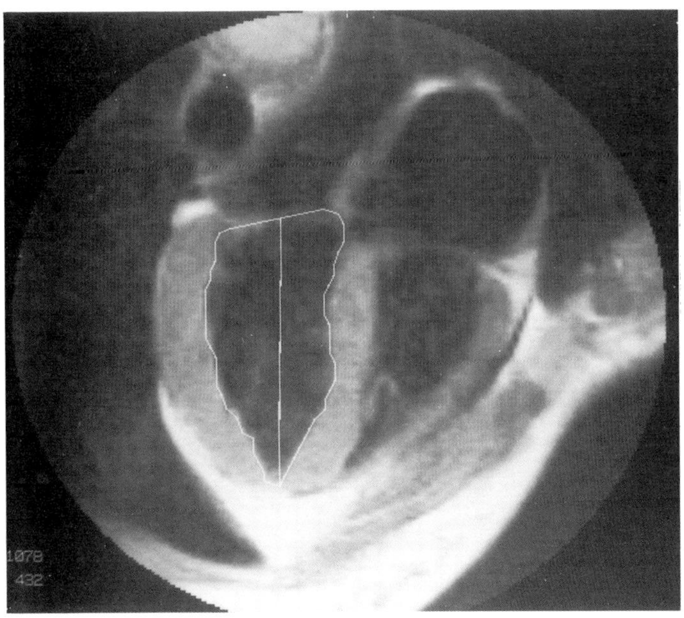

Figure 5.17. (b) Horizontal long axis image through the left ventricle. The area and long axis from which left ventricular volume can be calculated are indicated.

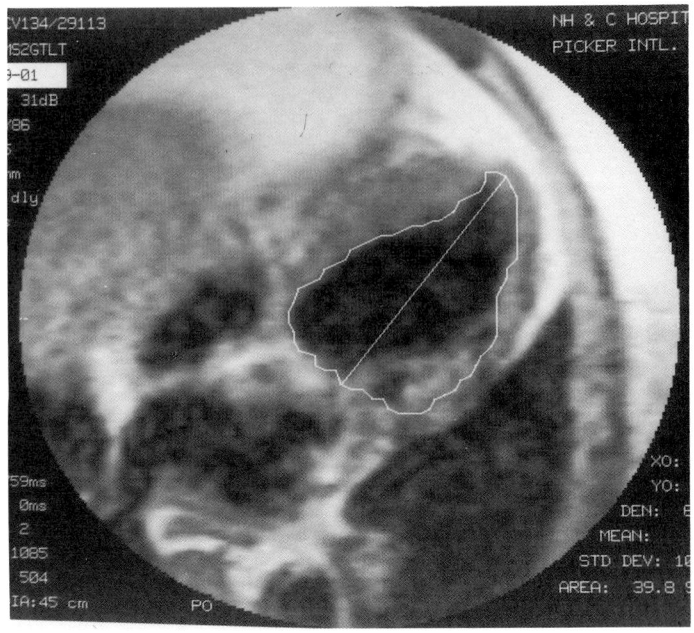

Figure 5.18. Systolic long axis image of a patient with previous anterolateral and apical infarction. There is thinning of the lateral wall and apex and there is intracavitary signal from blood close to the basal lateral wall. The area of the left ventricular cavity and its long axis are indicated and from these measurements the left ventricular volume was calculated to be 84 ml. (Reproduced with permission from *Br Heart J* 1988; **60**: 188–95.)

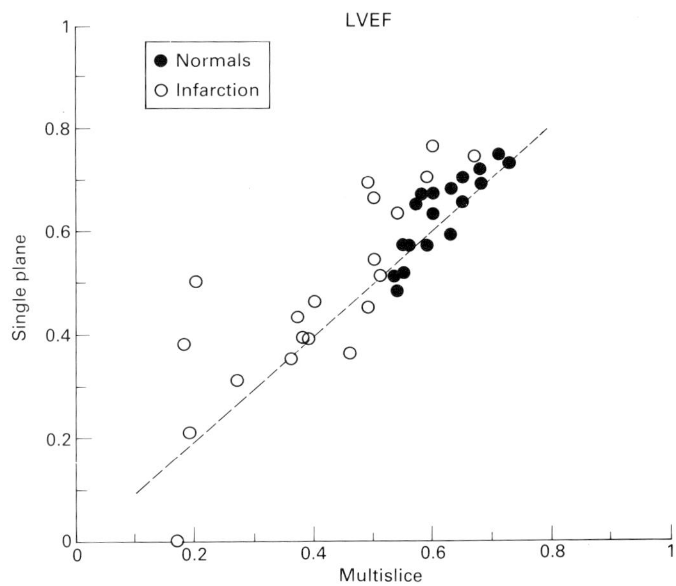

Figure 5.19. Left ventricular ejection fraction (LVEF) calculated from a single plane area-length measurement and by summing the areas of multiple slices. There is good agreement between the techniques in normal ventricles, but significant errors are made by the single plane method in some patients with previous infarction.

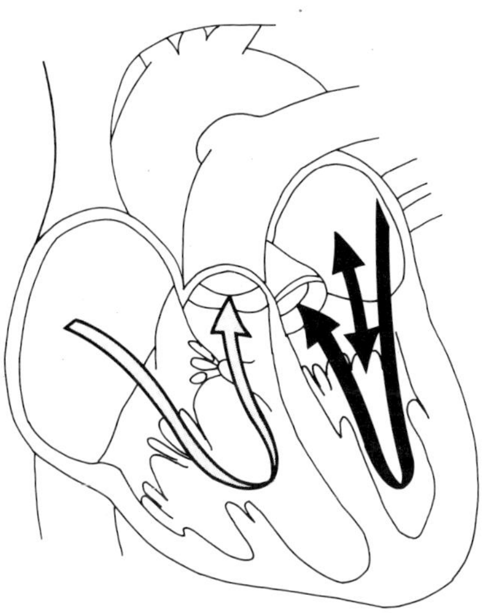

Figure 5.20. In mitral (and aortic) regurgitation the regurgitant volume increases the left ventricular stroke volume and comparison with the right ventricular stroke volume allows the regurgitant volume to be measured.

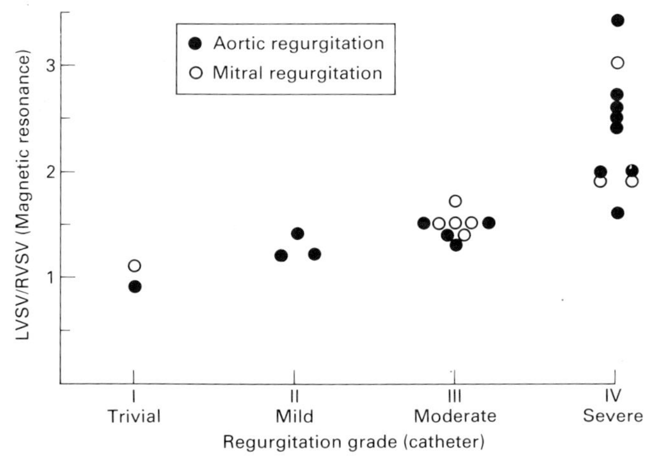

Figure 5.21. A comparison of the left to right ventricular stroke volume ratio measured by magnetic resonance compared with the grade of regurgitation assessed by X-ray contrast angiography in a group of patients with either aortic or mitral regurgitation. The group with grade IV regurgitation has a wide range of regurgitant fractions which are better assessed by magnetic resonance.

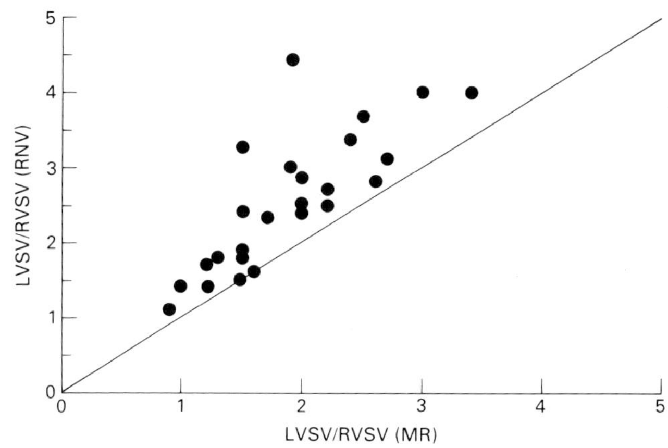

Figure 5.22. A comparison of left to right ventricular stroke volume ratio (LVSV/RVSV) measured by radionuclide ventriculography (RNV) and magnetic resonance (MR) in patients with left sided regurgitation shows that the radionuclide technique overestimates the ratio because of problems with the right heart when imaged in the left anterior oblique projection.

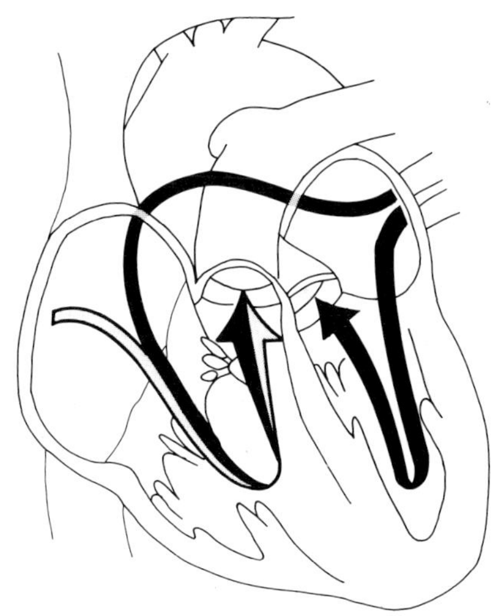

Figure 5.23. With left to right sided shunting through an atrial septal defect, the right ventricular stroke volume is augmented and the ratio of right to left ventricular stroke volumes equals the pulmonary to systemic flow ratio in the absence of valvular regurgitation or other shunting.

from T_1 relaxation still causes fading of the stripes after approximately 500 ms. Further experience is required with both of these techniques before their advantages over other methods in routine clinical practice can be assessed.

5.4.3 Myocardial hypertrophy

Using the same methods that are described above for the measurement of the cavity of the left ventricle, the volume of the myocardium can also be measured. The results have been extensively validated in animal experiments[98–101] and in humans,[102–104] and because of its accuracy magnetic resonance should now be the standard against which other techniques are judged. Increased muscle volume (and hence mass) can be observed in athletes[105] and patients with left ventricular hypertrophy, and the regression of hypertrophy following treatment of hypertension can be monitored.[106]

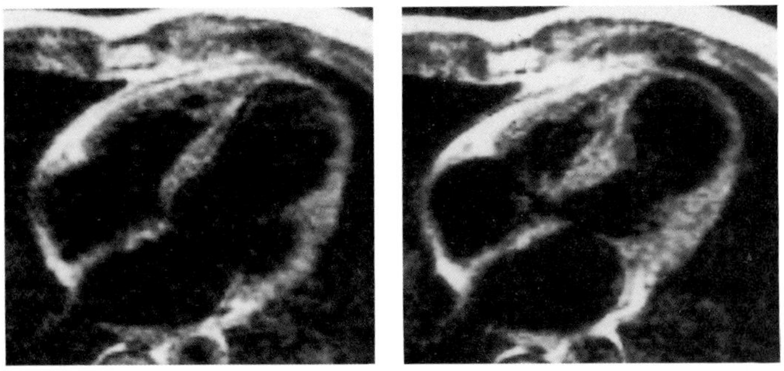

Figure 5.24. (a) Diastolic and (b) systolic transverse image through the left ventricle in a patient with previous infarction and an apical aneurysm. The basal myocardium thickens and contracts normally, but there is extensive apical thinning which is dyskinetic.

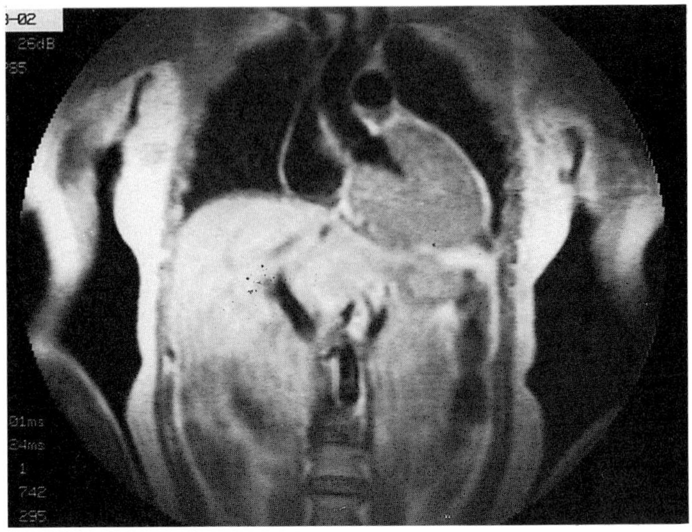

Figure 5.25. Coronal view at end systole in a West Indian lady with uncontrolled hypertension. There is severe symmetrical left ventricular hypertrophy and only a tiny left ventricular cavity remains.

It is not clear whether muscle that is hypertrophied secondary to increased afterload has different relaxation properties from myopathic muscle, but measurements of T_2 of hypertrophied muscle in a magnetic resonance spectrometer have shown it to be different from normal myocardium.[107] Figure 5.25 shows a patient with very severe symmetrical left ventricular hypertrophy.

Wall thickness in hypertrophic cardiomyopathy is better demonstrated than by echocardiography because the three dimensional distribution is more easily seen.[108–110] In some patients the abnormal muscle not only appears thickened but it also has a higher signal in spin echo images than the normal muscle. This most likely implies a lengthened T_2 although a contributing factor may be hypokinesis of the affected muscle which can also cause an increase in signal. Figure 5.26 shows an example of a patient with hypertrophic obstructive cardiomyopathy.

5.4.4 Myocardial disease

Non-coronary myocardial disease can manifest itself by abnormalities of global and regional left ventricular function or by abnormalities of relaxation times which lead to differential contrast within the myocardium. Myocardial sarcoidosis is an example where magnetic resonance may have an important clinical role. Cardiac involvement with sarcoidosis can be detected in 20–30% of patients at *post mortem* but it is only clinically evident in 5%. Thus there is a high incidence of sub-clinical involvement, detection of which is important because its first manifestation may be sudden death.[111] Conventional methods of detection include electrocardiography, echocardiography and thallium-201 or gallium-67 scintigraphy, but the sensitivity of all of these techniques is limited. In a study of 13 patients with documented cardiac sarcoidosis, magnetic resonance showed abnormalities of either the myocardium or pericardium in 11, and in the remaining 4 patients the disease was controlled on steroid therapy.[112,113] Although these were all patients with known involvement, the implication is that magnetic resonance may be sensitive in the detection of occult disease and that it may be possible to use magnetic resonance to control therapy. Figure 5.27 shows a patient with active myocardial and pericardial involvement.

The findings in dilated cardiomyopathy are not specific and a dilated left ventricle with generalised thinning and hypokinesis is usual. Thrombus is not uncommonly seen within the ventricle although care must be taken to distinguish it from static blood (see below). Figure 5.28 shows a patient with severe left ventricular dysfunction and a dilated cardiomyopathy.

Other myocardial diseases that can be detected by magnetic resonance include myocarditis (global and regional abnormalities with areas of high signal),[114] systemic lupus erythematosus (prolonged myocardial T_1 at 0.08 T),[115] amyloidosis (myocardial hypertrophy

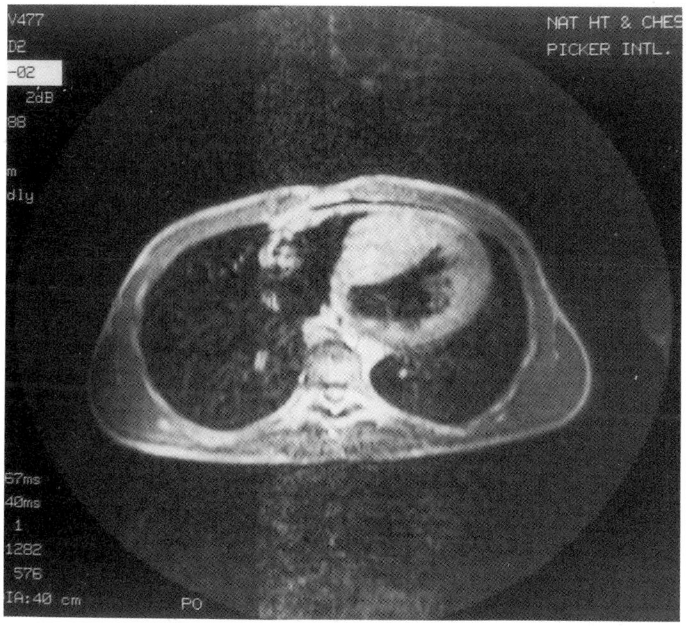

(a)

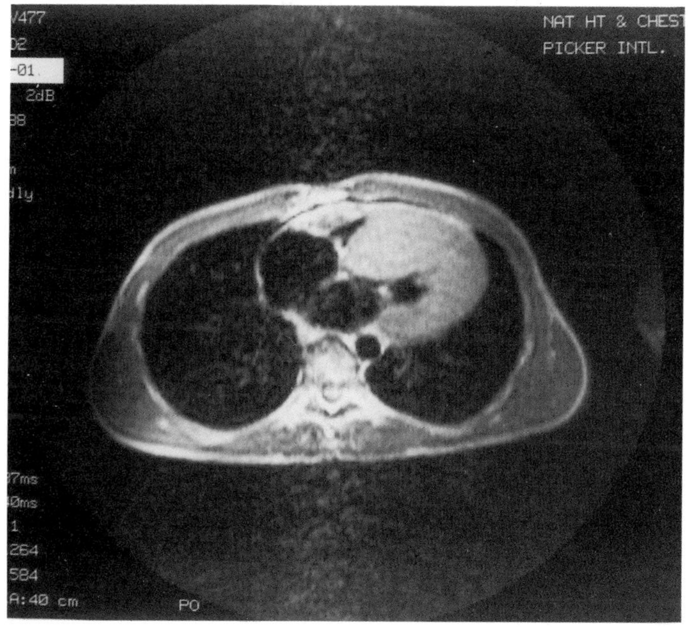

(b)

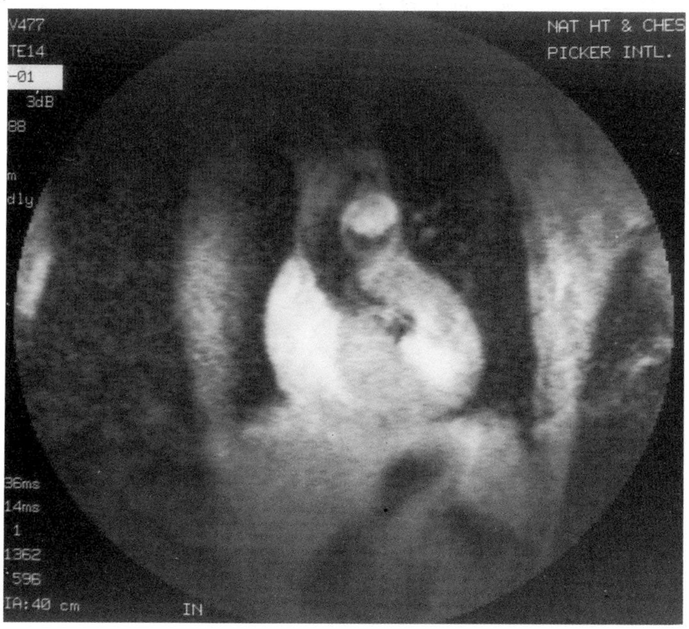

(c)

Figure 5.26. (a) Diastolic and (b) systolic spin echo images showing the asymmetric septal hypertrophy of hypertrophic cardiomyopathy. (c) A systolic frame from a coronal cine acquisition shows loss of signal originating in the left ventricular outflow tract indicating turbulence caused by outflow tract obstruction.

and restrictive physiology),[116] Pompe's disease,[117] and Fabry's disease.[118]

5.4.5 The right ventricle

As discussed above, it is possible to measure right ventricular volume very accurately without making any assumptions about its geometry. Regional abnormalities, however, are difficult to detect unless they are severe because of the complex motion of the right ventricle compared with the left. Despite this, it has been possible to demonstrate abnormalities of global function and of regional wall thickness in patients with arrhythmogenic right ventricular dysplasia, even when other imaging techniques such as echocardiography and X-ray contrast ventriculography suggest

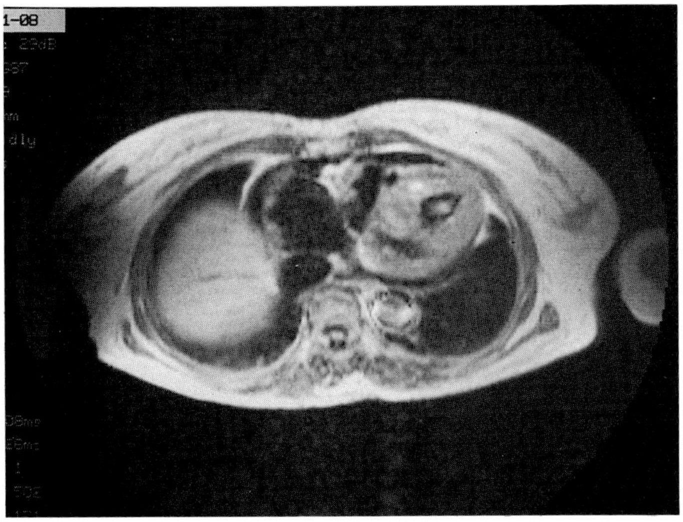

Figure 5.27. Transverse image of a patient with myocardial sarcoidosis. There is an area of high signal within the septum which suggests active disease and there is also pericardial thickening with a small effusion.

that the right ventricle is normal.[119] Figure 5.29 shows such a patient who presented with recurrent ventricular tachycardia of right ventricular origin.

5.5 The valves

Normal heart valves are thin, rapidly moving structures and they are poorly seen in spin echo images. Abnormal valves are more easily seen because they are thicker and they may be less mobile. Occasionally it is possible to obtain diagnostic information from spin echo images (figure 5.30) but cine gradient echo imaging is more informative and is covered in more detail in chapter 7. Valve calcification may show as a loss of signal, but the absence of this sign cannot rule out calcification.

Associated pathology can be seen including chamber dilatation and the presence of intracavitary thrombus. The measurement of left and right ventricular stroke volumes allows a calculation of the regurgitant fraction for single valve lesions and this has been discussed above. Cine imaging can also visualise regurgitant jets and jets distal to stenotic valves (chapter 7) and cine velocity mapping allows the peak velocity distal to a stenosed valve to be measured, hence the pressure gradient across the valve (chapter 10). At the time of writing (1990), echo times sufficiently short to avoid signal loss from turbulent jets and hence allow velocity mapping are not widely available, but the limitations

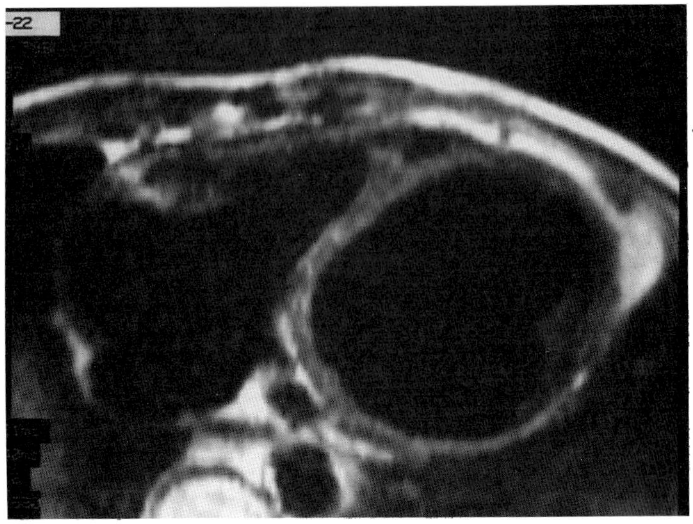

(a)

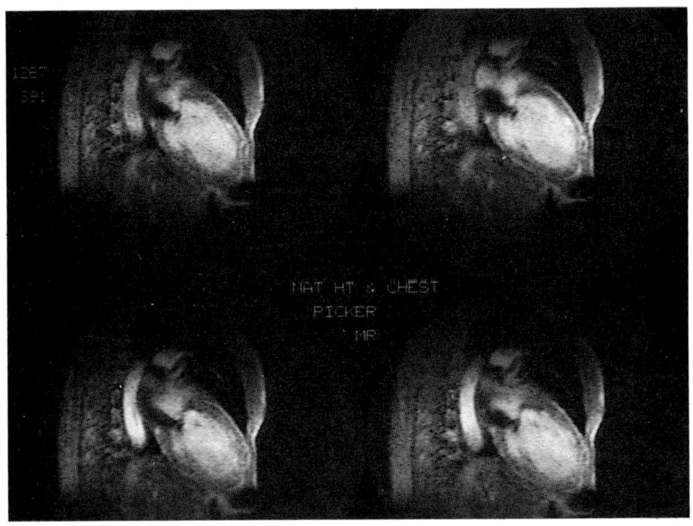

(b)

Figure 5.28. (a) Dilated and thinned left ventricle in a patient with dilated cardiomyopathy. The signal close to the lateral wall is static blood and not thrombus. (b) Four systolic frames in the vertical long axis plane from a cine field echo acquisition showing the global hypokinesis and a turbulent jet of mitral regurgitation.

are simply those of hardware and will not be long-lived.

Patients with prosthetic valves are commonly encountered but prostheses are not imaged because the alloy from which they are made contains no mobile hydrogen atoms and so does not give a magnetic resonance signal. There is distortion of the applied magnetic field by the difference of susceptibility between prosthesis and biological tissue and by eddy currents

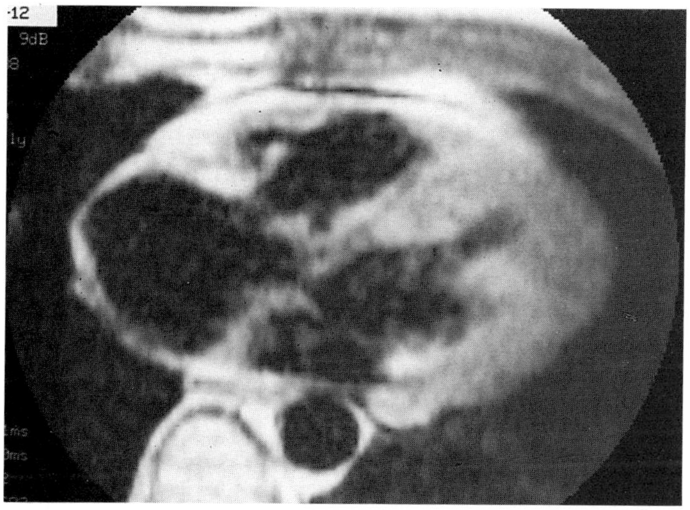

Figure 5.29. Spin echo image showing thinning of the anterior right ventricular wall in a patient with arrhythmogenic right ventricular dysplasia.

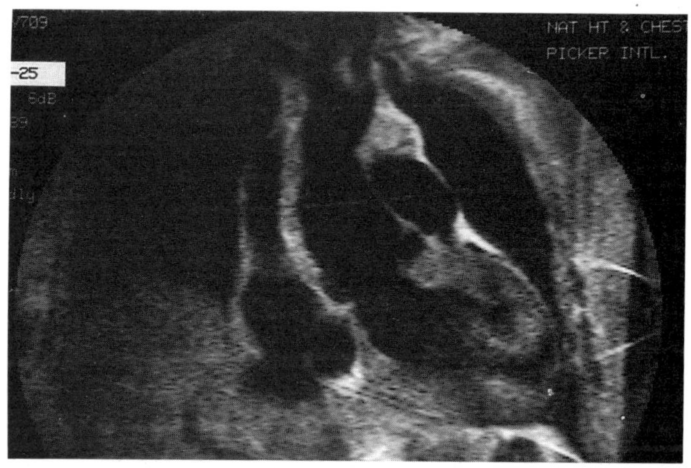

(a)

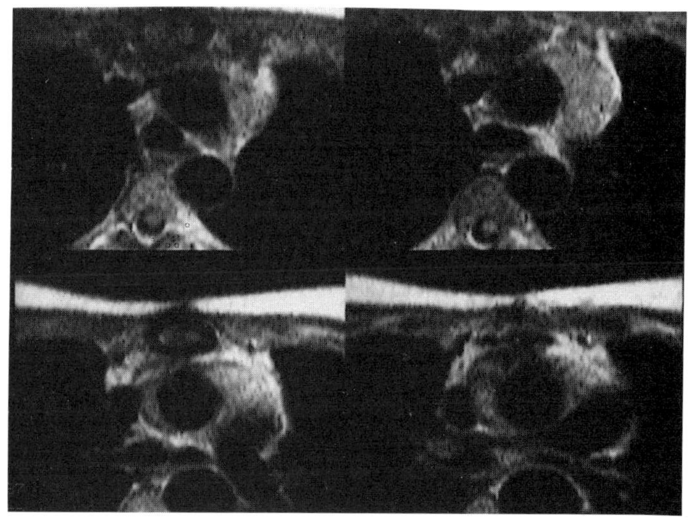

(b)

Figure 5.31. Coronal (a) and transverse (b) spin echo images in a patient who had undergone aortic root replacement including a prosthetic aortic valve. Postoperatively, he was febrile and responded poorly to antibiotics. A collection of pus is seen to the left of the aorta above the pulmonary artery and the collection extends around the root replacement to the right. Note that the metallic valve prosthesis is not seen, but surrounding structures can still be evaluated.

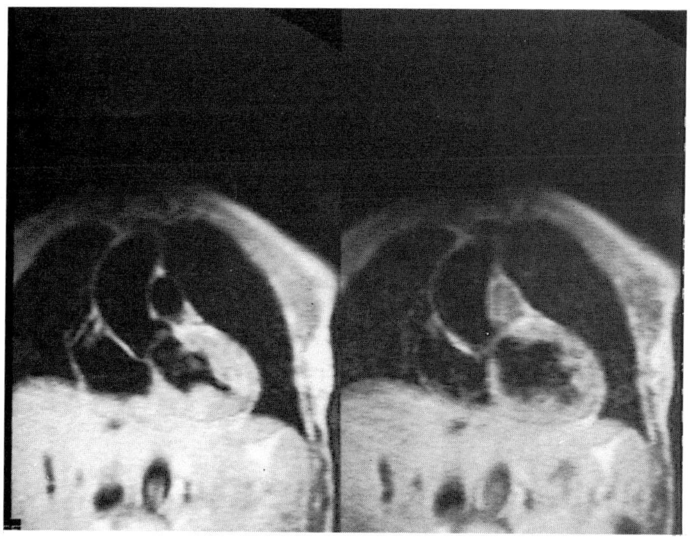

Figure 5.30. Coronal images through the aortic valve at end systole (left) and end diastole (right). A thickened aortic valve is seen at end diastole, but more importantly it does not open fully in systole and it is still seen in the aortic root. The patient had severe calcific aortic stenosis with a doming valve.

induced in the valve, and this leads to loss of signal from tissues for a variable distance around the prosthesis. This distance is small for spin echo images and neighbouring structures are seen normally (figure 5.31), but the defect in the image is much larger in gradient echo images making it difficult to assess turbulent jets in the region of the valve. Metal valves are not ferromagnetic however and at currently available magnetic field strengths there is no effect of the field upon the working of the valve.[120–123] The safety aspects of imaging prosthetic valves are more fully covered in chapter 14.

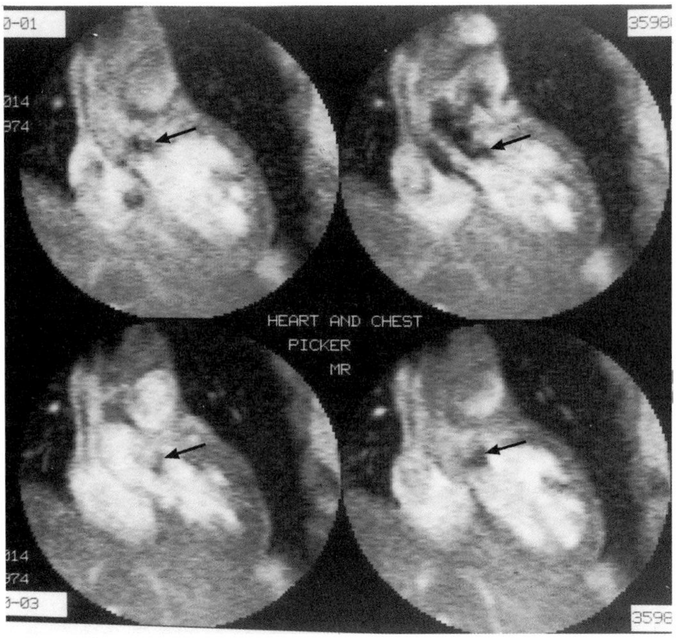

Figure 5.32. Cine gradient echo images in systole (top) and diastole (bottom) in a patient with systemic lupus erythematosus and Liebman–Sachs endocarditis. A large vegetation is seen as a constant filling defect in the region of the aortic valve (arrowed) and systolic turbulence is also seen in the aorta.

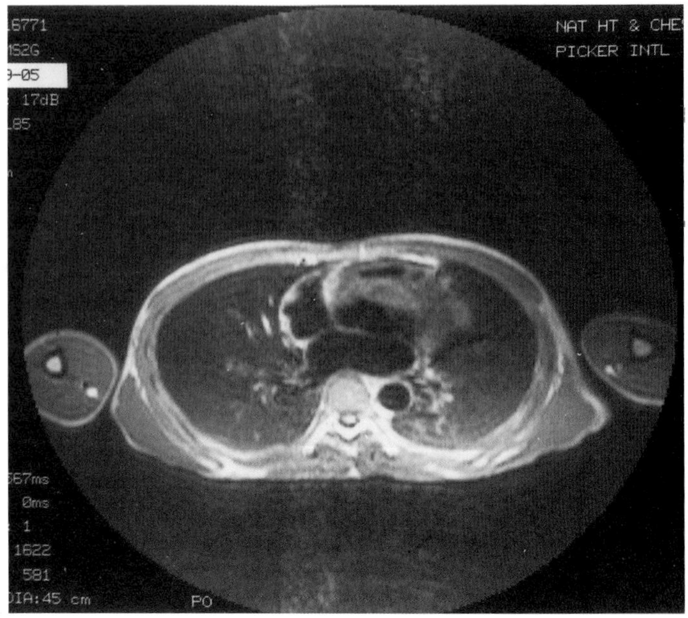

Figure 5.33. Transverse image through the base of the heart in a patient with Marfan's syndrome and infective endocarditis on a bicuspid aortic valve. There is an abscess between the aortic root and the right ventricular outflow tract, which is compressed. The abscess was not easily demonstrated by echocardiography.

5.6 The endocardium

The normal endocardium is too thin to be seen as a discrete structure, but a common clinical problem in patients with suspected infective endocarditis is to look for vegetations on the valves. Unfortunately, magnetic resonance can only demonstrate very large vegetations and it cannot rival echocardiography as a screening technique (figure 5.32). The same is not so if an abscess is suspected or if infection has spread outside the heart, and magnetic resonance is an ideal method of localising such infection (figure 5.33).[124]

Endomyocardial fibrosis is a rare disease but it sometimes causes diagnostic difficulty and it should be excluded in patients with restrictive cardiomyopathy. Obliteration of the apices of both ventricles by fibrous material and thrombus is characteristic and magnetic resonance can be helpful in cases of doubt (figure 5.34).

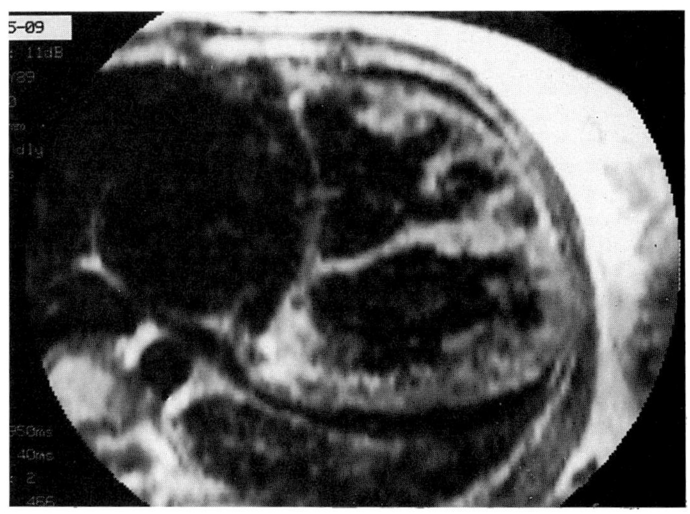

Figure 5.34. Endomyocardial fibrosis. Both ventricles are dilated and there is signal from fibrosis and thrombus at the apices of both ventricles. There is also a small pericardial effusion.

5.7 The pericardium

The normal fibrous pericardium appears as a thin dark line (not more than 1 mm) around the heart in spin echo images, and it is usually most easily seen anteriorly and postero-laterally in transverse images.[125,126] It is particularly easy to see when sandwiched between epicardial and pericardial fat, but at high field strengths

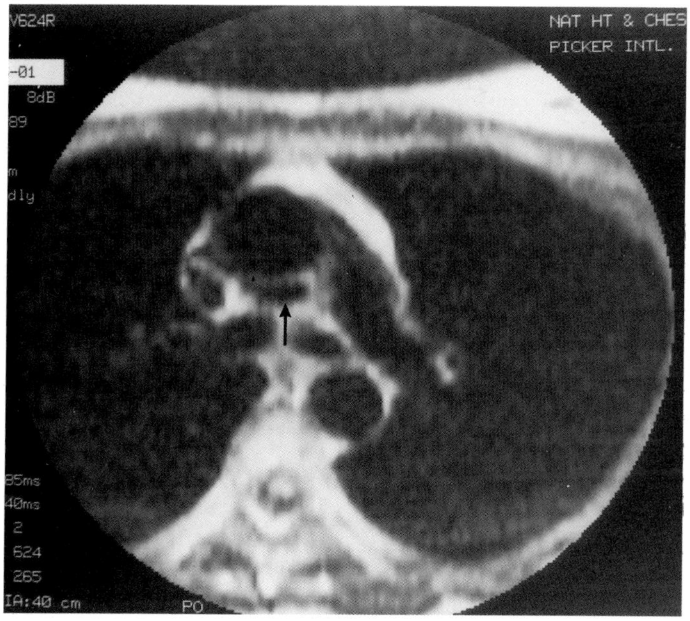

Figure 5.35. Transverse spin echo image of a woman following an episode of chest pain. The signal free space behind the ascending aorta (arrowed) is the posterior pericardial recess and could easily be mistaken for a localised aortic dissection.

chemical shift artefact can obscure it. It is important to be aware of the superior pericardial recesses which are the reflections of the pericardium upon itself both anteriorly and posteriorly around the great vessels.[127] Unless the normal anatomy of the pericardium is appreciated, it is possible to mistake these recesses for aortic dissection when a small signal free space is seen beside the aorta (figure 5.35).

Pericardial thickening and effusion can both be seen, but the appearance depends upon the pathology and can range from low, if the pericardium remains fibrous, to high, if there is active inflammation and infiltration.[128,129] In contrast to X-ray computed tomography, pericardial calcification is not seen, but a pericardial thickness greater than 4 mm distinguishes constrictive pericarditis from restrictive cardiomyopathy. Pericardial fluid has a high signal in the absence of motion but more often it loses signal because of flow within the pericardial space. It is not possible to distinguish exudate from transudate or haemorrhage, but with malignant effusions, metastatic nodules may be seen lining the pericardial space. Because of the variable signal of the pericardium and pericardial fluid it can be difficult to distinguish the two from fat in static images, but if there is confusion, then cine imaging is

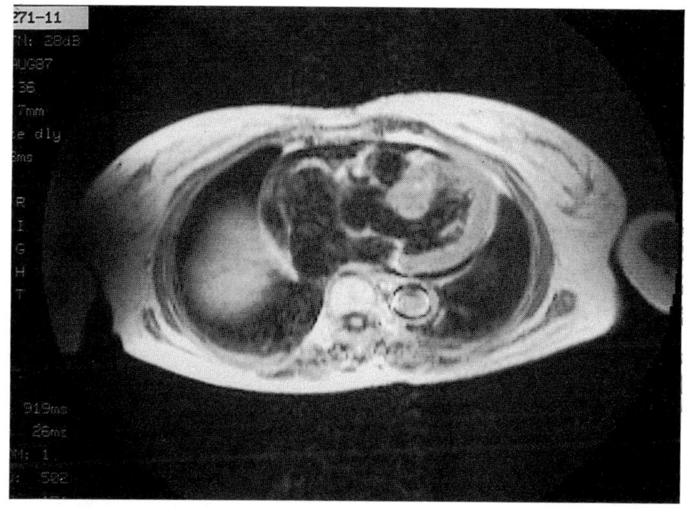

(a)

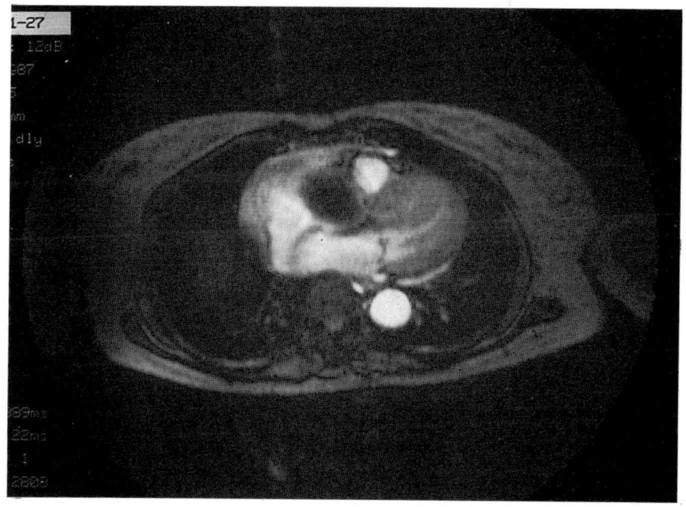

(b)

Figure 5.36. Transverse section using a spin echo sequence (a) and a field echo sequence (b) in a patient with sarcoidosis. The pericardial effusion gives no signal in the spin echo image because of motion of the fluid, but it gives a higher signal in the field echo image. Note also the high signal within the septum in the spin echo image indicating myocardial involvement in the inflammatory process.

helpful. With a cine display, the motion of the heart within a pericardial effusion is easily appreciated and a thickened and rigid pericardium is also more obvious (figure 5.36).

A common clinical problem is to rule out the presence of pericardial constriction in a patient with apparent heart failure. Whilst the presence of a normal pericardium rules out the possibility, a thickened peri-

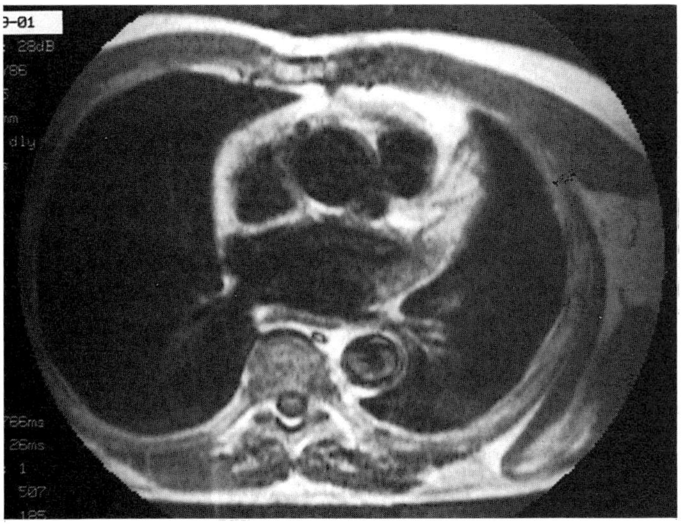

Figure 5.37. Transverse image in a patient with three vessel coronary artery disease and previous coronary bypass grafting. The graft to the right coronary artery is seen anterior to the ascending aorta, and the left anterior descending and circumflex arteries are also seen. The lesser cardiac vein runs alongside the anterior descending artery to enter the coronary sinus. Resolution is not sufficient to be confident of the presence of coronary stenoses.

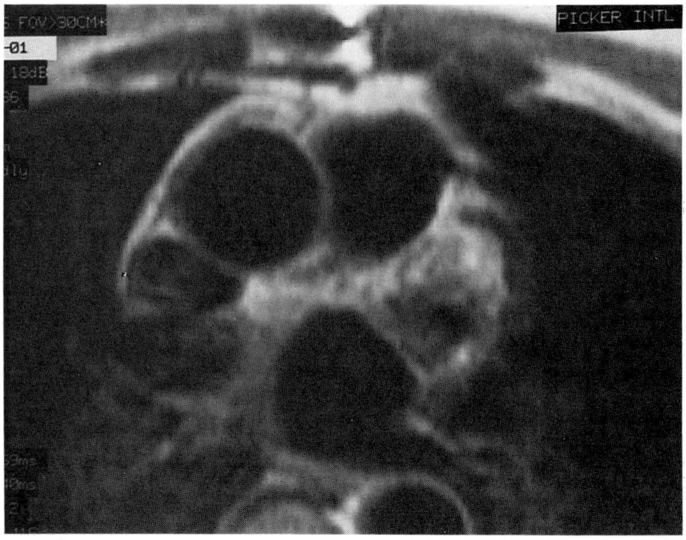

Figure 5.38. Transverse spin echo image showing two patent coronary bypass grafts that have arisen from the aorta at a higher level, have passed in front of the pulmonary artery, and are descending to the left coronary territory.

cardium cannot make the diagnosis of constriction, which is a functional one. Other features which help to make the functional diagnosis include small ventricular volumes with preserved ejection fraction and a dilated right atrium and caval veins, a motionless pericardium seen on cine imaging, and abnormal septal motion with a sudden stop or even reversal of motion in mid-diastole. Cine velocity mapping in the caval veins may also be valuable because any condition that impairs right ventricular filling will be reflected in reduced diastolic filling (see chapter 10).

5.8 The coronary arteries and bypass grafts

The coronary arteries are small, tortuous, and rapidly moving: three properties which conspire against successful imaging. Despite this, the proximal vessels can nearly always be identified and their appearance with low intraluminal signal implies that they contain moving blood and are patent. Unfortunately, resolution is not sufficient using current techniques to identify stenoses confidently,[130] although aneurysms are more reliably detected.[131,132] The transverse plane most commonly shows the left main coronary artery and its division to left anterior descending and circumflex vessels, and these vessels can often be followed distally in the anterior interventricular groove and the left atrioventricular groove respectively (figure 5.37). The right coronary artery can similarly be followed in the right atrioventricular groove. Alternative planes through which the coronary vessels can be seen to pass perpendicularly include the short axis plane, with the anterior and posterior descending arteries and the marginal and diagonal vessels, and the horizontal long axis plane, with the left circumflex artery and the right coronary artery in the left and right atrioventricular grooves respectively. In most cases a coronary vein runs beside the coronary artery, and potential confusion exists particularly because the vein is larger than the artery.

The two largest problems for more detailed imaging of the coronary arteries are the fact that a tomographic imaging technique is not ideal for tortuous structures, and a triggered technique that sums data from multiple cardiac cycles will generate artefact if the heart is not in an identical position with each cardiac cycle. It is in theory possible to overcome the first problem using three-dimensional acquisition and display,[133] but this would require unacceptable imaging times using conventional sequences. Real time imaging using an echo

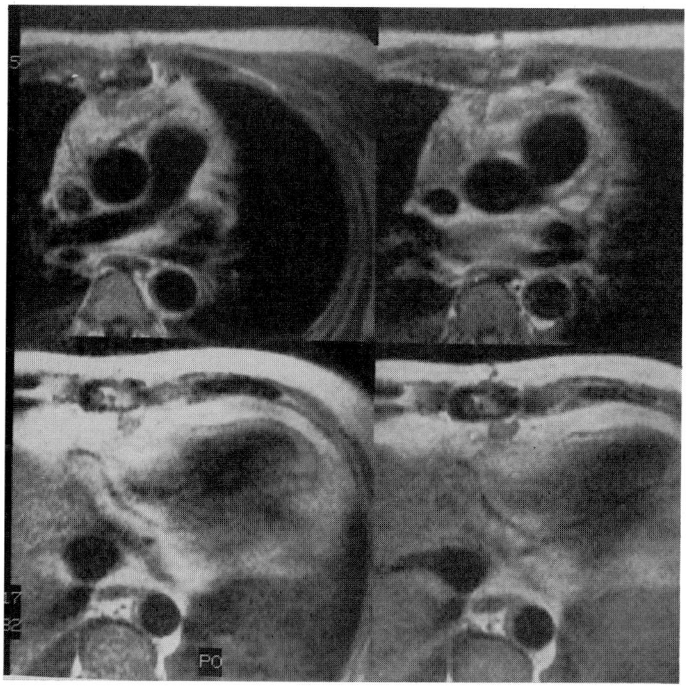

Figure 5.39. A patient with four patent coronary bypass grafts. The left anterior descending graft is seen arising from the aorta (top left) and grafts to the diagonal and marginal circumflex vessels are descending lateral to the pulmonary artery. On the inferior surface of the heart, a graft to the posterior descending artery is seen in the atrioventricular groove (bottom left) and it can be followed to its distal insertion (bottom right). The native coronary vessels are particularly well seen (top right).

Table 5.3 Results of a comparison of X-ray angiography against magnetic resonance imaging for the detection of patent coronary bypass grafts. These figures give a sensitivity of 86% and a specificity of 100%[139]

	Angiography	Magnetic resonance
Patent	29	25
Occluded	10	14

planar technique may overcome both problems and preliminary results are encouraging.[134]

Coronary artery bypass grafts are more easily imaged, mainly because they are less mobile proximally than coronary arteries. In spin echo images, the appearance of low intraluminal signal contrasting with the high signal of the surrounding fat or other soft tissue, implies that the graft contains moving blood and is patent (figure 5.38). It is also necessary to be able to follow the graft distally to its insertion to be confident of patency, although right coronary artery grafts can only rarely be followed as far as the posterior descending artery (figure 5.39). If a graft cannot be identified, or if its origin is seen but it cannot be followed distally, then it can be assumed to be occluded (figure 5.40). Using these criteria, sensitivity and specificity for the detection of patent grafts in the region of 90% can be achieved,[135–138] and our own experience is summarised in table 5.3.[139] Internal mammary artery grafts are more difficult to visualise than saphenous vein grafts, partly because of their smaller size and partly because they can be tortuous and are therefore more difficult to follow through multiple slices. The sensitivity of magnetic resonance for the detection of patent internal mammary grafts is much lower than 90% although large studies have not been performed.

Because bypass grafts are small and mobile a number of technical points need close attention. It is important to be familiar with the positioning of the grafts used by the surgeon because this is very variable and, as a rule, recently implanted grafts are more easily seen than older grafts that have become arterialised with consequent reduction in lumen. Magnetic resonance is therefore ideal for the early postoperative assessment of graft patency. For imaging strategy, a suitable starting plane is the transverse plane beginning high on the ascending aorta and descending at least as far as mid-ventricular level. Five millimetre slices are ideal, although at lower field strengths thicker slices may be required, in which case it is useful to interleave two acquisitions to acquire 10 mm slices at 5 mm spacing. A similar strategy in the sagittal plane often allows grafts to the left coronary territory to be identified arising anteriorly from the ascending aorta and passing in front of the pulmonary artery. Cine imaging can also be used to supplement spin echo imaging although, because it is time consuming to cover a large number of slices in this way, spin echo imaging is required in addition. Another drawback of cine imaging is that the artefact arising from sternal wire sutures is very much larger than in spin echo images and it often extends over the region where the grafts are best seen.

A number of artefacts can be mistaken for grafts. Figure 5.41 shows a spin echo image in the short axis plane with small artefacts from metal clips that could easily be mistaken for large patent grafts. Such clips

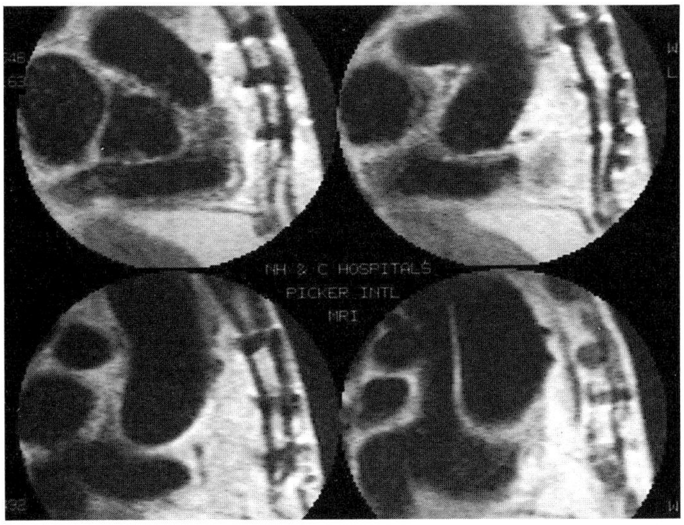

Figure 5.40. Contiguous sagittal images from left (top left) to right (bottom right). Two coronary bypass grafts are seen arising from the anterior wall of the ascending aorta (bottom right) and passing in front of the pulmonary artery. In the top left image, only one graft is seen because the second graft is occluded after its origin.

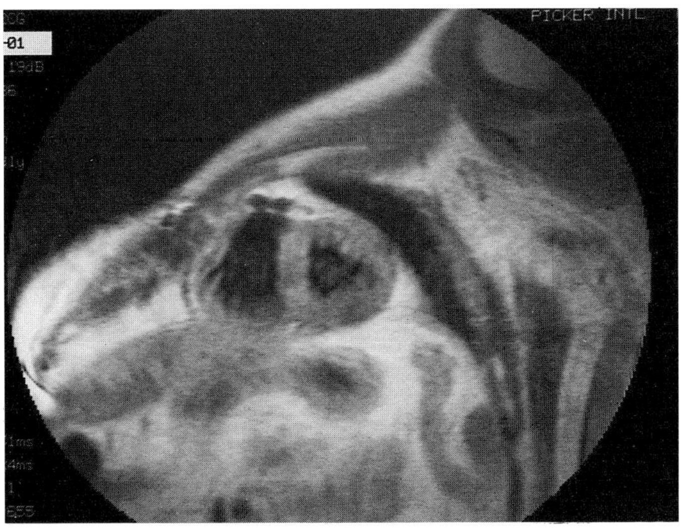

Figure 5.41. Short axis spin echo image showing two circular artefacts caused by metal clips in the anterior interventricular groove that could be mistaken for patent grafts.

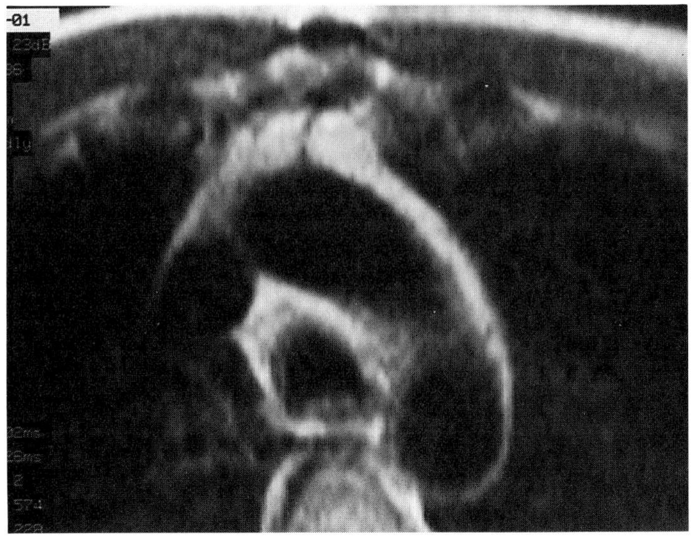

(a)

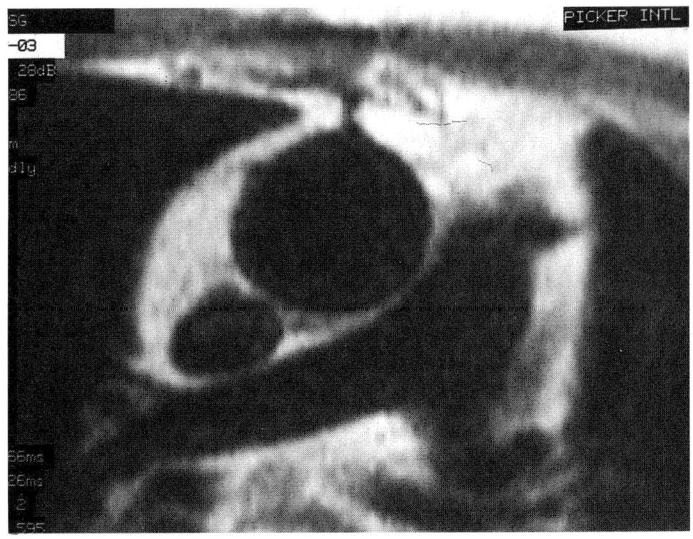

(b)

Figure 5.42. Transverse images at the level of the aortic arch (a) and the right pulmonary artery (b) in a patient with coronary artery bypass grafts. A patent right coronary graft is seen in the right hand image arising from the anterolateral aspect of the ascending aorta. The apparent graft arising in both images from the anterior wall is the fibrous scar following sternotomy.

are not ferromagnetic and imaging is perfectly safe,[140] but the artefacts can complicate interpretation of the images particularly cine gradient echo images which are much more sensitive to the field inhomogeneity caused by the clips. Also, the line of fibrosis in the anterior mediastinum which is formed by healing of the sternotomy scar can be mistaken for a graft, although the scar extends for the whole length of the ascending aorta, unlike a graft (figure 5.42).

In clinical cardiology it is not usually sufficient simply

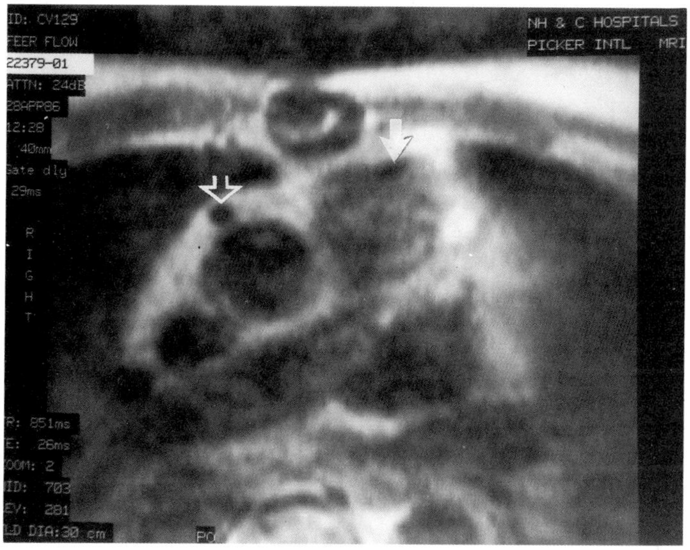

(a)

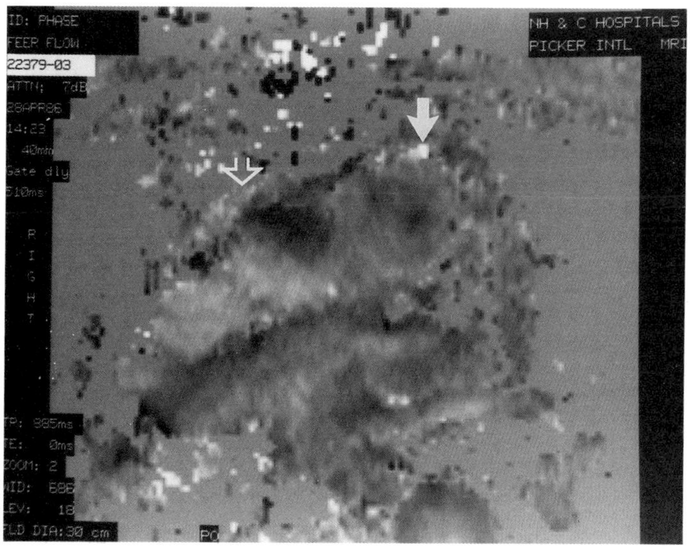

(b)

Figure 5.43. Transverse spin echo image (a) showing patent grafts to the right coronary artery anterior to the ascending aorta (open arrow), and to the left anterior descending artery anterior to the pulmonary artery (closed arrow). (b) The corresponding diastolic velocity map on the right shows high velocity in the left anterior descending graft (white) and very low velocity in the right coronary graft. The right coronary graft was confirmed by X-ray angiography to serve a vessel with distal disease and poor run-off. For a full description of the velocity mapping technique, see chapter 10.

to know whether a graft is patent because there may be disease of the graft or of the coronary vessel distal to the anastomosis, limiting flow down a patent graft. Magnetic resonance velocity mapping is a possible technique for the measurement of graft flow. This is covered in more detail in chapter 10. Velocity measurements have been achieved in vein grafts and have been compared with the adequacy of graft function assessed by conventional X-ray angiography (figure 5.43).[141] Peak velocities lower than 100 mm/s are an indication of poor graft function, but flow measurements throughout the cycle are more difficult to achieve, partly because of the small size of the grafts and partly because of their mobility. Velocity measurements can be obtained in approximately 50% of grafts and the factors which prevent a more complete assessment are the artefact from metal clips and sternal sutures, and the long imaging times needed for a complete study including spin echo imaging and cine velocity mapping in several planes.

References

1 Amparo EG, Higgins CB, Hoddick W, *et al*. Magnetic resonance imaging of aortic disease: preliminary results. *Am J Roentgenol* 1984; **143**: 1203–9.

2 Glazer HS, Gutierrez FR, Levitt RG, Lee JKT, Murphy WA. The thoracic aorta studied by MR imaging. *Radiology* 1985; **157**: 149–55.

3 Dooms GC, Higgins CB. The potential of magnetic resonance imaging for the evaluation of thoracic arterial disease. *J Thorac Cardiovasc Surg* 1986; **92**: 1088–95.

4 Mossard JM, Baruthio J, Germain P, *et al*. Apport de la résonance magnétique nucléaire dans le diagnostic des affections aortiques. *Arch Mal Coeur* 1986; **79**: 456–61.

5 Auffermann W, Olofsson P, Stoney R, Higgins CB. MR imaging of complications of aortic surgery. *J Comput Assist Tomogr* 1987; **11**: 982–9.

6 Lois JF, Gomes AS, Brown K, Mulder DG, Laks H. Magnetic resonance imaging of the thoracic aorta. *Am J Cardiol* 1987; **60**: 358–62.

7 Garbagnati F, Castoldi MC, Banchini E, *et al*. Risonanza magnetica dell'aorta toracica. *La Radiologica Medica* 1988; **75**: 433–8.

8 Amparo EG, Higgins CB, Hricak H, Sollitto R. Aortic dissection: magnetic resonance imaging. *Radiology* 1985; **155**: 399–406.

9 Geisinger MA, Risius B, O'Donnell JA, *et al*. Thoracic aortic dissections: magnetic resonance imaging. *Radiology* 1985; **155**: 407–12.

10 Dinsmore RE, Wedeen VJ, Miller SW, *et al*. MRI of dissection of the aorta: recognition of the intimal tear and differential flow velocities. *Am J Roentgenol* 1986; **146**: 1286–8.

11 Goldman AP, Kotler MN, Scanlon MH, Ostrum BJ, Parameswaran R, Parry WR. Magnetic resonance imaging and two dimensonal echocardiography. Alternative approach to aortography in diagnosis of aortic dissecting aneurysm. *Am J Med* 1986; **80**: 1225–9.

12 Goldman AP, Kotler MN, Scanlon MH, Ostrum B, Parameswaran R, Parry WR. The complementary role of magnetic resonance imaging, Doppler echocardiography, and computed tomography in the diagnosis of dissecting thoracic aneurysms. *Am Heart J* 1986; **111**: 970–81.

13 Akins EW, Hill JA, Carmichael MJ. MR imaging of blood pool signal variation with cardiac phase in aortic dissection. *J Comput Assist Tomogr* 1987; **11**: 543–5.

14 Barentsz JO, Ruijs JHJ, Heystraten FMJ, Buskens F. Magnetic resonance imaging of the dissected aorta. *Br J Radiol* 1987; **60**: 499–502.

15 Pernes JM, Grenier P, Desbleds MT, de Brux JL. MR evaluation of chronic aortic dissection. *J Comput Assist Tomogr* 1987; **11**: 975–81.

16 Kersting-Sommerhoff BA, Higgins CB, White RD, Sommerhoff CP, Lipton MJ. Aortic dissection: sensitivity and specificity of MR imaging. *Radiology* 1988; **166**: 651–5.

17 Bogren HG, Underwood SR, Firmin DN, *et al*. Magnetic resonance velocity mapping in aortic dissection. *Br J Radiol* 1988; **61**: 456–62.

18 Mitchell L, Jenkins JPR, Brownlee WC, Isherwood I. Aortic dissection: morphology and differential flow velocity patterns demonstrated by magnetic resonance imaging. *Clin Radiol* 1988; **39**: 458–61.

19 Yamada T, Tada S, Harada J. Aortic dissection without intimal rupture: diagnosis with MR imaging and CT. *Radiology* 1988; **168**: 347–52.

20 Moore EH, Webb WR, Verrier ED, *et al*. MRI of chronic posttraumatic false aneurysms of the thoracic aorta. *Am J Roentgenol* 1984; **143**: 1195–6.

21 Dinsmore RE, Liberthson RR, Wismer GL, *et al*. Magnetic resonance imaging of thoracic aortic aneurysms: comparison with other imaging methods. *Am J Roentgenol* 1986; **146**: 309–14.

22 Globits S, Neuhold A, Mayr H, Fezoulidis I, Wicke L, Glogar D. Magnetresonanztomographie in der abklarung von fraglichen aneurysmen der aorta thoracalis mit oder ohne dissektion der intima. *Zeitschrift für Kardiologie* 1989; **78**: 109–15.

23 Spielmann RP, Kung EE, Witte G, Heller M. Magnetic resonance imaging of ruptured aneurysm of the ascending aorta. *Br J Radiol* 1989; **62**: 373–5.

24 Amparo EG, Higgins CB, Shafton EP. Demonstration of coarctation of the aorta by magnetic resonance imaging. *Am J Roentgenol* 1984; **143**: 1192–4.

25 Boxer RA, LaCorte MA, Singh S, *et al*. Nuclear magnetic resonance imaging in evaluation and follow-up of children treated for coarctation of the aorta. *J Am Coll Cardiol* 1986; **7**: 1095–8.

26 von Schulthess GK, Higashino SM, Higgins SS, Didier D, Fisher MR, Higgins CB. Coarctation of the aorta: MR imaging. *Radiology* 1986; **158**: 469–75.

27 Bank ER, Aisen AM, Rocchini AP, Hernandez RJ. Coarctation of the aorta in children undergoing angioplasty: pretreatment and posttreatment MR imaging. *Radiology* 1987; **162**: 235–40.

28 Simpson IA, Chung KJ, Glass RF, Sahn DJ, Sherman FS, Hesselink J. Cine magnetic resonance imaging for evaluation of anatomy and flow relations in infants and children with coarctation of the aorta. *Circulation* 1988; **78**: 142–8.

29 Pucillo AL, Schechter AG, Kay RH, Herman MV. Magnetic resonance imaging of vascular conduits in coarctation of the aorta. *Am Heart J* 1989; **117**: 482–5.

30 Boxer RA, Fishman MC, LaCorte MA, Singh S, Parnell VA Jr. Diagnosis and postoperative evaluation of supravavular aortic stenosis by magnetic resonance imaging. *Am J Cardiol* 1986; **58**: 367–8.

31 Coscina WF, Kressel HY, Gefter W, Axel L. MR imaging of double aortic arch. *J Comput Assist Tomogr* 1986; **10**: 673–5.

32 Guit GL, Bluemm R, Rohmer J, *et al*. Levotransposition of the aorta: identification of segmental cardiac anatomy using MR imaging. *Radiology* 1986; **161**: 673–9.

33 Bisset GS, Strife JL, Kirks DR, Bailey WW. Vascular rings: MR imaging. *Am J Roentgenol* 1987; **149**: 251–6.

34 Brown K, Batra P. MR imaging of aneurysm of an aberrant right subclavian artery. *J Comput Assist Tomogr* 1987; **11**: 1071–3.

35 Gomes AS, Lois JF, George B, Alpan G, Williams RG. Congenital abnormalities of the aortic arch: MR imaging. *Radiology* 1987; **165**: 691–5.

36 Bernard C, Galloy MA, Marcon F, Prevot J, Hoeffel JC, Pernot C. Contribution of MRI to the diagnosis of double aortic arch. *Arch Mal Coeur* 1988; **81**: 1277–80.

37 Boxer RA, LaCorte MA, Singh S, Davis J, Goldman M, Stein HL. Evaluation of the aorta in the Marfan syndrome by magnetic resonance imaging. *Am Heart J* 1986; **111**: 1001–2.

38 Kersting-Sommerhoff BA, Sechtem UP, Schiller NB, Lipton MJ, Higgins CB. MR imaging of the thoracic aorta in Marfan patients. *J Comput Assist Tomogr* 1987; **11**: 633–9.

39 Schaefer S, Peshock RM, Mallot CR, Katz J, Parkey RW, Willerson JT. Nuclear magnetic resonance imaging in Marfan's syndrome. *J Am Coll Cardiol* 1987; **9**: 70–4.

40 Soulen RL, Fishman EK, Pyeritz RE, Zerhouni EA, Pessar ML. Marfan syndrome: evaluation with MR imaging versus CT. *Radiology* 1987; **165**: 697–701.

41 Winkler M, Higgins CB. MRI of perivalvular infectious pseudoaneurysms. *Am J Roentgenol* 1986; **147**: 253–6.

42 Miller SW, Palmer EL, Dinsmore RE, Brady TJ. Gallium-67 and magnetic resonance imaging in aortic root abscess. *J Nucl Med* 1987; **28**: 1616–9.

43 Amparo EG, Hoddick WK, Hricak H, *et al*. Comparison of magnetic resonance imaging and ultrasonography in the evaluation of abdominal aortic aneurysms. *Radiology* 1985; **154**: 451–6.

44 Flak B, Li DKB, Ho BYB, *et al*. Magnetic resonance imaging of aneurysms of the abdominal aorta. *Am J Roengenol* 1985; **144**: 991–6.

45 Miller DL, Reinig JW, Volkman DJ. Vascular imaging with MRI: inadequacy in Takayasu's arteritis compared with angiography. *Am J Roentgenol* 1986; **146**: 949–54.

46 Erdman WA, Weinreb JC, Cohen JM, Buja LM, Chaney C, Peshock RM. Venous thrombosis: clinical and experimental MR imaging. *Radiology* 1986; **161**: 233–8.

47 Rapoport S, Sostman HD, Pope C, Camputaro CM, Holcomb W, Gore JC. Venous clots: evaluation with MR imaging. *Radiology* 1987; **162**: 527–30.

48 Spritzer CE, Sussman SK, Blinder RA, Saeed M, Herfkens RJ. Deep venous thrombosis evaluation with limited-flip-angle, gradient-refocused MR imaging: preliminary experience. *Radiology* 1988; **166**: 371–5.

49 Gamsu G, Hirji M, Moore EH, Webb WR, Brito A. Experimental pulmonary emboli detected using magnetic resonance. *Radiology* 1984; **153**: 467–70.

50 Moore EH, Gamsu G, Webb WR, Stulbarg MS. Pulmonary embolus: detection and followup using magnetic resonance. *Radiology* 1984; **153**: 471–2.

51 Stein MG, Crues JV, Bradley WG, *et al*. MR imaging of pulmonary emboli: an experimental study in dogs. *Am J Roentgenol* 1986; **147**: 1133–7.

52 Fisher MR, Higgins CB. Central thrombi in pulmonary arterial hypertension detected by MR imaging. *Radiology* 1986; **158**: 223–6.

53 Posteraro RH, Sostman HD, Spritzer CE, Herfkens RJ. Cine-gradient-refocussed MR imaging of central pulmonary emboli. *Am J Roentgenol* 1989; **152**: 465–8.

54 Fisher MR, Higgins CB, Andereck W. MR imaging of an intrapericardial pheochromocytoma. *J Comput Assist Tomogr* 1985; **9**: 1103–5.

55 Pizzarello RA, *et al*. Tumour of the heart diagnosed by magnetic resonance imaging. *J Am Coll Cardiol* 1985; **5**: 989–91.

56 Conti VR, Saydjari R, Amparo EG. Paraganglioma of the heart. The value of magnetic resonance imaging in the preoperative evaluation. *Chest* 1986; **90**: 604–6.

57 Applegate PM, Tajik AJ, Ehman RL, Julsrud PR, Miller FA Jr. Two-dimensional echocardiographic and magnetic resonance imaging observations in massive lipomatous hypertrophy of the atrial septum. *Am J Cardiol* 1987; **59**: 489–91.

58 Dichek DA, Holmvang G, Fallon JT, *et al*. Angiosarcoma of the heart: three-year survival and follow-up by nuclear magnetic resonance imaging. *Am Heart J* 1988; **115**: 1323–4.

59 Gindea AJ, Gentin B, Naidich DP, Freedberg RS, McCauley D, Kronzon I. Unusual cardiac metastasis in hypernephroma: the complementary role of echocardiography and magnetic resonance imaging. *Am Heart J* 1988; **116**: 1359–61.

60 Gossinger HD, Siostrzonek P, Zangeneh M, *et al*. Magnetic resonance imaging findings in a patient with pericardial mesothelioma. *Am Heart J* 1988; **115**: 1321–2.

61 Johnson DE, Vacek J, Gollub SB, Wilson DB, Dunn M. Comparison of gated cardiac magnetic resonance imaging and two-dimensional echocardiography for the evaluation of right ventricular thrombi: a case report with autopsy correlation. *Cath Cardiovasc Diagn* 1988; **14**: 266–8.

62 Magherini A, Bartolozzi C, Petacchi D. Magnetic resonance and echocardiography in the investigation of cardiac tumour in an infant. *Int J Cardiol* 1988; **18**: 263–6.

63 Amparo EG, Higgins CB, Farmer D, Gamsu G, McNamara M. Gated MRI of cardiac and paracardiac masses: initial experience. *Am J Roentgenol* 1984; **143**: 1151–6.

64 Boxer RA, LaCorte MA, Singh S, *et al*. Diagnosis of cardiac tumours in infants by magnetic resonance imaging. *Am J Cardiol* 1985; **56**: 831–2.

65 Conces DJ, Vix VA, Klatte EC. Gated MR imaging of left atrial myxomas. *Radiology* 1985; **156**: 445–7.

66 Go RT, O'Donnell JK, Underwood DA, *et al*. Comparison of gated cardiac MRI and 2D echocardiography of intracardiac neoplasms. *Am J Roentgenol* 1985; **145**: 21–5.

67 Grötz J, Steiner G, Josephs W, Sorge B, Wiechmann W, Beyer HK. Darstellung intra- und parakardialer raumfordernder Prozesse mit der magnetischen Resonanztomographie. *Dtsch Med Wochenschr* 1986; **111**: 1594–8.

68 von Schulthess GK, McMurdo K, Tscholakoff D, de Geer G, Gamsu G, Higgins CB. Mediastinal masses: MR imaging. *Radiology* 1986; **158**: 289–96.

69 Winkler M, Higgins CB. Suspected intracardiac masses: evaluation with MR imaging. *Radiology* 1987; **165**: 117–22.

70 Freedberg RS, Kronzon I, Rumancik WM, Liebeskind D. The contribution of magnetic resonance imaging to the evaluation of intracardiac tumours diagnosed by echocardiography. *Circulation* 1988; **77**: 96–103.

71 Barakos JA, Brown JJ, Higgins CB. MR imaging of secondary cardiac and paracardiac lesions. *Am J Roentgenol* 1989; **153**: 47–50.

72 Dooms GC, Higgins CB. MR imaging of cardiac thrombi. *J Comput Assist Tomogr* 1986; **10**: 415–20.

73 Dooms GC, Hricak H, Solitto R, Higgins CB. Lipomatous tumors and tumors with fatty component: MR imaging potential and comparison of MR and CT results. *Radiology* 1985; **157**: 479–83.

74 Sunderam M, McGuire MH, Schajowicz F. Soft-tissue masses: histologic basis for decreased signal (short T_2) on T_2-weighted MR images. *Am J Roentgenol* 1987; **148**: 1247–50.

75 Mogelvang J, Thomsen C, Mehlsen J, Brackle G, Stubgaard M, Henriksen O. Evaluation of left ventricular volumes measured by magnetic resonance imaging. *Eur Heart J* 1986; **7**: 1016–21.

76 Markiewicz W, Sechtem U, Kirby R, Derugin N, Caputo GC, Higgins CB. Measurement of ventricular volumes in the dog by nuclear magnetic resonance imaging. *J Am Coll Cardiol* 1987; **10**: 170–7.

77 Mogelvang J, Stubgaard M, Thomsen C, Henriksen O. Evaluation of right ventricular volumes measured by magnetic resonance imaging. *Eur Heart J* 1988; **9**: 529–33.

78 Van Rossum AC, Visser FC, Sprenger M, van Eenige MJ, Valk J, Roos JP. Evaluation of magnetic resonance imaging for determination of left ventricular ejection fraction and comparison with angiography. *Am J Cardiol* 1988; **62**: 628–33.

79 Longmore DB, Klipstein RH, Underwood SR, *et al*. Di-

mensional accuracy of magnetic resonance in studies of the heart. *Lancet* 1985; **i**: 1360–2.
80 Buckwalter KA, Aisen AM, Dilworth LR, Mancini GBJ, Buda AJ. Gated cardiac MRI: ejection fraction determination using the right anterior oblique view. *Am J Roentgenol* 1986; **147**: 33–7.
81 Osbakken M, Yuschok T. Evaluation of ventricular function with gated cardiac magnetic resonance imaging. *Cath Cardiovasc Diag* 1986; **12**: 156–60.
82 Statemeier EJ, Thompson R, Brady TJ, *et al*. Ejection fraction determination by MR imaging: Comparison with left ventricular angiography. *Radiology* 1986; **158**: 775–7.
83 Just H, Holubarsch C, Friedburg H. Estimation of left ventricular volume and mass by magnetic resonance imaging: comparison with quantitative biplane angiography. *Cardiovasc Intervent Radiol* 1987; **10**: 1–4.
84 Van Rossum AC, Visser FC, van Eenige MJ, Valk J, Roos JP. Magnetic resonance imaging of the heart for determination of ejection fraction. *Int J Cardiol* 1988; **18**: 53–63.
85 Underwood SR, Gill CRW, Firmin DN, *et al*. Left ventricular volume measured rapidly by oblique magnetic resonance imaging. *Br Heart J* 1988; **60**: 188–95.
86 Underwood SR, Klipstein RH, Firmin DN, *et al*. Magnetic resonance assessment of aortic and mitral regurgitation. *Br Heart J* 1986; **56**: 455–62.
87 Underwood SR, Klipstein RH, Firmin DN, *et al*. Magnetic resonance assessment of the accuracy of radionuclide methods for the quantification of valvular regurgitation and atrial shunting. In: Hoefer R, Bergman H (eds). *Radioactive Isotopes in Medicine and Research*. Vienna: Verlag H Egerman 1986; **17**: 299–305.
88 Byrd BF III, Schiller NB, Botvinick EH, Higgins CB. Normal cardiac dimensions by magnetic resonance imaging. *Am J Cardiol* 1985; **55**: 1440–2.
89 Fisher MR, von Schulthess GK, Higgins CB. Multiphasic cardiac magnetic resonance imaging: normal regional left ventricular wall thickening. *Am J Roentgenol* 1985; **145**: 27–30.
90 Kaul S, Wismer GL, Brady TJ, *et al*. Measurement of normal left heart dimensions using optimally oriented MR images. *Am J Roentgenol* 1986; **146**: 75–9.
91 Underwood SR, Rees RSO, Savage PE, *et al*. The assessment of regional left ventricular function by magnetic resonance. *Br Heart J* 1986; **56**: 334–40.
92 Akins EW, Hill JA, Sievers KW, Conti CR. Assessment of left ventricular wall thickness in healed myocardial infarction by magnetic resonance imaging. *Am J Cardiol* 1987; **59**: 24–8.
93 Sechtem U, Sommerhoff BA, Markiewicz W, White RD, Cheitlin MD, Higgins CB. Regional left ventricular wall thickening by magnetic resonance imaging: evaluation in normal persons and patients with global and regional dysfunction. *Am J Cardiol* 1987; **59**: 145–51.
94 White RD, Cassidy MM, Cheitlin MD, *et al*. Segmental evaluation of left ventricular wall motion after myocardial infarction: magnetic resonance imaging versus echocardiography. *Am Heart J* 1988; **115**: 166–75.
95 White RD, Holt WW, Cheitlin MD, *et al*. Estimation of the functional and anatomic extent of myocardial infarction using magnetic resonance imaging. *Am Heart J* 1988; **115**: 740–8.
96 Zerhouni E, Parish D, Rogers WJ, Yang A, Shapiro EP. Human heart: tagging with MR imaging—a method for noninvasive assessment of myocardial motion. *Radiology* 1988, **169**: 59–63.
97 Axel L, Dougherty L. Heart wall motion improved method of spatial modulation of magnetization for MR imaging. *Radiology* 1989, **172**, 349–50.
98 Florentine MS, Grosskreutz CL, Chang W, *et al*. Measurement of left ventricular mass in vivo using gated nuclear magnetic resonance imaging. *J Am Coll Cardiol* 1986; **8**: 107–12.
99 Keller AM, Peshock RM, Malloy CR, *et al*. In vivo measurement of myocardial mass using nuclear magnetic resonance imaging. *J Am Coll Cardiol* 1986; **8**: 113–7.
100 Caputo GR, Tscholakoff D, Sechtem U, Higgins CB. Measurement of canine left ventricular mass by using MR imaging. *Am J Roentgenol* 1987; **148**: 33–8.
101 Maddahi J, Crues J, Berman DS, *et al*. Noninvasive quantification of left ventricular myocardial mass by gated proton nuclear magnetic resonance imaging. *J Am Coll Cardiol* 1987; **10**: 682–92.
102 Katz J, Milliken MC, Stray-Gundersen J, *et al*. Estimation of human myocardial mass with MR imaging. *Radiology* 1988; **169**: 495–8.
103 Ostrzega E, Maddahi J, Honma H, *et al*. Quantification of left ventricular myocardial mass in humans by nuclear magnetic resonance imaging. *Am Heart J* 1989; **117**: 444–52.
104 Shapiro EP, Rogers WJ, Beyar R, *et al*. Determination of left ventricular mass by magnetic resonance imaging in hearts deformed by acute infarction. *Circulation* 1989; **79**: 706–11.
105 Milliken MC, Stray-Gundersen J, Peshock RM, Katz J, Mitchell JH. Left ventricular mass as determined by magnetic resonance imaging in male endurance athletes. *Am J Cardiol* 1988; **62**: 301–5.
106 Eichstädt HW, Felix R, Langer M, *et al*. Use of nuclear magnetic resonance imaging to show regression of hypertrophy with ramipril treatment. *Am J Cardiol* 1987; **59**: 98D–103D.
107 Fried R, Boxt LM, Miller RH, *et al*. Nuclear magnetic resonance spectroscopy of rat ventricles following supravalvar aortic banding. A model of left ventricular hypertrophy. *Invest Radiol* 1986; **21**: 622–5.
108 Berghöfer G, Köhler D, Schmutzler H, Schneider R, Felix R. Die magnetresonanztomographische Darstellung bei hypertropher Kardiomyopathie im Vergleich zur Echokardiographie. *Herz/Kreisl* 1987; **19**: 135–9.
109 Suzuki J-I, Sakamoto T, Takenaka K, *et al*. Assessment of the thickness of the right ventricular free wall by magnetic resonance imaging in patients with hypertrophic cardiomyopathy. *Br Heart J* 1988; **60**: 440–5.
110 Casolo GC, Trotta F, Rostagno C, *et al*. Detection of apical hypertrophic cardiomyography by magnetic resonance imaging. *Am Heart J* 1989; **117**: 468–72.

111 Fleming HA. Sarcoid heart disease. *Br Heart J* 1974; **36**: 54–68.
112 Underwood SR, Prigent F, Mohiaddin RH, Rees RSO, Longmore DB. Magnetic resonance imaging of cardiac sarcoidosis. *Br Heart J* 1989; **61**: 103–4 (Abstract).
113 Riedy K, Fisher MR, Belic N, Koenigsberg DI. MR imaging of myocardial sarcoidosis. *Am J Roentgenol* 1988; **151**: 915–6.
114 Buran-Kilian B, Hombach V, Arnold G, *et al*. Correlation of NMR imaging and histomorphological findings in patients with inflammatory heart disease and with cardiomyopathy. *Eur Heart J* 1987; **8**: 125–8.
115 Been M, Smith MA, Ridgway JP, *et al*. Myocardial involvement in systemic lupus erythematosus detected by magnetic resonance imaging. *Eur Heart J* 1988; **9**: 1250–6.
116 Sechtem U, Higgins CB, Sommerhoff BA, Lipton MJ, Huycke EC. Magnetic resonance imaging of restrictive cardiomyopathy. *Am J Cardiol* 1987; **59**: 480–2.
117 Boxer RA, Fishman M, LaCorte MA, Singh S, Cooper RS. Cardiac MR imaging in Pompe disease. *J Comput Assist Tomogr* 1986; **10**: 857–9.
118 Matsui S, Murakami E, Takekoshi N, Nakatou H, Enyama H, Takeda F. Myocardial tissue characterization by magnetic resonance imaging in Fabry's disease. *Am Heart J* 1989; **117**: 472–4.
119 Underwood SR, Burman ED, Rowlands E, Mohiaddin RH, Rees RSO, Longmore DB. Global and regional right ventricular function in arrhythmogenic right ventricular dysplasia studied by magnetic resonance imaging. *Magn Reson Imag* 1990; **8**: 72 (Abstract).
120 Soulen R, Higgins CB, Budinger TF. Magnetic resonance imaging of prosthetic heart valves. *Radiology* 1985; **154**: 705–7.
121 Randall PA, Kohman LJ, Scalzetti EM, Szeverenyi NM, Panicek DM. Magnetic resonance imaging of prosthetic cardiac valves in vitro and in vivo. *Am J Cardiol* 1988; **62**: 973–6.
122 Shellock FG. MR imaging of metallic implants and materials: a compilation of the literature. *Am J Roentgenol* 1988; **151**: 811–4.
123 Shellock FG, Crues JV. High-field-strength MR imaging and metallic biomedical implants: an ex vivo evaluation of deflection forces. *Am J Roentgenol* 1988; **151**: 389–92.
124 Winkler M, Higgins CB. MRI of perivalvular infectious pseudoaneurysms. *Am J Roentgenol* 1986; **147**: 253–6.
125 Stark DD, Higgins CB, Lanzer P, *et al*. Magnetic resonance imaging of the pericardium: normal and pathologic findings. *Radiology* 1984; **150**: 469–74.
126 Sechtem U, Tscholakoff D, Higgins CB. MRI of the normal pericardium. *Am J Roentgenol* 1986; **147**: 239–44.
127 McMurdo KK, Webb WR, von Schultess GK, Gamsu G. Magnetic resonance imaging of the superior pericardial recesses. *Am J Roentgenol* 1985; **145**: 985–8.
128 Soulen RL, Stark DD, Higgins CB. Magnetic resonance imaging of constrictive pericardial disease. *Am J Cardiol* 1985; **55**: 480–4.
129 Sechtem U, Tscholakoff D, Higgins CB. MRI of the abnormal pericardium. *Am J Roentgenol* 1986; **147**: 245–52.
130 Paulin S, von Schulthess GK, Fossel E, Krayenbuehl HP. MR imaging of the aortic root and proximal coronary arteries. *Am J Radiol* 1987; **148**: 665–70.
131 Bisset GS, Strife JL, McCloskey J. Case report. MR imaging of coronary artery aneurysms in a child with Kawasaki disease. *Am J Roentgenol* 1989; **152**: 805–7.
132 Sherry CS, Harms SE. MR imaging of pseudoaneurysms in aortocoronary bypass graft. *J Comput Assist Tomogr* 1989; **13**: 426–9.
133 Alfidi RJ, Haacke EM, Lenz GW, *et al*. MR angiography of peripheral, carotid, and coronary arteries. *Am J Roentgenol* 1987; **149**: 1097–109.
134 Stehling M, Chapman B, Glover P, *et al*. Real-time NMR imaging of coronary vessels. *Lancet* 1987; **ii**: 964–5.
135 Gomes AS, Lois JF, Drinkwater DC Jr, Corday SR. Coronary artery bypass grafts: visualization with MR imaging. *Radiology* 1987; **162**: 175–9.
136 Rubinstein RI, Askenase AD, Thickman D, Feldman MS, Agarwal JB, Helfant RH. Magnetic resonance imaging to evaluate patency of aortocoronary bypass grafts. *Circulation* 1987; **76**: 786–91.
137 White RD, Caputo GR, Mark AS, Modin GW, Higgins CB. Coronary artery bypass graft patency: noninvasive evaluation with MR imaging. *Radiology* 1987; **164**: 681–6.
138 Jenkins JPR, Love HG, Foster CJ, Isherwood I, Rowlands DJ. Detection of coronary artery bypass graft patency as assessed by magnetic resonance imaging. *Br J Radiol* 1988; **61**: 2–4.
139 Underwood SR, Firmin DN, Klipstein RH, Rees RSO, Longmore DB. Towards magnetic resonance flow measurements in the coronary arteries and coronary artery bypass grafts. *Radiology* 1986; **161(P)**: 224 (Abstract).
140 Shellock FG. MR imaging of metallic implants and materials: a compilation of the literature. *Am J Roentgenol* 1988; **151**: 811–4.
141 Underwood SR, Firmin DN, Klipstein RH, Rees RSO, Longmore DB. The assessment of coronary artery bypass grafts using magnetic resonance imaging with velocity mapping. *Br Heart J* 1987; **57**: 93 (Abstract).

Chapter 6
Imaging of Congenital Heart Disease

SIMON REES

Gated spin echo imaging is particularly suitable for the display of anatomy in congenital heart disease.[1-3] Venous, atrial, ventricular, outlet and arterial anatomy and connections can all be shown with the acquisition of multiple 10 mm slices in the three orthogonal as well as oblique planes. These can be supplemented with a second acquisition offset by 5 mm if required. The images have a striking clarity which is superior to cross sectional echocardiography and less dependent on operator skill and experience. However in practical terms, the examinations are complementary and magnetic resonance should not be regarded as a potential replacement for echocardiography but as a method of completing the anatomical assessment and rendering catheterisation and angiography unnecessary. Image acquisition is still relatively slow and it is essential to have a cooperative patient who will lie still for the 3–4 minutes that it takes to acquire each set of data. Imaging of the small heart in an infant requires the acquisition of multiple thin slices preferably no more than 3 mm thick to display the anatomy properly. At low field strength of 0.5 T, the signal to noise ratio in slices less than 5 mm is inadequate to produce images of acceptable quality. However excellent results have been obtained at field strengths of 1.5 T (figure 6.1)[4].

Cine imaging (see chapter 7) using gradient echo sequences can give important functional information.[5-8] Sequences with longer echo times can detect areas of turbulence which can be exploited for the identification of abnormal valve function, abnormalities of the vascular lumen, which may only be minor, and abnormal flow created by shunts.[9-11] Sequences with shorter echo times are less sensitive to turbulence and have been used successfully to measure flow velocities by phase mapping (see chapter 10). This has been applied to quantify absolute flow in the aorta, pulmonary trunk and other vessels,[12] and to measure peak velocities above 1 m/s in and distal to a stenosis, enabling a prediction of pressure gradients to be made by principles similar to those applied to Doppler echocardiography.[13,14]

6.1 Septal defects

The atrial septum is a thin structure and much of it lies oblique to conventional planes so that it is common on spin echo images to have signal drop out mimicking a defect.[15,16] Echocardiography is usually more reliable,[17] but others claim higher sensitivity and specificity for magnetic resonance imaging.[18] In cases of doubt, cine velocity mapping will show flow through the defect (figure 6.2). Ventricular septal defects are easier to see on spin echo images,[19] and excellent results have been reported in infants using a high field strength.[20] Cine imaging to display turbulent jets is also of value should there be doubt (figure 6.3). Ostium primum defects, atrioventricular canal defects and left ventricular to right atrial shunts are easy to recognise on spin echo images, including the common area of attachment of the mitral and tricuspid valves to the septum (figure 6.4),[21] and in the case of complex shunting cine imaging is of great value in identifying the origin and destination of each jet (figure 6.5).

The volume of atrial shunts is reflected in the ventricular stroke volume difference which can be measured by the transverse multislice method.[22] Alternatively, flow can be measured directly in the aorta and pulmonary trunk by velocity mapping, and this also can be applied to ventricular shunts (figure 6.6).[12] It is also possible in some cases to measure flow directly within a defect (figure 6.7). Prediction of the pulmonary artery pressure is also possible from cine velocity mapping in the pulmonary trunk using principles which have been applied in Doppler echocardiography.[13]

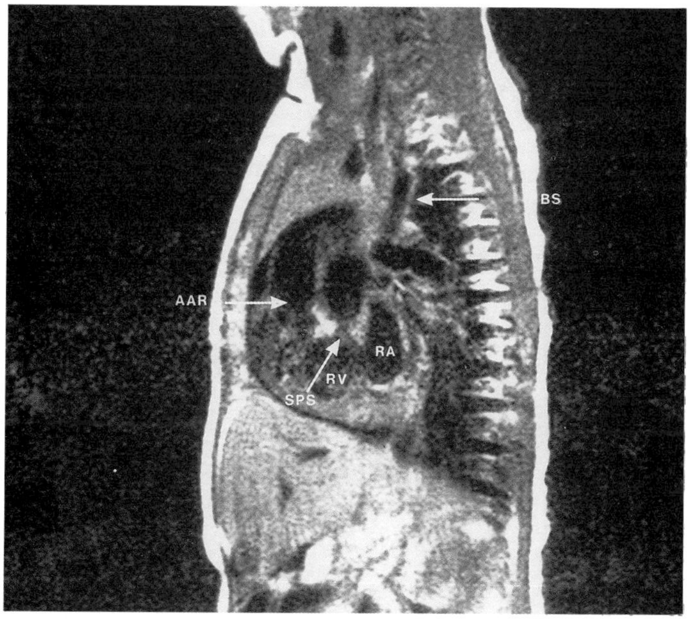

(a)

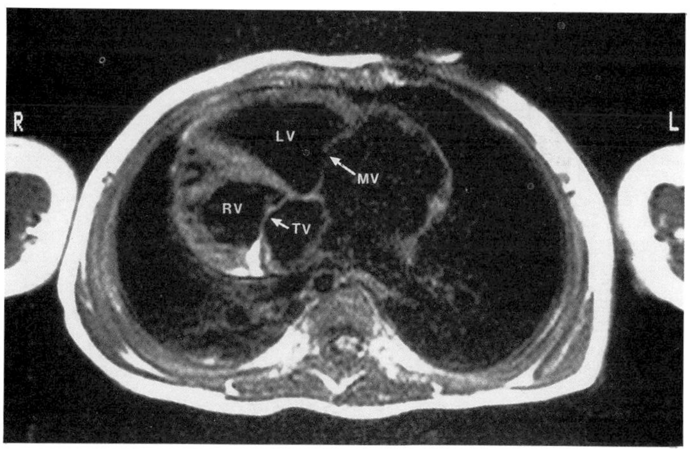

(b)

Figure 6.1. (a) Sagittal image 5 mm thick in a 3-month old infant with double outlet of the right ventricle. It shows the two great arteries arising anteriorly from the right ventricle (RV). The ascending aorta (AAR) is anterior and there is subpulmonary stenosis (SPS). The image also shows the right atrium (RA) and a modified Blalock shunt (BS) anatomosed to the left pulmonary artery. (b) A transverse image, 5 mm thick, from a 7-month old infant with atrioventricular discordance. The apex of the heart is directed to the right. The anterior ventricle is morphologically left sided (LV) with a mitral valve (MV) connected to the right atrium. The atrial septum is not well seen because it is oblique to the plane and the left atrium is divided by a membrane behind the tricuspid valve (TV). The pulmonary veins drain to the left atrium. The posterior ventricle has the trabecular pattern of a right ventricle (RV) and is connected to the left atrium by the tricuspid valve. (Courtesy of Dr E Baker, Guy's Hospital, London)

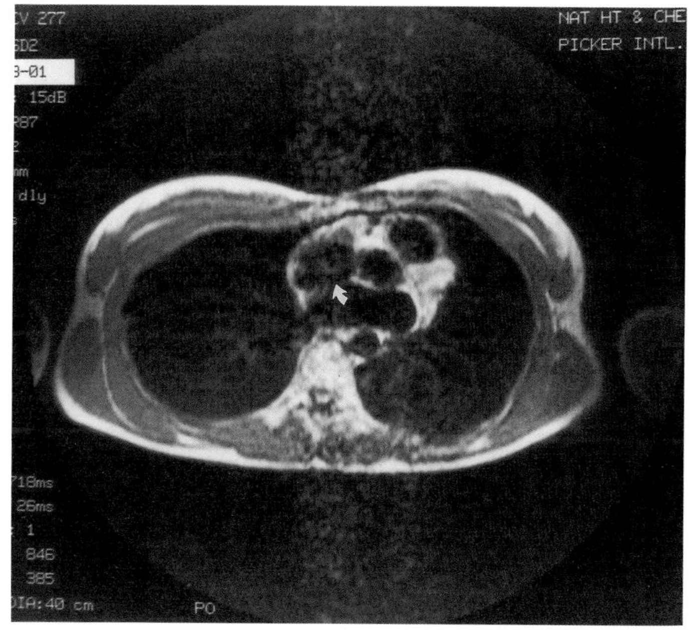

(a)

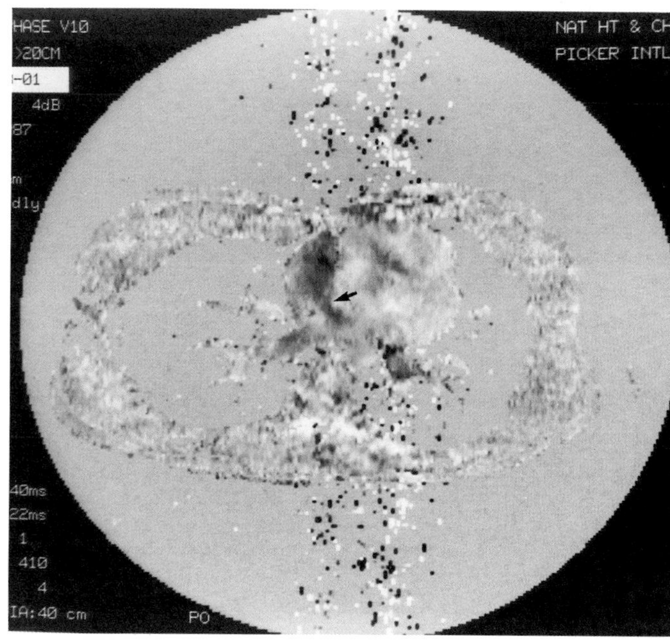

(b)

Figure 6.2. (a) Transverse spin echo image through the atrial septum showing a secundum defect (arrow). To ensure that this was not signal drop-out, cine velocity mapping was performed (b). A diastolic frame encoded from bottom to top of the image shows flow through the defect (arrow).

6.2 Other shunts

Similar principles apply to the demonstration and functional assessment of other lesions resulting in

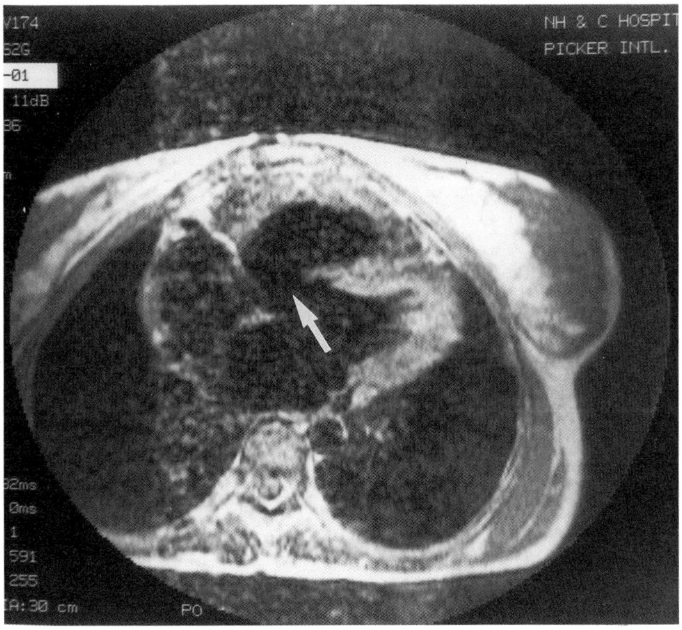

(a)

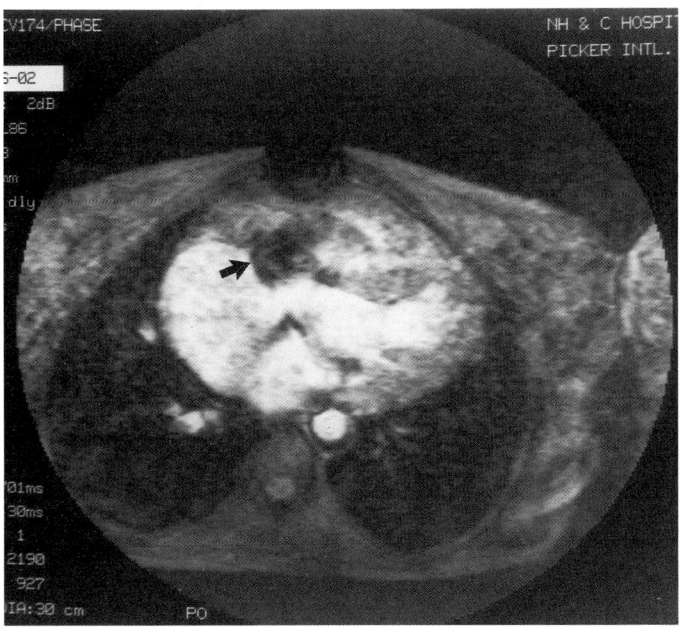

(b)

Figure 6.3. Transverse spin echo image showing a ventricular septal defect (arrow). (b) Systolic gradient echo image in the same, showing single loss caused by turbulence on the right side of the defect (arrow).

shunts. Not only can the anatomy be displayed, but the flow can be measured using velocity mapping to build up a complete picture of the functional con-

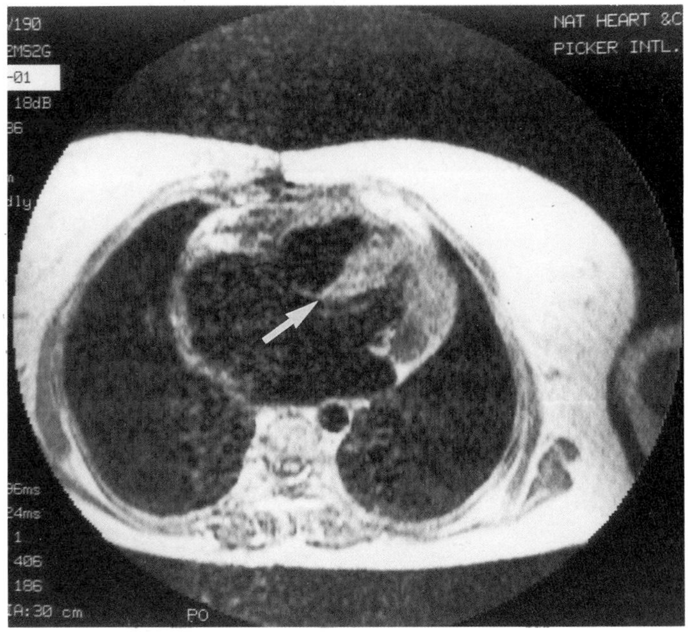

Figure 6.4. Transverse spin echo image in atrioventricular canal. The anterior mitral valve cusp and the septal tricuspid cusp are attached to the same point on the free edge of the ventricular septum (arrow).

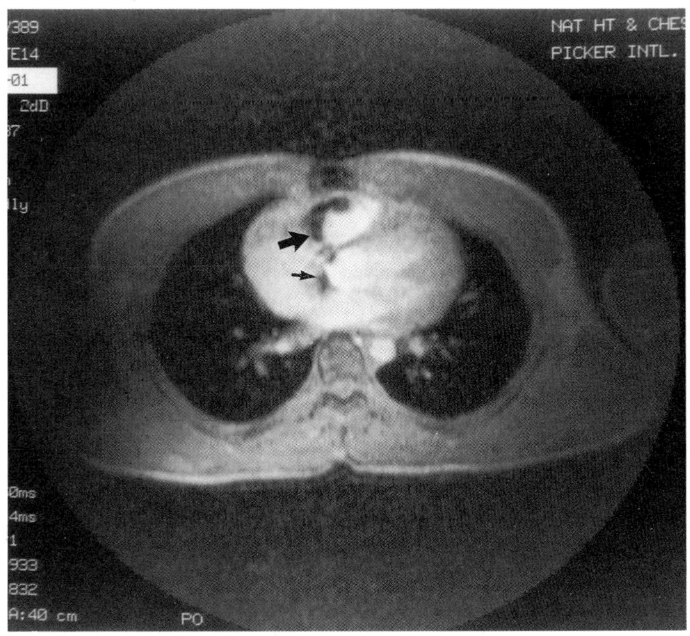

Figure 6.5. Transverse gradient echo image from a 16 frame cine sequence in a patient 20 years after repair of a left ventricular to right atrial shunt. A persistent shunt was suspected. The image is early systole, 111 ms after the R wave. It shows two areas of signal loss caused by turbulence arising from the proximal ventricular septum. One (larger arrow, top) indicates residual shunt into the right ventricle and the other (smaller arrow) a shunt into the right atrium. These findings were confirmed at subsequent surgery.

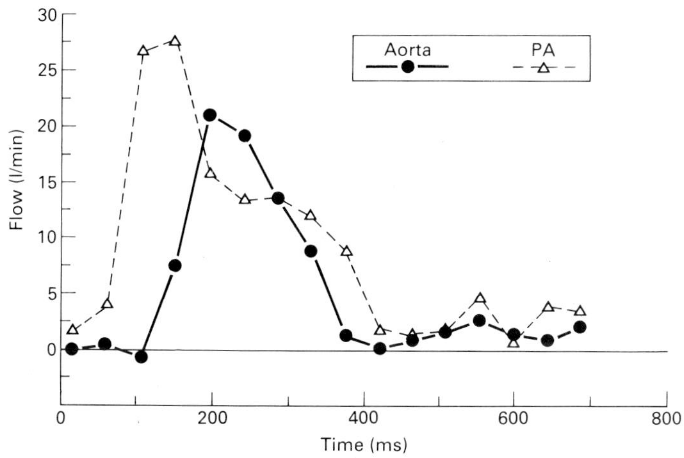

Figure 6.6. The measurement of shunting across a ventricular septal defect. Cine velocity mapping provides a plot of flow in the aorta and pulmonary artery. Pulmonary flow was 6.9 l/min and aortic flow 4.0 l/min, giving a Qp/Qs of 1.7.

sequences of the abnormal morphology. Examples are illustrated of a ductus with pulmonary hypertension (figure 6.8) and a coronary artery fistula (figure 6.9).

6.3 Valve disease

Congenital bicuspid aortic valve and aortic valve stenosis have been identified on spin echo images in some instances, but cross sectional echocardiography gives more reliable information about the anatomy. Early studies with long echo time gradient echo sequences showed that turbulence was generated distal to a bicuspid valve in the absence of a gradient and diastolic signal loss proximal to the valve indicated regurgitation. However it is now possible to measure the peak systolic velocity with a short echo time sequence and the results are showing good correlation with Doppler predictions and catheter gradients (see chapter 10).

6.4 Coarctation of the aorta

Spin echo images are ideal for showing the anatomy of coarctation.[23] A set of transverse images 10 mm thick with an interleaved set offset by 5 mm is ideal, but they can be supplemented by oblique slices acquired by the three point method, using points defined in the arch and the ascending and descending aorta (figure 6.10). Cine imaging using an echo time of 14 ms in an oblique slice displaying the whole of the aorta shows that signal loss is commonly generated at the aortic valve, confirming the high incidence of bicuspid or other abnormality of the aortic valve which is usually of trivial haemodynamic significance.[24] Cine imaging has also been used to assess the severity of the obstruction, relying on the maximum area of the signal loss in the descending aorta to predict the gradient.[25] However short echo time cine sequences now allow accurate peak velocity measurements to be obtained directly and pressure gradients can be computed from these (figure 6.11). Magnetic resonance imaging is also ideal for displaying the anatomy of other congenital lesions of the aorta, such as aortic arch anomalies.

6.5 Cyanotic heart disease

Multislice spin echo imaging in the three orthogonal planes can display the anatomy of any lesion, however complex, and this can be supplemented by cine imaging and velocity mapping as appropriate. Most patients will have had cross sectional echocardiography, but there are some areas where echocardiographic methods are unsatisfactory. For example, patients with pulmonary atresia depend upon branches of the systemic circulation to provide a pulmonary blood supply. Development of pulmonary arteries centrally and segmentally is variable, as is the size and number of the systemic collateral arteries, and there tends to be an inverse relationship between the two.[26] Successful palliative or radical reparative surgery depends on complete demonstration of both, and currently this information cannot be obtained non-invasively, but requires angiography with multiple contrast injections and selective catheterisation of individual collateral arteries.[27–29] Transverse spin echo slices show hypoplastic arteries particularly well and agree with surgical and angiographic data.[29] The origin and proximal course of large collaterals can also be identified (figure 6.12)[30] although their distal connections cannot be established and if such information is required, angiography will still be needed. Other complex lesions are readily studied and again data complementary to echocardiography is provided (figure 6.13).

6.6 Postoperative studies

Magnetic resonance imaging has proved to be of great value as a method of assessing the progress of patients following surgery and interventional procedures. For

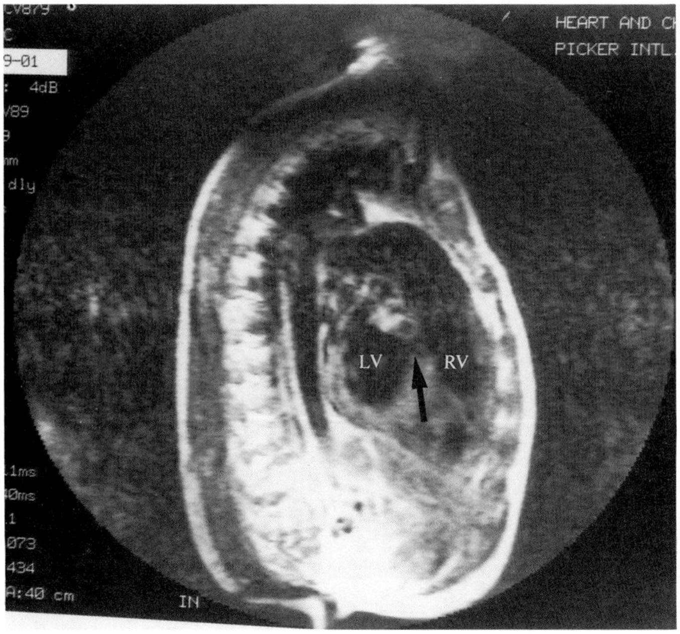

(a)

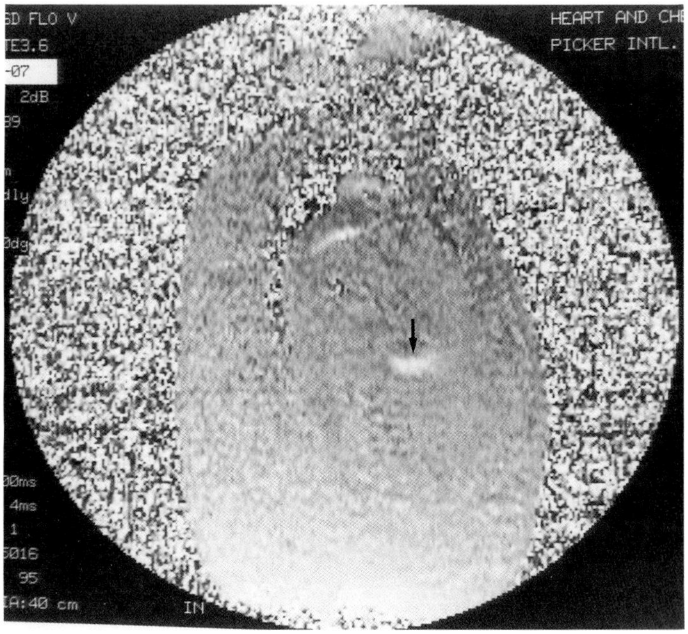

(b)

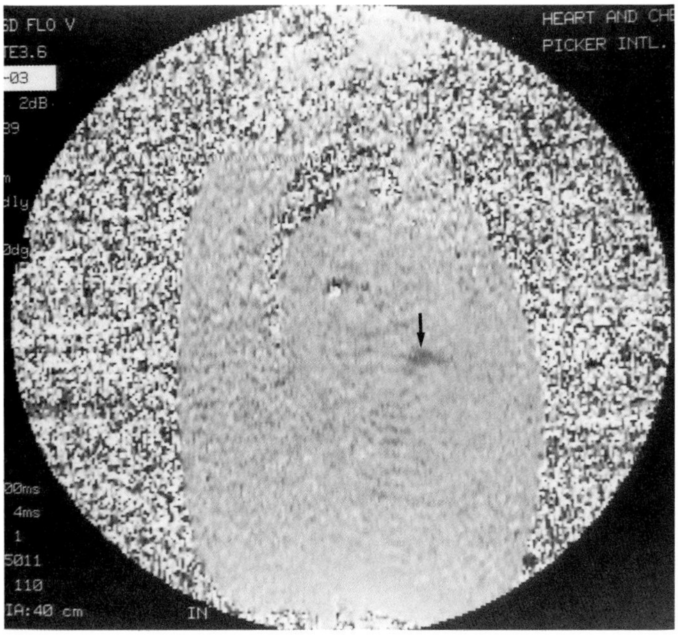

(c)

Figure 6.7. Flow across an Eisenmenger ventricular septal defect. (a) Oblique spin echo image showing the defect (arrow) left ventricle (LV), right ventricle (RV). (b) Cine velocity mapping in the same plane encoded from right to left of the image shows flow from left ventricle to right ventricle in early systole, and (c) flow reversal in late systole.

example, after resection of coarctation[31] and aortoplasty,[32] the isthmus can be studied non-invasively on spin echo images and diameters can be measured. It has been shown that if the minimal diameter is less than 50% of the mean diameter of the mid ascending and descending aorta, a pressure gradient may be expected.[24] The introduction of short echo time cine sequences now enables peak velocity to be measured

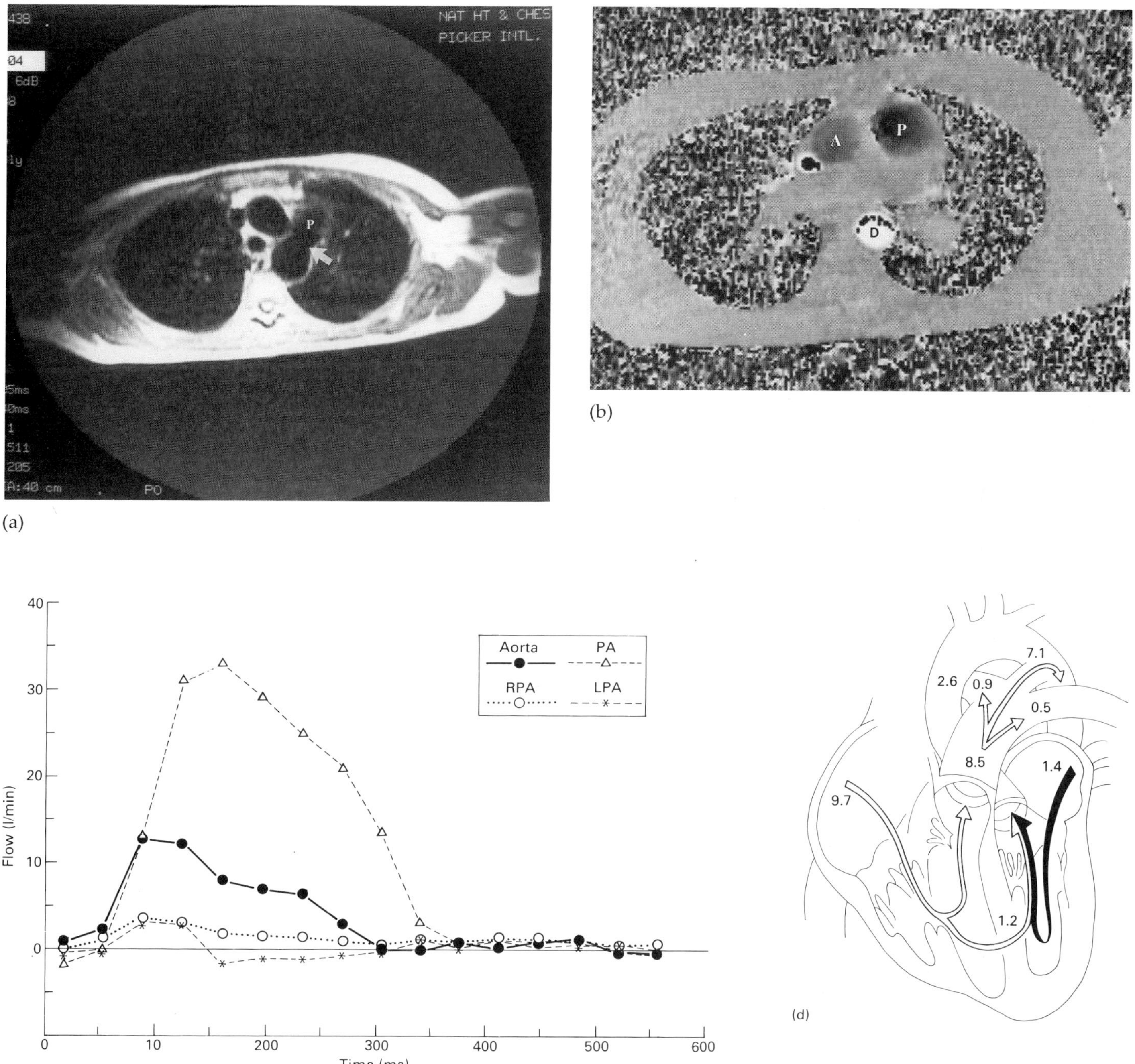

Figure 6.8. Shunt direction and volume measurement in a patient with an Eisenmenger patent ductus arteriosus and a small ventricular septal defect. (a) Transverse spin echo image through the aortic arch showing the ductus (arrow) connecting to the roof of the pulmonary trunk (P).
(b) Systolic velocity map in transverse slice showing cranial flow in the ascending aorta (A), pulmonary trunk (P) and caudal flow in the descending aorta (D). There is some aliasing in the descending aorta and superior caval vein because the velocity window has been optimised for cranial flow. (c) From similar velocity maps, flow in the major vessels was measured pulmonary trunk (PA), left pulmonary artery (LPA), right pulmonary artery (RPA). (d) Diagram showing flow in litres per minute extrapolated to the rest of the circulation showing a net right to left shunt of 7.1 l/min through the duct and 1.2 l/min through the VSD. Systemic venous return was 9.7 l/min compared with pulmonary venous return of 1.4 litres per minute.

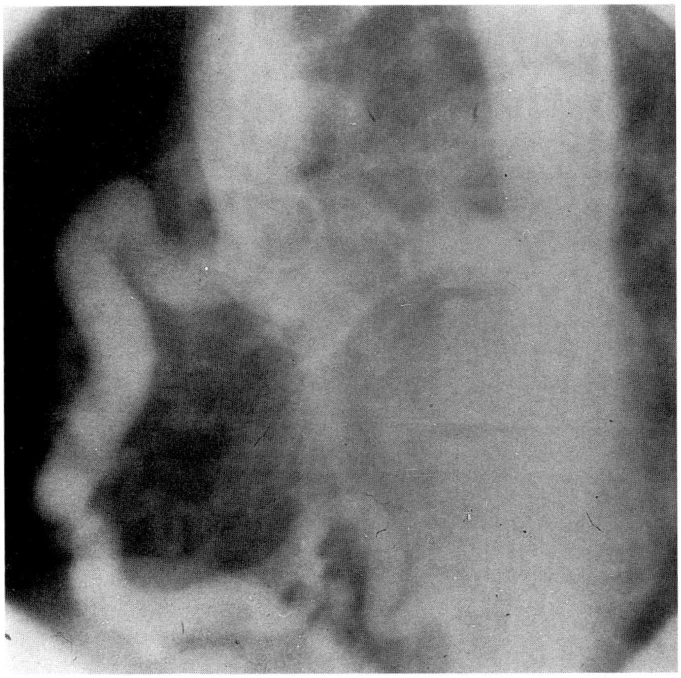

(a)

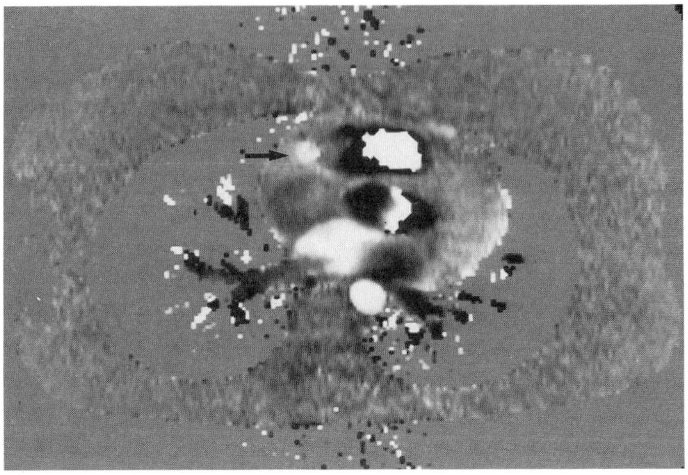

(b)

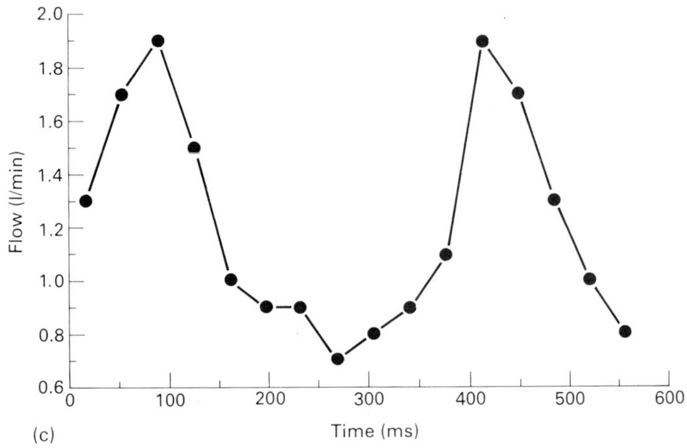

(c)

Figure 6.9. Flow in a patient with an anomalous left main coronary artery from the pulmonary trunk. (a) Right coronary arteriogram showing the dilated artery which was shunting around the apex into the low pressure left coronary artery system. (b) Systolic velocity map in a transverse slice through the mid right atrioventricular groove showing caudal flow in the dilated right coronary artery (arrow). There is aliasing in the aorta and pulmonary artery because a narrow velocity window has been used. (c) Flow throughout the cycle showed a normal diastolic peak corresponding to myocardial flow, but an abnormal systolic peak corresponding to the shunt.

giving a more precise method of predicting restenosis, which correlates well with Doppler measurements. Aneurysm formation may complicate Dacron patch angioplasty,[33] and be difficult to predict from the chest radiograph, but is readily visible on spin echo images (figure 6.14). It has also been observed that aortic compliance measured from systolic and diastolic spin echo images[34] is abnormally low following resection of coarctation. The mechanism of systolic hypertension after successful coarctation repair is uncertain, but does not appear to be related to abnormalities in the sympathetic nervous system or the angiotensin-aldosterone axis and is more likely to be due to primary baroreceptor alterations or structural changes in the arterial wall.[35,36] This finding of abnormal compliance suggests a possible mechanism for persistent systolic hypertension which is so commonly found in these patients, despite an apparently satisfactory repair.[24]

Patients who have had surgical procedures to alleviate complex lesions require continual clinical

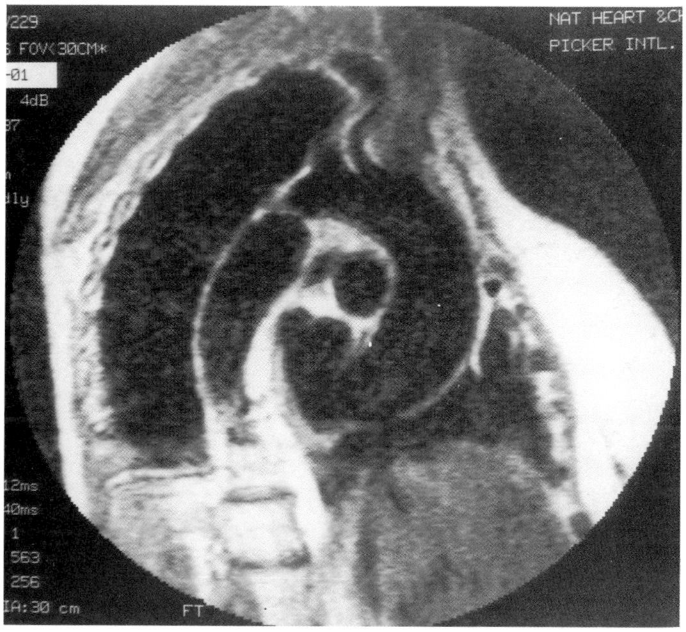

Figure 6.10. An oblique spin echo image through the thoracic aorta showing coarctation at the isthmus.

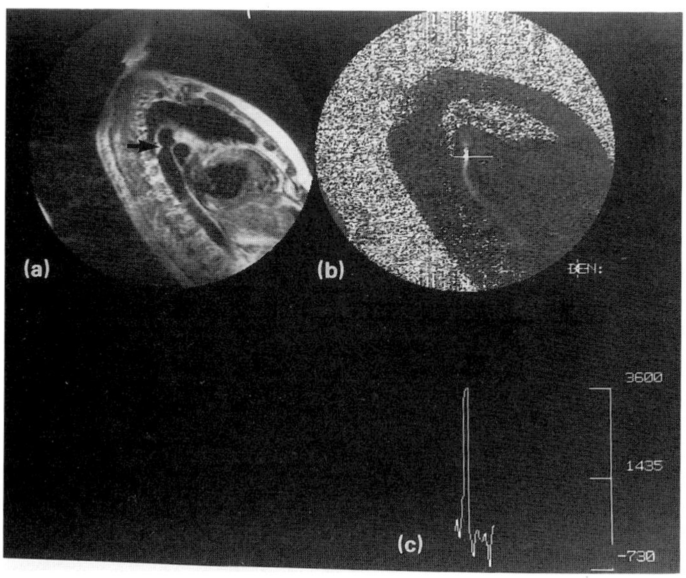

Figure 6.11. Peak velocity measurement through a coarctation. (a) Oblique spin echo image showing the coarctation (arrow). (b) Systolic velocity map showing a high velocity jet distal to the coarctation. (c) Velocity profile through the jet in (b) showing a peak velocity of 3.6 m/s. Using the modified Bernoulli equation, this corresponds to a pressure gradient of 50 mm of mercury.

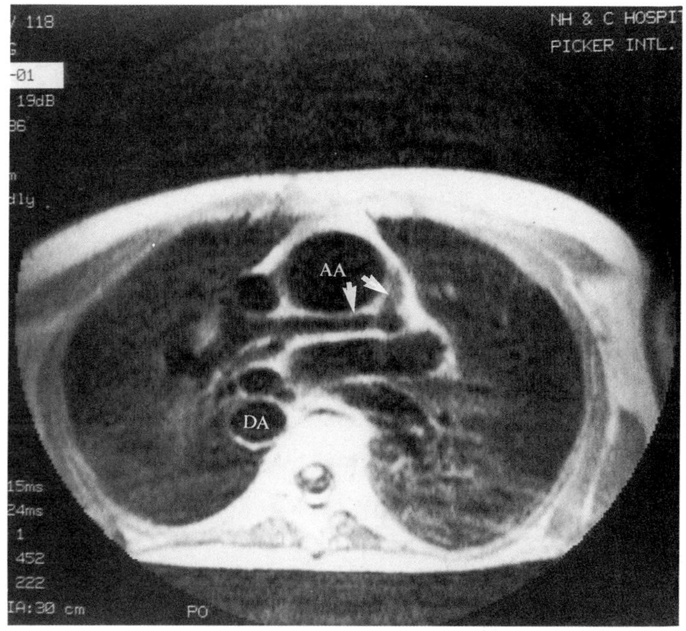

(a)

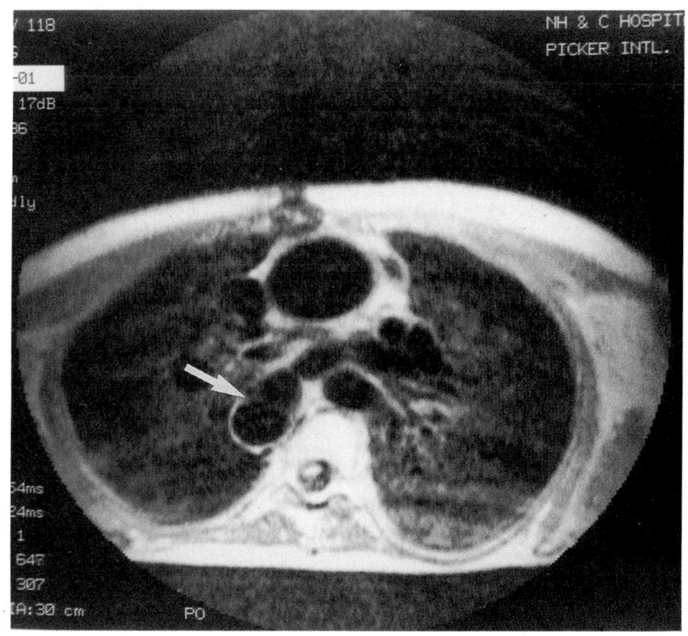

(b)

Figure 6.12. Anatomy of the pulmonary blood supply in pulmonary atresia. (a) Transverse image showing hypoplastic pulmonary arteries (arrow). Ascending aorta (AA), descending aorta on right (DA). (b) Transverse slice at a different level in the same patient showing the origin of a large collateral vessel from the descending aorta (arrow).

follow-up and assessment for which non-invasive imaging methods are indispensable. Cross sectional and Doppler echocardiography provide important data but there are many areas in which magnetic resonance can give complementary information, and some in which it is the only method short of catheterisation.

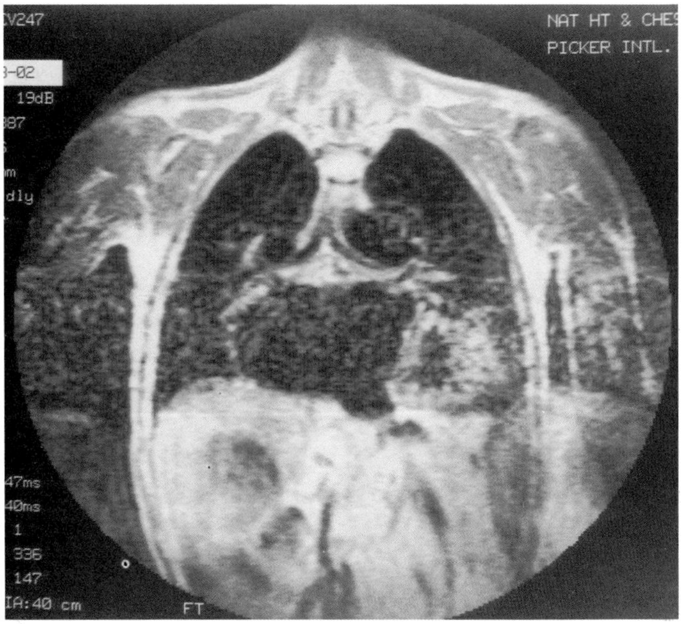

(a)

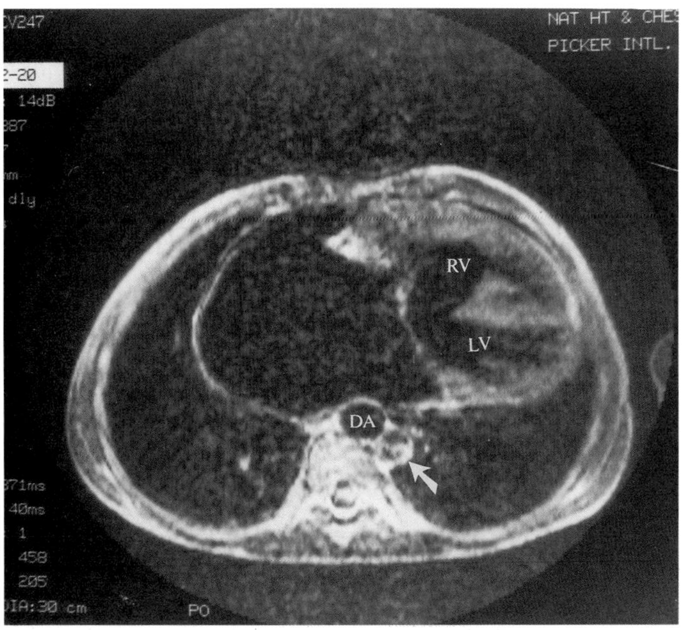

(b)

Figure 6.13. Isomerism with complex congenital heart disease. (a) Coronal spin echo image through the carina in a patient with left isomerism. The bronchi branch symmetrically within the hila which are both morphologically left with the hilar artery above the bronchus. Below is a single large atrial cavity. (b) Transverse spin echo image through the atrioventricular valve showing a common atrioventricular canal and a single atrium. Posteriorly, the azygos continuation of the inferior vena cava (arrow) lies behind and to the left of the descending aorta. Descending aorta (DA), left ventricle (LV), right ventricle (RV).

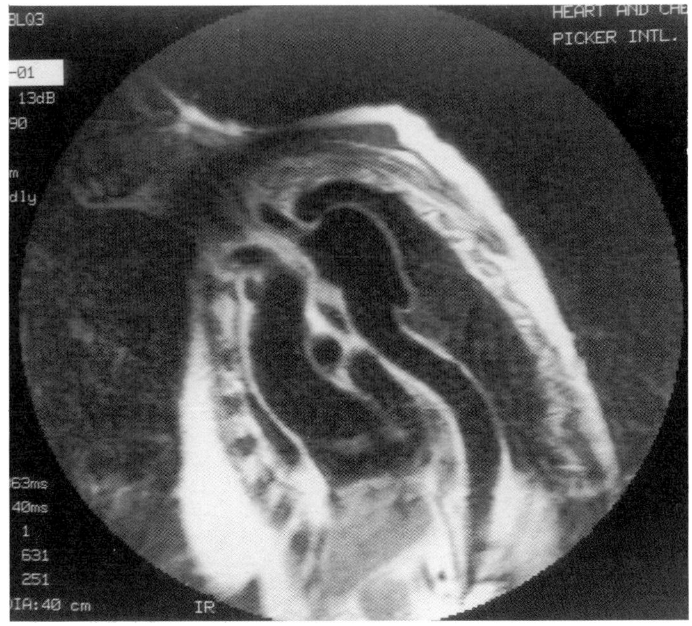

Figure 6.14. Oblique spin echo image showing a posterior aneurysm at the site of a Dacron patch repair of aortic coarctation.

For example, accurate measurement of ventricular function is needed. This is not the place to discuss the relative accuracy of the various imaging modalities, but for volume measurements of both right and left ventricles, magnetic resonance is almost certainly the most accurate.[22] Valve regurgitation can be assessed by Doppler echocardiography, but this can be supplemented by cine magnetic resonance in which turbulence upstream gives qualitative data and the stroke volume difference adds quantitative information. For example in patients after Mustard's procedure for atrial correction of the circulation in transposition, the right ventricle supports the systemic circulation and repeated accurate assessment of right ventricular function is essential to monitor progress. Dilatation may lead to tricuspid regurgitation and vice versa so that vigorous therapy needs to be instituted at the earliest sign of deterioration.[37]

Another area where magnetic resonance has proved to be useful is in assessing atriopulmonary and ventriculopulmonary connections, usually with valved conduits. These include operations for Fallot's tetralogy, pulmonary atresia, tricuspid atresia, single ventricle, complete transposition with VSD, corrected transposition with pulmonary stenosis, double outlet ventricle and truncus arteriosus. Conduits may be fashioned

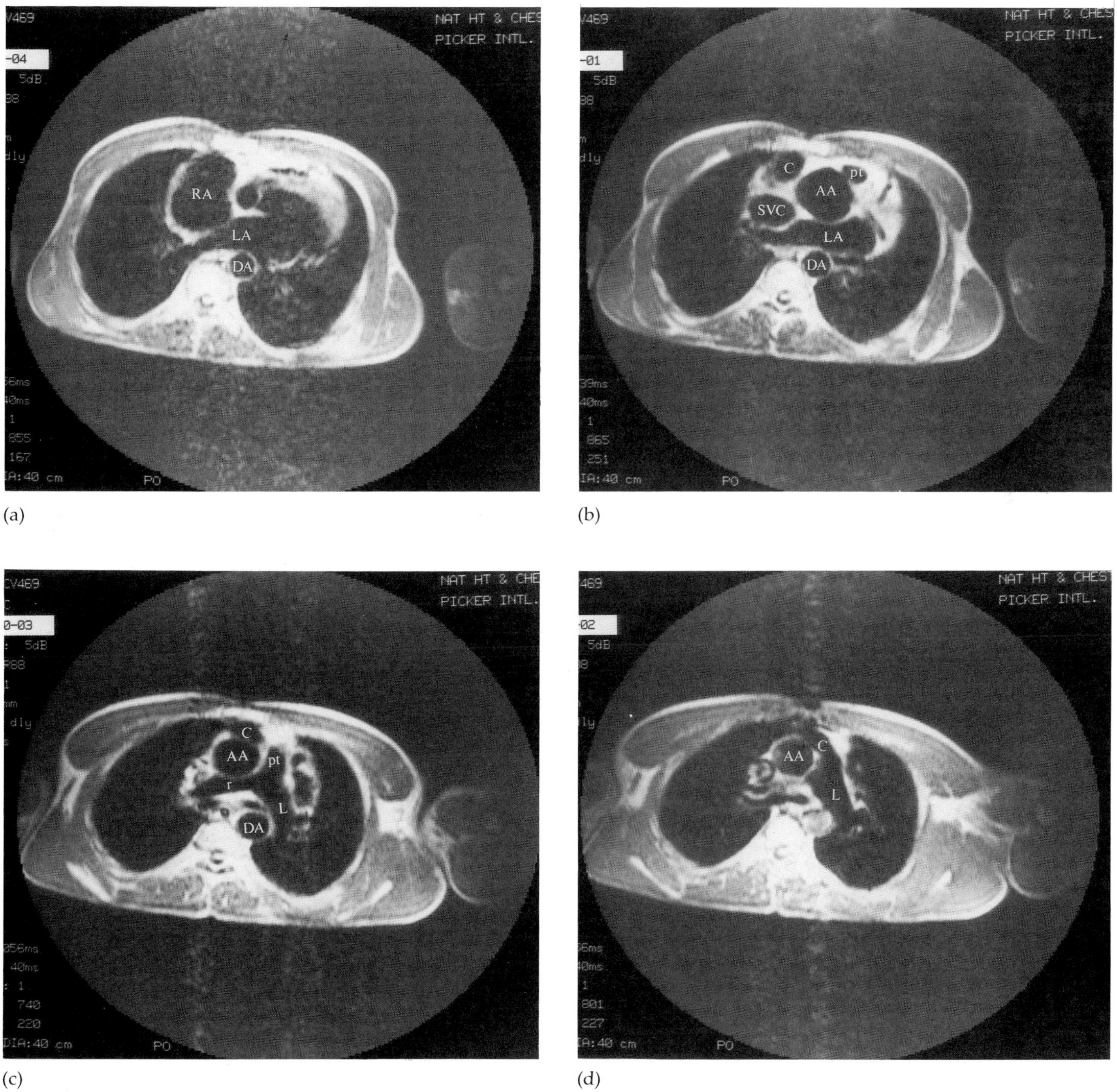

Figure 6.15. Assessment of a Fontan conduit. The conduit (C) connects the right atrial appendix to the pulmonary trunk. The diameter can be measured in successive transverse slices (a to d). Ascending aorta (AA), descending aorta (DA), left pulmonary artery (L), left atrium (LA), pulmonary trunk (PT), right pulmonary artery (R), right atrium (RA), superior vena cava (SVC).

from various materials including Dacron, fascia lata and pericardium, and the valves are mainly homografts but occasionally autografts or heterografts. They commonly calcify, although the deposits are usually confined to the wall and rarely encroach on the lumen. Stenosis is common and may occur by contraction of either suture line or in the valve itself due to cusp thickening and fusion or shrinkage of the valve ring or

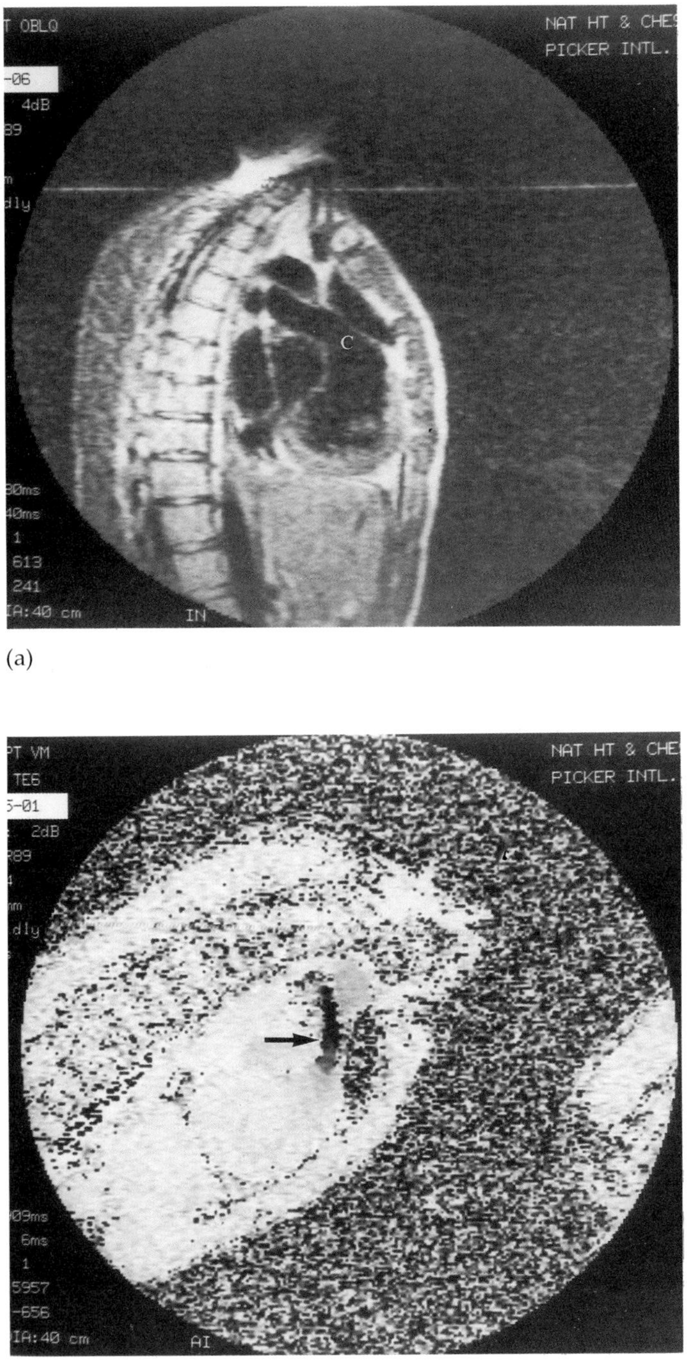

(a)

(b)

Figure 6.16. Measurement of peak velocity distal to a calcified and stenosed homograft valve in the right ventricular outflow tract. (a) An oblique spin echo image through the homograft conduit (C) shows a wide lumen containing no signal and suggesting the absence of obstruction. (b) Systolic velocity map showing a peak velocity of over 4 m/s corresponding to a predicted pressure gradient 60 mm of mercury (arrow). The spin echo image was misleading as the obstructing calcific material gave no signal.

both. The valve may also become regurgitant and there are often stenoses in the right or left pulmonary arteries related to a previous systemic to pulmonary shunt which has been closed. Tomographic spin echo images can display these conduits with great accuracy and allow diameter measurements to be made (figure 6.15).[38] At suspected areas of narrowing, velocity maps can be obtained and the peak velocity measured to assess severity (figure 6.16). Such data can sometimes be obtained by echocardiography, but the combination of a previous sternotomy and the frequent incidence of chest deformities make finding a window difficult in most patients and this is compounded by the position of the conduit which is often mainly retrosternal and hidden from the probe. The availability of magnetic resonance imaging for these patients has greatly reduced the need for catheterisation and angiography.

References

1 Fletcher BD, Jacobstein MD, Nelson AD, Riemenschneider TA, Alfidi RJ. Gated magnetic resonance imaging of congenital cardiac malformations. *Radiology* 1984; **150**: 137–40.
2 Boxer RA, Singh S, LaCorte MA, Goldman *M*, Stein HL. Cardiac magnetic resonance imaging in children with congenital heart disease. *J Paediatr* 1986; **109**: 460–4.
3 Didier D, Higgins CB, Fisher MR, Osaki L, Silverman NH Cheitlin MD. Congenital heart disease: gated MR Imaging in 72 Patients. *Radiology* 1986; **158**: 227–35.
4 Smith MA, Baker EJ, Ayton VT, Parsons JM, Ladusans EJ, Maisey MN. Magnetic resonance imaging of the infant heart at 1.5 T. *Br J Radiol* 1989; **62**: 367–70.
5 Underwood SR, Klipstein RH, Firmin DN, *et al.* Magnetic resonance quantification of atrial shunting and valvular regurgitation. *Br Heart J* 1985; **54**: 61 (Abstract).
6 Waterton JC, Jenkins JPR, Zhu XP, Love HG, Isherwood I, Rowlands DJ. Magnetic resonance cine imaging of the human heart. *Br J Radiol* 1985; **58**: 711–6.
7 Underwood SR, Klipstein RH, Firmin DN, *et al.* Magnetic resonance assessment of aortic and mitral regurgitation. *Br Heart J* 1986; **56**: 455–62.
8 Underwood SR, Firmin DN, Klipstein RH, Rees RSO, Longmore DB. Magnetic resonance velocity mapping: clinical application of a new technique. *Br Heart J* 1987; **57**: 404–12.
9 Schiebler M, Axel L, Reichek N, *et al.* Correlation of cine MR imaging with two-dimensional pulsed Doppler echocardiography in valvular insufficiency. *J Comput Assist Tomogr* 1987; **11**: 627–32.
10 Sechtem U, Pflugfelder PW, Cassidy MM, *et al.* Mitral or aortic regurgitation: quantification of regurgitant volumes with cine MR imaging. *Radiology* 1988; **167**: 425–30.
11 Sechtem U, Pflugfelder PW, White RD, *et al.* Cine MR imaging: potential for the evaluation of cardiovascular function. *Am J Roentgenol* 1987; **148**: 239–46.

12 Rees S, Firmin DN, Mohiaddin R, Underwood SR, Longmore DB. Application of flow measurements by magnetic resonance to congenital heart disease. *Am J Cardiol* 1989; **64**: 953–6.

13 Kilner PJ, Firmin DN, Mohiaddin RH, Underwood SR, Rees RSO, Longmore DB. Magnetic resonance measurement of post stenotic jet velocities in vitro and in vivo. *Proceedings of the Eighth Annual Meeting of the Society of Magnetic Resonance in Medicine*, 1989; 320 (Abstract).

14 Firmin DN, Kilner PJ, Pennell DJ, *et al*. Short echo time (3.5 to 6 ms) field even echo rephasing sequences for improved accuracy and reliability of blood flow velocity and acceleration measurements. *Proceedings of the Eighth Annual Meeting of the Society of Magnetic Resonance in Medicine* 1989: 888 (Abstract).

15 Dinsmore RE, Wismer GL, Guyer D, *et al*. Magnetic resonance imaging of the interatrial septum and atrial septal defects. *Am J Roentgenol* 1985; **145**: 697–703.

16 Sakakibara M, Kobayashi S, Imai H, Watanabe S, Masuda Y, Inagaki Y. Diagnosis of atrial septal defect using magnetic resonance imaging. *J Cardiol* 1987; **17**: 817–29.

17 Lowell DG, Turner DA, Smith SM, *et al*. The detection of atrial and ventricular septal defects with electrocardiographically synchronised magnetic resonance imaging. *Circulation* 1986; **73**: 89–94.

18 Diethelm L, Déry R, Lipton MJ, Higgins CB. Atrial-level shunts: sensitivity and specificity of MR in diagnosis. *Radiology* 1987; **162**: 181–6.

19 Didier D, Higgins CB. Identification and localisation of ventricular septal defect by gated magnetic resonance imaging. *Am J Cardiol* 1986; **57**: 1363–8.

20 Baker EJ, Ayton V, Smith MA, *et al*. Magnetic resonance imaging at high field strength of ventricular septal defects in infants. *Br Heart J* 1989; **62**: 305–10.

21 Jacobstein MD, Fletcher BD, Goldstein S, Riemenschneider TA. Evaluation of atrioventricular septal defect by magnetic resonance imaging. *Am J Cardiol* 1985; **55**: 1158–61.

22 Longmore DB, Klipstein RH, Underwood SR, *et al*. Dimensional accuracy of magnetic resonance in studies of the heart. *Lancet* 1985; **i**: 1360–2.

23 Amparo EG, Higgins CB, Shafton EP. Demonstration of coarctation of the aorta by magnetic resonance imaging. *Am J Roentgenol* 1984; **143**: 1192–4.

24 Rees S, Somerville J, Ward C, *et al*. Coarctation of the aorta: MR imaging in late postoperative assessment. *Radiology* 1989; **173**: 499–502.

25 Simpson IA, Chung KJ, Glass RF, Sahn DJ, Sherman FS, Hesselink J. Cine magnetic resonance imaging for evaluation of anatomy and flow relations in infants and children with coarctation of the aorta. *Circulation* 1988; **78**: 142–8.

26 Jefferson KE, Rees S, Somerville J. Systemic arterial supply to the lungs in pulmonary atresia and its relation to pulmonary artery development. *Br Heart J* 1972; **34**: 418–27.

27 Somerville J. Management of pulmonary atresia. *Br Heart J* 1970; **32**: 641–51.

28 Somerville J, Saravalli O, Ross D. Complex pulmonary atresia with congenital systemic collaterals: classification and management. *Arch Mal Coeur* 1978; **71**: 322–28.

29 Chesler E, Beck W, Shrire V. Selective catheterization of pulmonary or bronchial arteries in the pre-operative assessment of pseudo-truncus arteriosus type IV. *Am J Cardiol* 1970; **26**: 20–4.

30 Rees RSO, Somerville J, Underwood SR, *et al*. Magnetic resonance imaging of pulmonary arteries and their systemic connections in pulmonary atresia: comparison with angiographic and surgical findings. *Br Heart J* 1987; **58**: 621–6.

31 Boxer RA, LaCorte MA, Singh S, *et al*. Nuclear magnetic resonance imaging in evaluation and follow-up of children treated for coarctation of the aorta. *J Am Coll Cardiol* 1986; **7**: 1095–8.

32 Bank ER, Aisen AM, Rocchini AP, Hernandez RJ. Coarctation of the aorta in children undergoing angioplasty: pretreatment and posttreatment MR imaging. *Radiology* **162**: 235–40.

33 Rheuban KS, Gutgesell HP, Carpenter MA, *et al*. Aortic aneurysm after patch angioplasty for aortic isthmic coarctation in childhood. *Am J Cardiol* 1986; **58**: 178–9.

34 Mohiaddin RH, Underwood SR, Bogren HG, *et al*. Regional aortic compliance studied by magnetic resonance imaging: the effects of age, training, and coronary artery disease. *Br Heart J* 1989; **62**: 90–6.

35 Simsolo R, Grunfeld B, Giminez M, *et al*. Long-term systemic hypertension in children after successful repair of coarctation of the aorta. *Am Heart J* 1988; **115**: 1268.

36 Somerville J. Fate of survivors of successfully treated congenital heart disease. Problems for the adult physician. In, Harper PS, Muir JR (eds), *Advanced Medicine* 15. Tunbridge Wells: Pitman Medical Publishing 1979: 14–26.

37 Rees RSO, Somerville J, Warnes C, *et al*. Comparison of magnetic resonance imaging with echocardiography and radionuclide angiography in assessing cardiac function and anatomy following Mustard's operation for transposition of the great arteries. *Am J Cardiol* 1988; **61**: 1316–22.

38 Sampson C, Martinez J, Rees S, Somerville J, Underwood SR, Longmore DB. Evaluation of Fontan's operation by magnetic resonance imaging. *Am J Cardiol* 1990; **65**: 819–21.

Chapter 7
Cine Imaging of the Heart

RICHARD SEMELKA, STEFAN WAGNER, PETER BUSER AND CHARLES HIGGINS

Conventional magnetic resonance imaging using spin echo sequences produces static images at chosen points of the cardiac cycle. These images demonstrate cardiac anatomy well, but some aspects of function are better evaluated by cine imaging. Cine imaging is available on most commercial scanners and it is being used increasingly for the assessment of cardiac function, valvular function, and for the measurement of blood flow.

7.1 Technical considerations

As described in chapter 2, magnetic resonance images are constructed from a number of data acquisitions, each with a different phase encoding gradient. A typical number of acquisitions for cardiac imaging is 128 and these may be acquired twice and averaged. Each acquisition contributes to a line of the image, although the line is in frequency or K-space and not in real space. For cardiac imaging, only one acquisition can be triggered per cycle since all the acquisitions must correspond to the same part of the cycle. Total imaging time is therefore 256 cycles or 3–4 minutes depending upon heart rate.

For cine acquisition, the selected plane is excited many times per cycle but each excitation contributes to a different image. At the end of 256 cycles a number of images is produced corresponding to different parts of the cycle. The repetition time of the sequence must equal the required temporal resolution and is typically between 10 and 50 ms. If the usual 90° excitation pulse is used, the imaging plane would become magnetically saturated and little or no signal would be obtained, but by reducing the excitation flip angle to between 20 and 45° this problem can be overcome. Using this technique, cine spin echo images have been acquired with a temporal resolution of 12 frames per cardiac cycle.[1]

The spin echo sequence is not ideal for such rapid repetition and much greater success has been achieved using variants of the field echo (or gradient refocussed echo) sequence, which have become known by acronyms such as FEER, GRASS, FAST, and FLASH. In these sequences, magnetic field gradients are used to dephase and then rephase the protons following an excitation pulse, and an echo is produced much more rapidly than by using a 180° pulse. Reduced flip angles are used for the initial exciting pulse to avoid saturation. An additional manoeuvre to maintain signal from moving blood is to make use of the 'even echo rephasing' phenomenon and to acquire the second echo rather than the first. Echo times of 6 ms and repeat times of 10 ms can be attained in commercial magnetic resonance scanners and in experimental small bore machines echo times of 1 ms and repeat times of 3 ms have been achieved.

For clinical imaging, 32 frames per cardiac cycle are adequate but 16 frames are often used so that the repeat time is not greater than 30 or 50 ms. Excitation need not be in a single plane and, for instance, with 48 excitations per cardiac cycle 4 different planes can be imaged with 12 frames per cycle in each.

One of the main features of spin echo images is the high contrast between soft tissues. With the very rapid repetition times of cine field echo sequences this contrast is lost because adequate time for longitudinal relaxation (and hence T_1 contrast) is not available. Contrast between blood and myocardium is maintained, however, because fresh unmagnetised blood is continuously flowing through the plane. If flow is inadequate then contrast is lost and this occurs particularly in the vertical and horizontal long axis planes where flow is mainly in the plane of the image. Contrast in the short axis and transverse planes is usually good.

The choice of plane depends upon the information

required. Left ventricular function is best assessed in the long axis or short axis planes but because of the reduced contrast between blood and myocardium in the long axis, a limited number of frames per cycle may be required. The mitral valve is best imaged in the transverse plane and either of the long axis planes, the aortic valve in the coronal or horizontal long axis, the tricuspid valve in the transverse plane, and the pulmonary valve in the sagittal or oblique sagittal plane.

7.2 Image analysis

Rapid cine display of the images on the computer screen allows a subjective assessment of cardiac motion. For left ventricular function it is usual to consider myocardial thickness, changes in thickness between diastole and systole, the extent of endocardial motion and its timing. With training, abnormalities of any of these parameters can be detected reliably and, depending upon the application, quantitative analysis may not be necessary. The end systolic frame can usually be selected from the cine display for further analysis, although end systole is strictly at the point of minimum left ventricular volume and this cannot easily be judged from a single slice, particularly if different regions of the myocardium contract at different times. In cases of pericardial disease it may also be helpful to assess the motion of the epicardial surface of the heart. Motion of the heart within a pericardial effusion can be seen and this aids the distinction of effusion from pericardial thickening. Pericardial constriction is suggested by a thickened and immobile pericardium with restricted myocardial relaxation.

The intensity of signal from the blood also gives important information. Blood flowing rapidly through the plane of imaging gives high signal and blood remaining within the plane becomes magnetically saturated and produces lower signal. Filling defects such as thrombus are seen as areas of reduced signal and the constancy of shape and position usually helps to distinguish thrombus from loss of signal for other reasons. Areas of turbulence lead to loss of signal and this is valuable in the qualitative assessment of valvular disease as discussed later.

7.3 Ventricular volumes

Chamber sizes can be assessed subjectively from the cine display but a more objective measurement is to calculate ventricular volumes by summing the areas in multiple contiguous sections. This can be done at any point in the cardiac cycle that has been acquired but most commonly only the end diastolic and end systolic volumes are computed. The volumes so calculated are very accurate and several studies have successfully compared the results with angiography[2] and with echocardiography.[3,4] In theory, it does not matter which plane is used for the measurements, but the short axis plane appears to be the best because of the good contrast between blood and myocardium. In a comparison of the transverse and short axis planes for the measurement of left ventricular volumes, good agreement has been obtained (figure 7.1).[5] Further validation comes from a comparison of left and right ventricular stroke volumes in normal subjects since the two should be the same (figure 7.2).

The technique is time consuming, however, since definition of the blood pool in each image has to be performed manually. Much more rapid measurements can be made using the area-length technique in either a single plane or in two perpendicular planes. The area-length technique assumes that the ventricle is an ellipsoid of revolution about its long axis and although this is a reasonable assumption in normal ventricles, significant errors can be made in ventricles with regional abnormalities.[6]

7.4 Ventricular muscle mass

In the same way that the volume of the ventricular cavities can be computed, ventricular muscle volume and hence mass can also be measured. The accuracy of the results has been demonstrated by comparing muscle mass measured at end diastole and at end systole. Interobserver variability is also good, as is the reproducibility in sequential studies.[5]

7.5 Regional left ventricular function

Cine display of the left ventricular images allows systolic function to be evaluated subjectively from wall motion and wall thickening. Figure 7.3 shows diastolic and systolic images in the short axis plane in a normal subject. Wall thickening is uniform and motion is concentric, but there is a gradient of wall thickening which decreases from apex to base (figure 7.4).[5]

In patients with coronary artery disease and previous infarction myocardial thinning, failure to thicken in systole, and motion abnormalities such as hypokinesis,

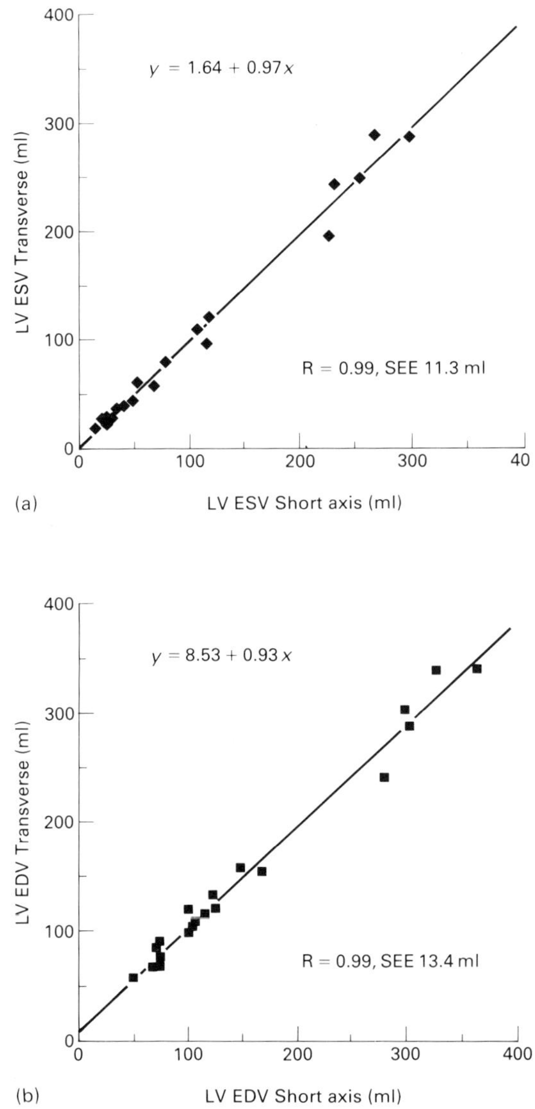

Figure 7.1. In a comparison between the transverse and short axis planes for the calculation of left ventricular volume, good agreement is seen at end diastole (a) and end systole (b). The volumes were calculated by summing the areas of the chamber in multiple contiguous sections. (Reproduced with permission from Buser *et al.*[5].)

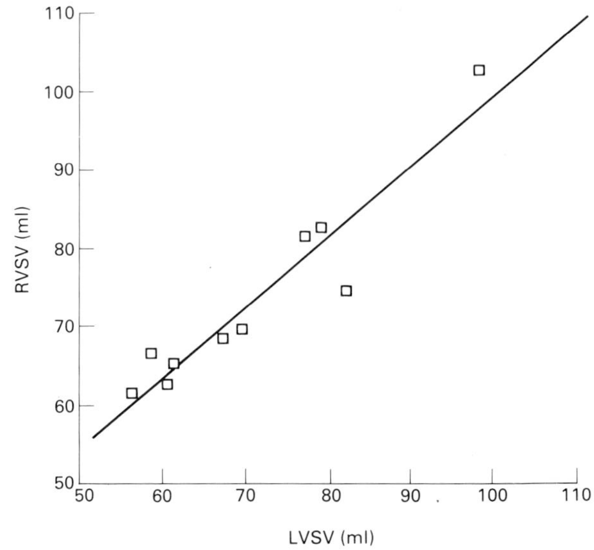

Figure 7.2. Validation of ventricular volume measurements from cine imaging comes from the good agreement between left and right ventricular stroke volumes in normal subjects. Right ventricular stroke volume (RVSV), left ventricular stroke volume (LVSV). (Reproduced with permission from Sechtem *et al.*[4].)

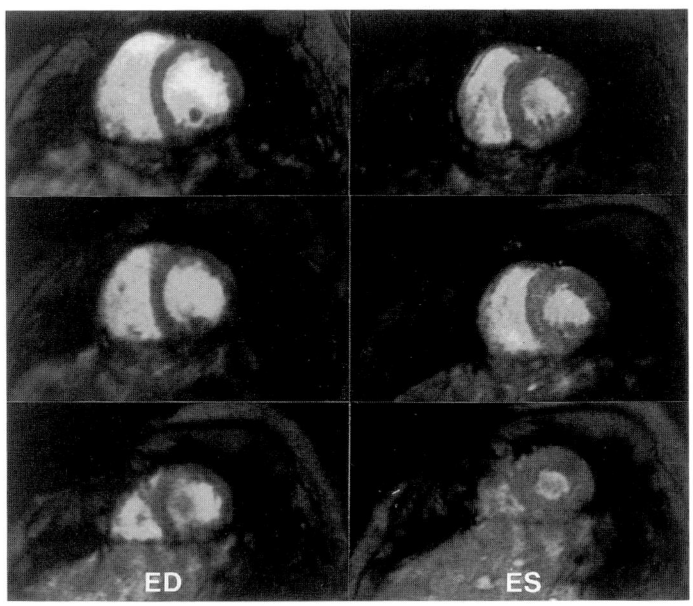

Figure 7.3. End diastolic (ED) and end systolic images (ES) in the short axis plane at basal, midcavity, and apical levels (top to bottom) in a normal subject. Note the symmetrical contraction and wall thickening.

akinesis or dyskinesis are seen (figure 7.5). Failure to thicken in systole is the most specific indicator of disease, and in a comparison of patients with previous infarction and normal subjects, mean thickening in the infarcted territories was 0.3 mm compared with 4 mm in the normal segments (figure 7.6).[3]

In the absence of previous infarction, wall motion is often normal but abnormalities can be induced by intravenous dipyridamole which is a powerful coronary arterial dilator increasingly used as an adjunct to dynamic exercise in thallium-201 myocardial perfusion

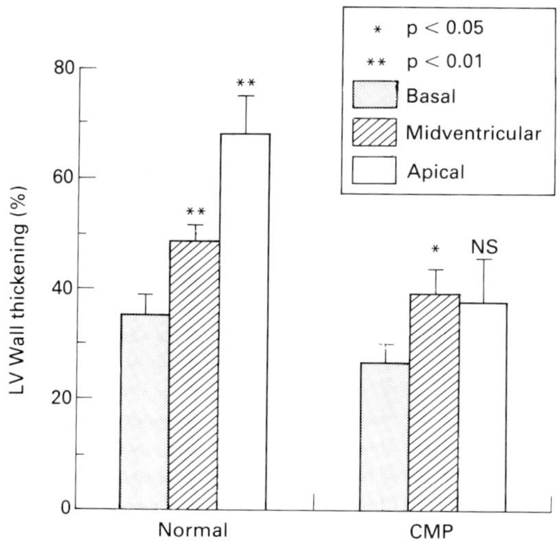

Figure 7.4. Left ventricular wall thickening in normal subjects and patients with dilated cardiomyopathy (CMP). There is a gradient of wall thickening from base to apex in the normal subjects which is absent in the patients. (Reproduced with permission from Buser *et al.*[5].)

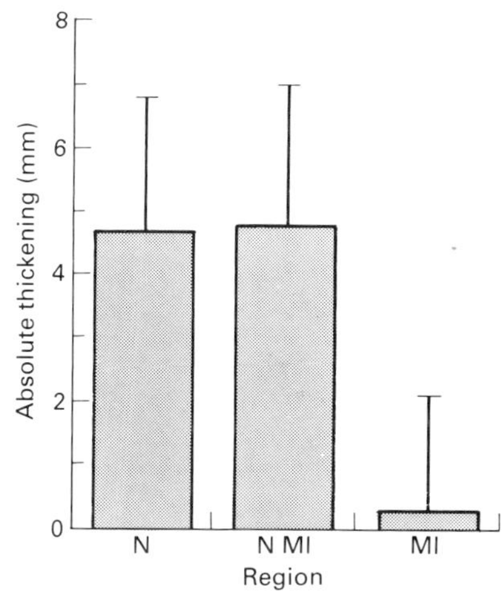

Figure 7.6. Mean left ventricular myocardial thickening in normal subjects (N), normal areas in subjects with previous infarction (NMI), and infarcted areas (MI). (Reproduced with permission from Higgins *et al.*[3].)

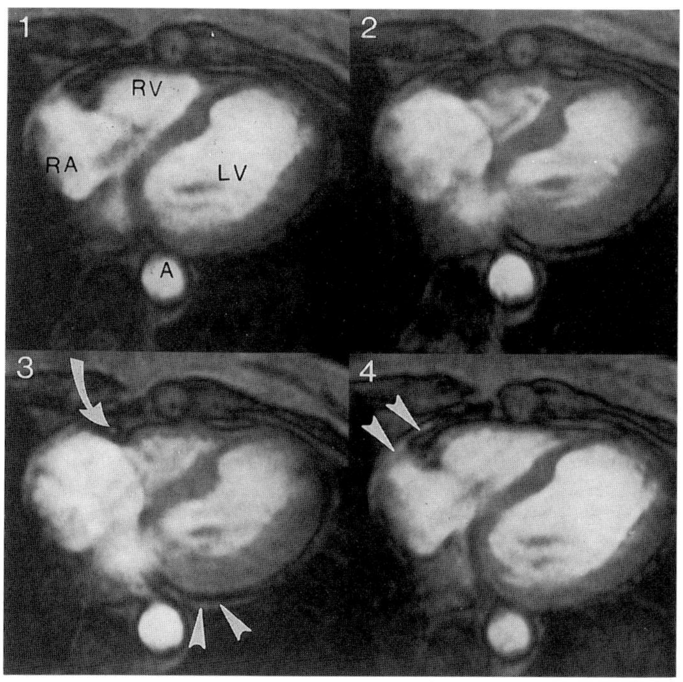

Figure 7.5. Transverse cine images 3 months after anteroseptal infarction. Frames 1–4 span the cycle from early systole to late diastole. There is anteroseptal thinning in diastole and failure to thicken in systole. There is also a small pericardial effusion with high signal intensity over the right atrium and behind the left ventricle (arrowheads). Note the right coronary artery within right atrioventricular groove (curved arrow). (Reproduced with permission from Utz *et al.*[2].)

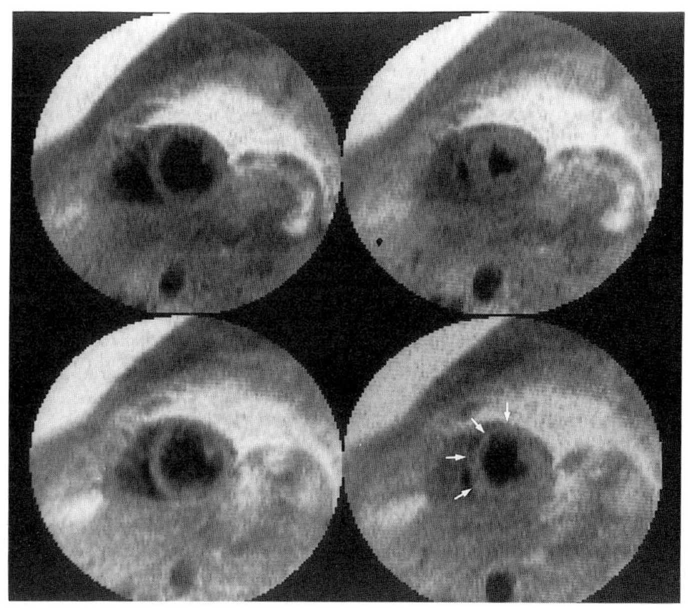

Figure 7.7. Diastolic (left) and systolic (right) short axis images in a patient with coronary artery disease without previous infarction, before (above) and following (below) intravenous dipyridamole. Hypokinesis and failure to thicken are induced in the anterolateral wall (arrows). (Reproduced with permission from Pennell *et al.*[7].)

imaging. Although the mechanism is complex, it may induce ischaemia and wall motion abnormalities in a proportion of patients with coronary artery disease.[7,8] Figure 7.7 shows an example.

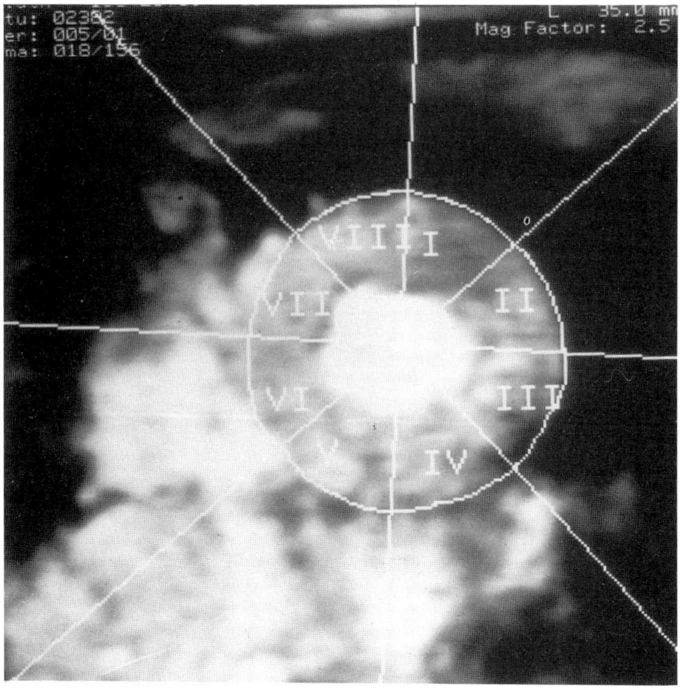

Figure 7.8. The end diastolic and end systolic frames are selected from a short axis cine acquisition in order to measure regional wall thickness. An end systolic image is shown and the left ventricle is divided into eight radial sections. Mean wall thickness is calculated in each segment.

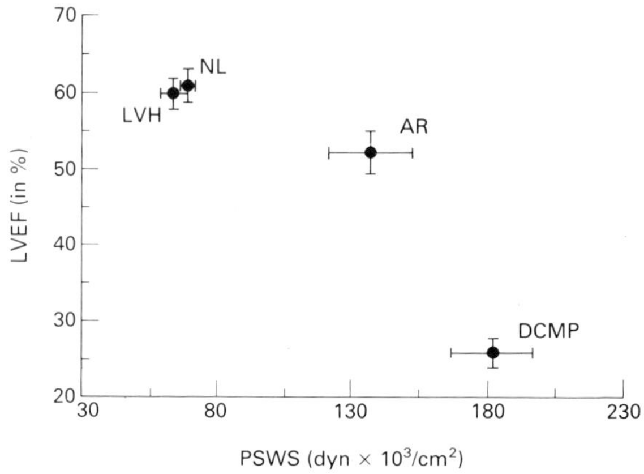

Figure 7.9. Peak systolic wall stress (PSWS) plotted against left ventricular ejection fraction (LVEF) in normal subjects (NL), patients with secondary left ventricular hypertrophy (LVH), aortic regurgitation (AR) and dilated cardiomyopathy (DCMP). The bars represent one standard deviation.

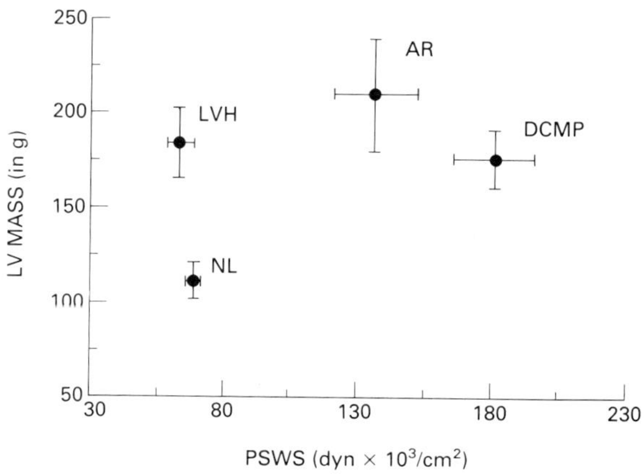

Figure 7.10. Peak systolic wall stress (PSWS) plotted against left ventricular (LV) mass in normal subjects (NL), patients with secondary left ventricular hypertrophy (LVH), aortic regurgitation (AR) and dilated cardiomyopathy (DCMP).

For quantitative analysis of wall thickness and motion it is necessary to define an endocardial boundary. This has been achieved using automatic computer programs and thresholding or second derivative techniques, but the quality of the cine images is not always adequate for reliable automatic edge detection. Wall thickening can be calculated in four to eight radial sections, depending on the available software and clinical application (figure 7.8) and measurements in three short axis planes (basal, midventricular, and apical) gives reasonable coverage of the ventricle without prolonging the acquisition unduly.

An important problem when studying regional left ventricular wall motion is the distinction between active contraction and passive motion caused by translation and rotation. Many different methods have been used and whilst none is ideal, the centre-line technique is probably the best. This uses a fixed external reference system and measures motion along a line perpendicular to the centre-line between the diastolic and the systolic endocardial contours. Because of these problems, wall thickening between diastole and systole is preferable to wall motion alone when considering regional function.[9] The short axis plane is ideal and the effect of previous infarction is readily detected and quantified.[10]

7.6 Left ventricular wall stress

More sophisticated measures of left ventricular function can also be derived by calculating wall stress. End systolic stress can be calculated as:

$$Stress = \frac{1.35 \cdot PD}{4h(1+h/\mathrm{D})}$$

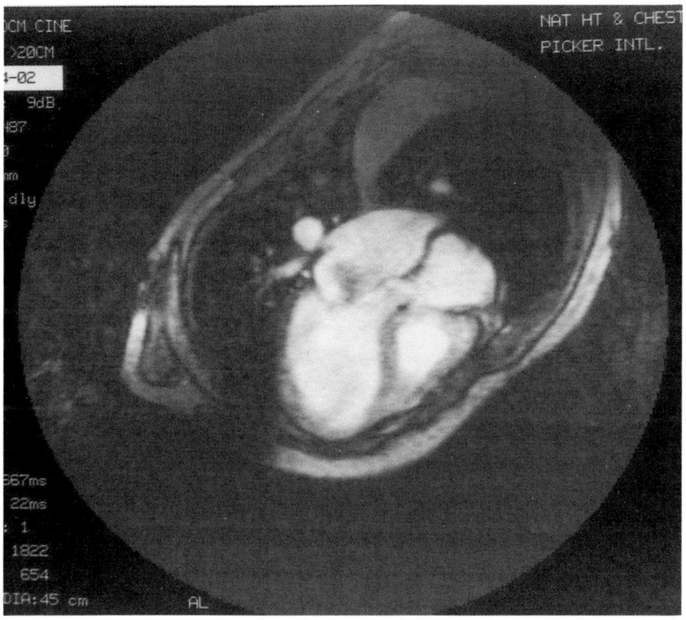

(a)

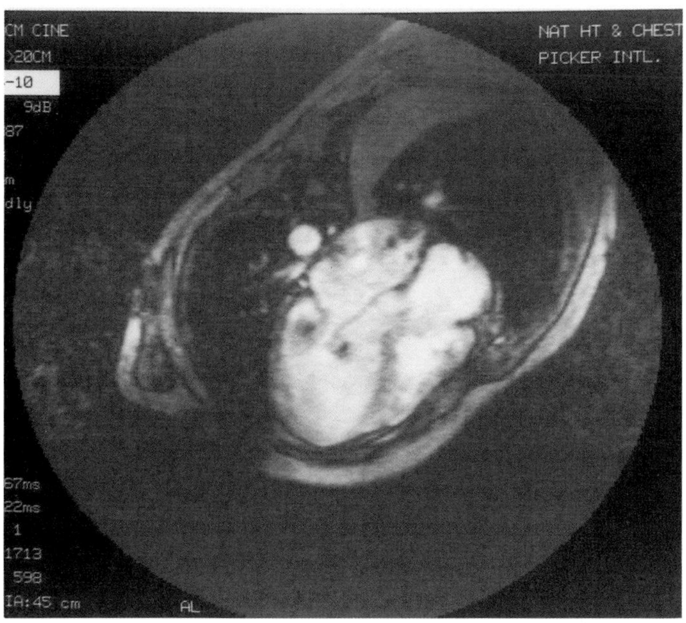

(b)

Figure 7.11. (a) Systolic and (b) diastolic frames from a cine acquisition in the horizontal long axis plane in a patient with a dilated cardiomyopathy. The mitral valve leaflets are thin and are seen to open normally in diastole. There is a small area of turbulence (signal loss) in the left atrium indicating trivial mitral regurgitation, and vortices of turbulence are seen being shed from the tips of the valve in diastole. (With thanks to Dr SR Underwood.)

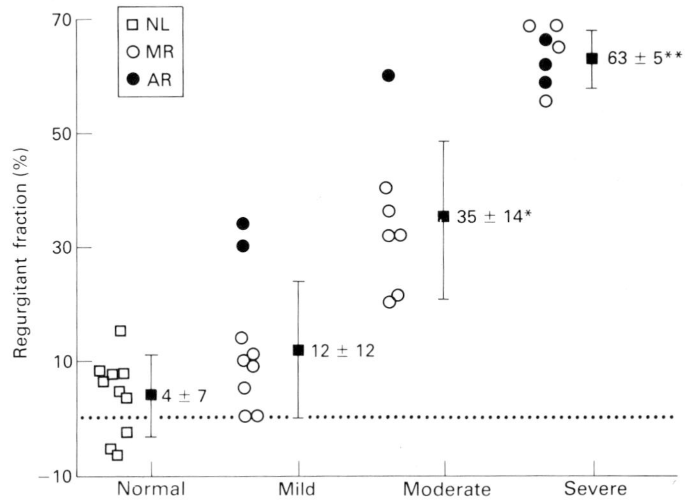

Figure 7.12. Regurgitant fraction calculated from left and right ventricular stroke volumes in normal subjects and patients with mild, moderate, and severe left-sided regurgitation. Mitral regurgitation (MR), aortic regurgitation (AR), $^*p < 0.01$ compared with normals and mild regurgitation; $^{**}p < 0.001$ compared with the other three groups. (Reproduced with permission from Sechtem *et al.*[14].)

where P is the end systolic left ventricular pressure in millimetres of mercury which is calculated from systolic blood pressure corrected for the time of the dichrotic notch on a carotid pulse tracing, D is the end systolic diameter of the ventricle in centimetres, and h is the end systolic wall thickness in centimetres. Such measurements in patients with a variety of conditions have provided interesting results, which may be valuable for assessing therapeutic responses. Patients with secondary left ventricular hypertrophy have wall stress comparable with that of normal subjects, but patients with valvular regurgitation have high stress in proportion to the severity of regurgitation. In dilated cardiomyopathy, wall stress is also increased but ejection fraction is much less than in patients with regurgitation and comparable wall stress (figure 7.9).[11] Similar relationships can be defined between wall stress and myocardial mass and these may prove useful for characterising the state of the myocardium and following its response to therapy (figure 7.10).

7.7 Valvular function

Static spin echo magnetic resonance images do not have sufficient resolution to show valve anatomy in detail although it is possible to see both atrioventricular

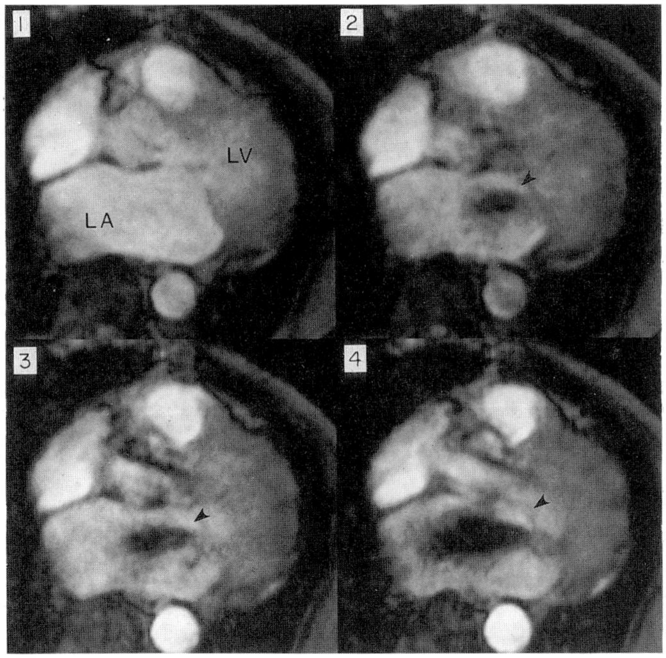

(a)

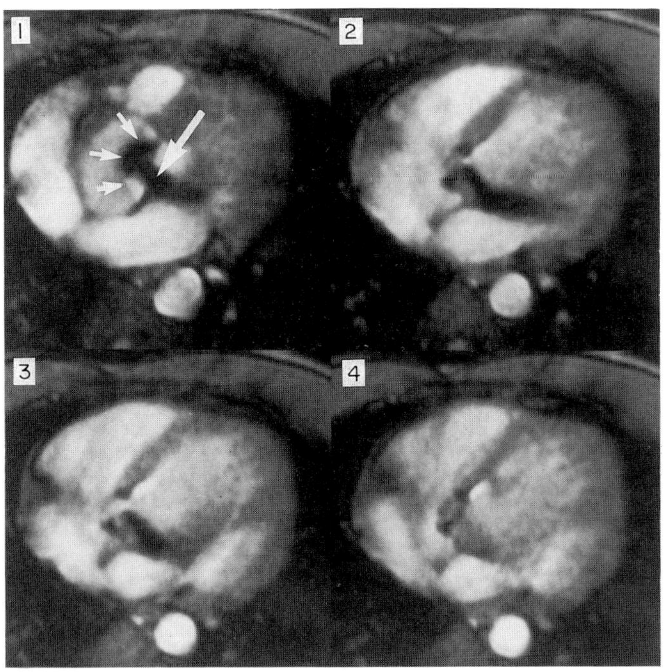

(b)

Figure 7.13. (a) Transverse cine images in one plane showing mitral regurgitation. There is an area of signal loss arising from the mitral valve and extending into the left atrium throughout systole. (b) Diastolic images in multiple planes showing aortic regurgitation. The turbulent jet arises from the valve (small arrows) and extends into the left ventricle. It is possible to distinguish aortic regurgitation from turbulent left ventricular filling across the mitral valve because of the origin of the jet.

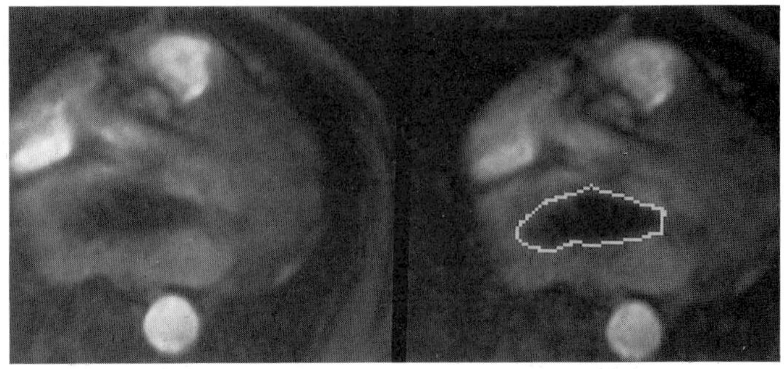

(a)

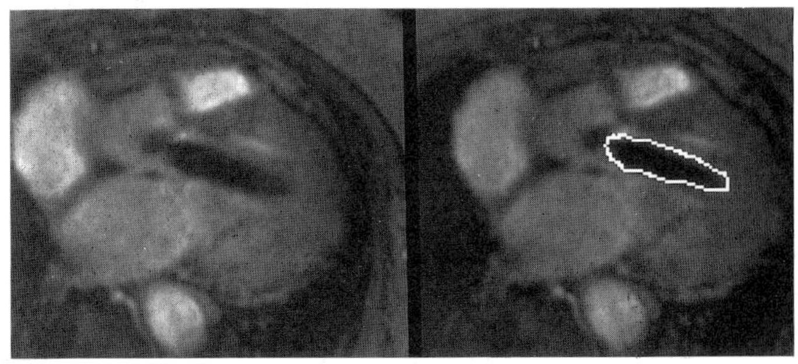

(b)

Figure 7.14. Cine images of a patient with moderate mitral regurgitation with a systolic signal void in the left atrium (a) and a patient with moderate aortic regurgitation with a diastolic signal void in the left ventricle (b). The signal void can be outlined on the computer screen and the total volume of the turbulent area calculated.

and semilunar valves in some images. Abnormal and thickened valves are more easily seen, and calcification may be revealed as loss of signal in a thickened valve. Valve morphology is slightly better seen in cine images because the human eye is capable of integrating the information in a series of images and compensating for inadequacies in any individual image (figure 7.11). Magnetic resonance cannot therefore replace echocardiography for the demonstration of valve anatomy.

A number of methods is available however for assessing valvular function. If left and right ventricular volumes are measured at end diastole and end systole, any discrepancy between the stroke volumes must be due to regurgitation and the regurgitant fraction can be calculated as (LVSV-RVSV)/LVSV (figure 7.12).[12] This is a particularly accurate technique, as has been shown by a comparison of stroke volumes in normal subjects where left and right ventricular stroke volumes should be almost identical.[13] If more than one valve is regurgitant then the regurgitant fraction is the mean of

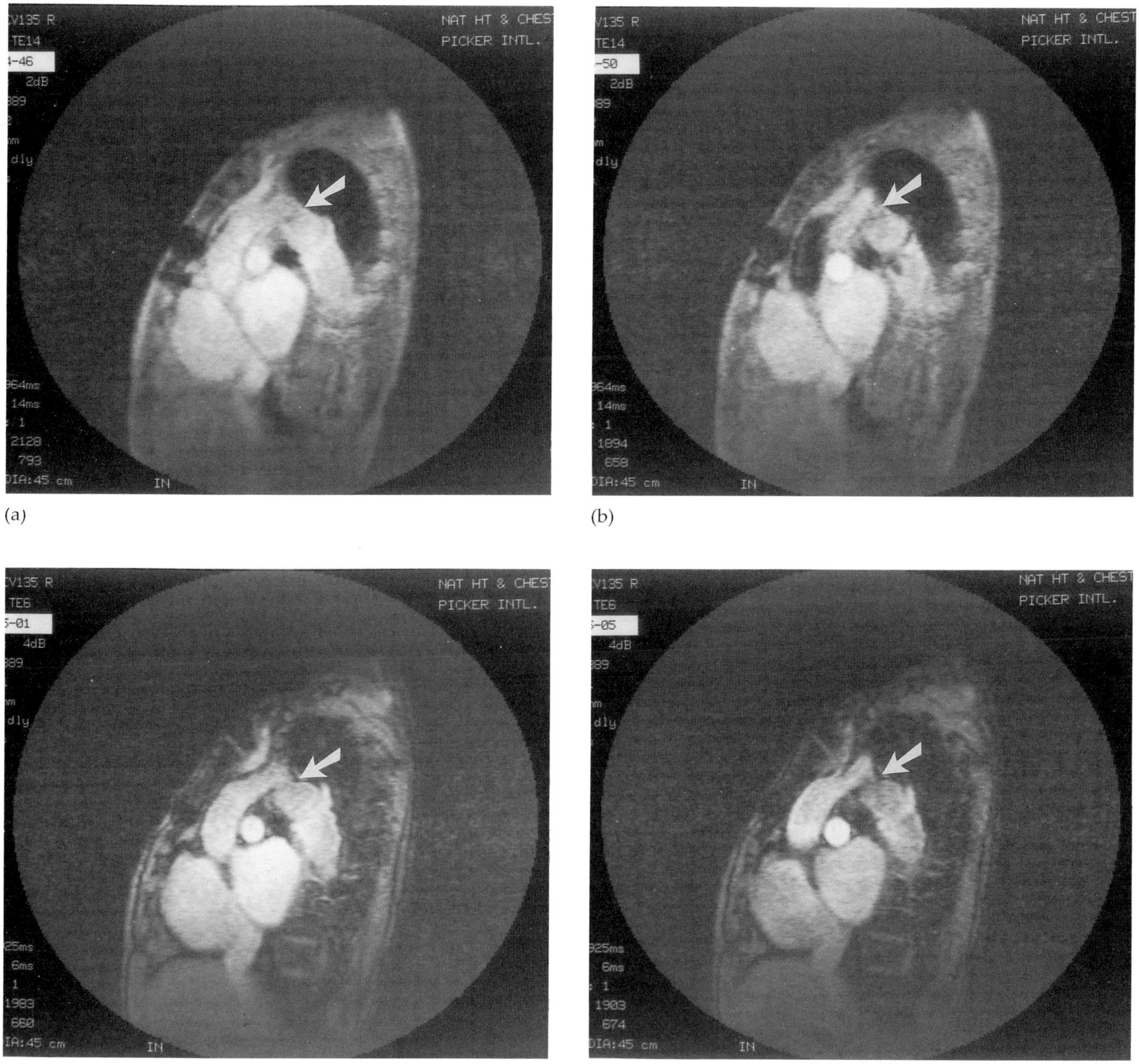

(a) (b) (c) (d)

Figure 7.15. This patient has aortic coarctation (arrowed) and a bicuspid but unstenosed aortic valve. (a) and (c) are diastolic frames and (b) and (d) are systolic. (a) and (b) had an echo time of 14 ms and (c) and (d) 6 ms. There is systolic signal loss using the longer echo time in the ascending aorta and also distal to the coarctation at the entry of a collateral vessel. With the 6 ms sequence signal is preserved throughout the aorta. No turbulence is seen distal to the coarctation because it was very tight with little flow across it. (With thanks to Dr SR Underwood.)

that from both valves, unless they are on opposite sides when accurate quantification is impossible. The technique appears to be equally accurate whether spin echo images[12] or cine field echo images[14] are used.

A second method by which valvular regurgitation can be assessed is measurement of the area of signal loss produced by the turbulent jet. As discussed above, cine field echo sequences give high signal from blood unless it is turbulent, when signal is lost. The mechanisms leading to signal loss are complicated and they are discussed in detail in chapter 10. The presence of a range of values of acceleration and other higher orders of motion in a single pixel produces the signal loss, and these higher orders are present in the turbulent vortices of regurgitant jets or distal to a stenosis or other vascular abnormality (figure 7.13). Although the signal loss may not correspond exactly with turbulence, its size has been used to provide a semi-quantitative estimate of regurgitation through individual valves (figure 7.14).[15,16] The extent of turbulence can either be expressed as an absolute volume or more conveniently by grading the size of the jet. It has been shown that a simple grading system agrees approximately with the conventional grading system used in angiocardiography, with grade 1 being signal loss close to the valve, grade 2 extending into the proximal chamber, grade 3 filling the whole of the proximal chamber, and grade 4 if the receiving chamber has signal loss throughout the whole of the relevant half of the cardiac cycle.[15]

It was hoped that the same method of quantifying regurgitation could be used to measure valvular stenosis, but results have been unreliable. Although in phantom experiments the size of the turbulent area downstream from a stenosis is related to the gradient across it, in clinical applications other factors may lead to turbulence.[17] A bicuspid but unstenosed aortic valve, for instance, may produce marked turbulence. The area of signal loss also depends upon the sequence used and sequences with shorter echo times are much less susceptible to turbulence. This is illustrated in figure 7.15 where there is marked systolic signal loss distal to a bicuspid aortic valve using the FEER sequence with an echo time of 14 ms, but no signal loss using 6 ms. As discussed in chapter 10, the development of sequences with very short echo times allows velocity mapping across stenoses and the significance of a stenosis can then be assessed from the pressure gradient across it.

References

1 Waterton JC, Jenkins JPR, Zhu XP, Love HG, Isherwood I, Rowlands DJ. Magnetic resonance (MR) cine imaging of the human heart. *Br J Radiol* 1985; **58**: 711–6.

2 Utz JA, Herfkens RJ, Heinsimer JA, *et al*. Cine MR determination of left ventricular ejection fraction. *Am J Roentgenol* 1987; **148**: 839–43.

3 Higgins CB, Holt W, Pflugfelder P, Sechtem U. Functional evaluation of the heart with magnetic resonance imaging. *Magn Reson Med* 1988; **6**: 121–39.

4 Sechtem U, Pflugfelder PW, Gould RG, Cassidy MM, Higgins CB. Measurement of right and left ventricular volumes in healthy individuals with cine MR imaging. *Radiology* 1987; **163**: 697–702.

5 Buser PT, Auffermann W, Holt WW, *et al*. Noninvasive evaluation of global left ventricular function using cine MR imaging. *J Am Coll Cardiol* 1989; **13**: 1294–1300.

6 Underwood SR, Gill CRW, Firmin DN, *et al*. Left ventricular volume measured rapidly by oblique magnetic resonance imaging. *Br Heart J* 1988; **60**: 188–95.

7 Pennell DP, Underwood SR, Ell PJ, Swanton RH, Walker JM, Longmore DB. Magnetic resonance imaging using dipyridamole: the establishment of a new technique and a comparison with thallium-201 emission tomography. *Br Heart J* 1990; (In press).

8 Pennell DJ, Underwood SR, Ell PJ. The detection of coronary artery disease by magnetic resonance imaging using dipyridamole. *J Comput Assist Tomogr* 1990; **14**: 167–70.

9 Underwood SR, Rees RSO, Savage PE, *et al*. The assessment of regional left ventricular function by magnetic resonance. *Br Heart J* 1986; **56**: 334–40.

10 Pflugfelder PW, Sechtem UP, White RD, *et al*. Cine MRI: quantitation of regional myocardial function by rapid cine MR imaging. *Am J Roentgenol* 1988; **150**: 523–9.

11 Holt WW, Wolfe C, Pflugfelder P, *et al*. *Quantitation of Left Ventricular Function by Cine MR: Wall Stress Measurement in Normal and Cardiomyopathic Subjects* (Abstract). Society of Magnetic Resonance in Medicine, San Francisco, 1988: p. 136.

12 Underwood SR, Klipstein RH, Firmin DN, *et al*. Magnetic resonance assessment of aortic and mitral regurgitation. *Br Heart J* 1986; **56**: 455–62.

13 Longmore DB, Klipstein RH, Underwood SR, *et al*. Dimensional accuracy of magnetic resonance in studies of the heart. *Lancet* 1985; **i**: 1360–2.

14 Sechtem U, Pflugfelder PW, Cassidy MM, *et al*. Mitral or aortic regurgitation: Quantification of regurgitant volumes with cine MR imaging. *Radiology* 1988; **167**: 425–30.

15 Underwood SR, Firmin DN, Mohiaddin RH, *et al*. *Cine Magnetic Resonance Imaging of Valvular Heart Disease* (Abstract). Society of Magnetic Resonance Imaging, New York, 1987; p. 723.

16 Wagner S, Auffermann W, Buser P, *et al*. *The Signal Void in Cine MR Accurately Detects and Grades Severity of Valvular Regurgitation* (Abstract). Society of Magnetic Resonance in Medicine, San Francisco, 1988; p. 201.

17 de Roos A, Reichek N, Axel L, Kressel HY. Cine MR imaging in aortic stenosis. *J Comput Assist Tomogr* 1989; **13**: 421–5.

Chapter 8
Relaxation Measurements and Contrast Media

UDO SECHTEM AND CHARLES HIGGINS

8.1 Relaxation times

When magnetic resonance imaging first became available, much of the enthusiasm it engendered was based on the hope that the relaxation times of different tissues would differ sufficiently to provide histological information. The hope has not entirely been fulfilled and although relaxation time measurements provide some important information about tissues, they do not allow unique identification of pathology.[1] It is possible however to achieve some degree of tissue specificity using measurements of relaxation times and signal intensities.

Myocardial characterisation is of enormous clinical interest and *in vitro* magnetic resonance proton spectrometry has suggested that ischaemic myocardium can be differentiated from normal myocardium because of significant prolongation of relaxation times. Relaxation measurements may also be helpful for the identification of viable myocardium within an infarct, the distinction of reversibly from irreversibly ischaemic myocardium, and the verification of successful reperfusion after thrombolysis. Noninvasive tissue diagnosis would also influence clinical decisions in patients with intracardiac or paracardiac tumours and those with cardiac transplants.

The physical basis of relaxation has been described in chapter 1 but it is relevant to summarise some of the details here. After a 90° radio-frequency pulse, longitudinal magnetisation recovers from zero to its original value exponentially. This process has a time constant, T_1, which is the time required for the longitudinal magnetization to reach 0.63 of its original value. Longitudinal relaxation is thus a measure of how rapidly the sample can release the radio-frequency energy that it absorbed from the exciting radio-frequency pulse to the surrounding environment. After the same 90° pulse, transverse magnetisation in the *xy* plane is initially high because the protons that have jumped between parallel and anti-parallel energy states are in phase. They subsequently lose phase coherence, however, and the transverse magnetisation decays exponentially with a time constant T_2.

These relaxation times are determined by the physical and chemical environment of the relaxing protons, and protons in different tissues have different relaxation times. Although T_1 and T_2 depend upon a variety of variables, the concentration of water is an important determinant. When the water content of a tissue rises, such as in the oedema following infarction, both relaxation times rise or, in other words, the relaxation rates decrease.[2] Dehydration, however, reduces relaxation times and increases the rates. In contrast, the low fat content of most tissues does not noticeably influence relaxation times.[1] Other tissue variables which may influence longitudinal relaxation include the motion of the nuclei, regional temperature, the viscosity of tissue, and the magnetic effects of nearby nuclei.[3] T_1 is also affected by the chemical state and site of water in tissues.[4]

In general, a shortening of T_1 leads to an increase in signal intensity whereas a shortening of T_2 has the opposite effect. Because the presence of pathology usually alters T_1 and T_2 in the same direction, there are opposing effects on signal intensity, and for this to alter noticeably, one relaxation process must have a dominant influence. It is usually possible to stress the influence of each relaxation process by choosing appropriate imaging parameters, but in cardiac imaging T_1 weighting is limited because of the requirement for electrocardiographic gating which restricts the sequence repetition time to multiples of the cardiac cycle. By introducing additional excitation pulses into a gated spin echo sequence, the repetition time can be effectively reduced to a fractional value of the R—R interval which results in more pronounced T_1 weighting and an improvement in the precision of T_1 measurements.[5]

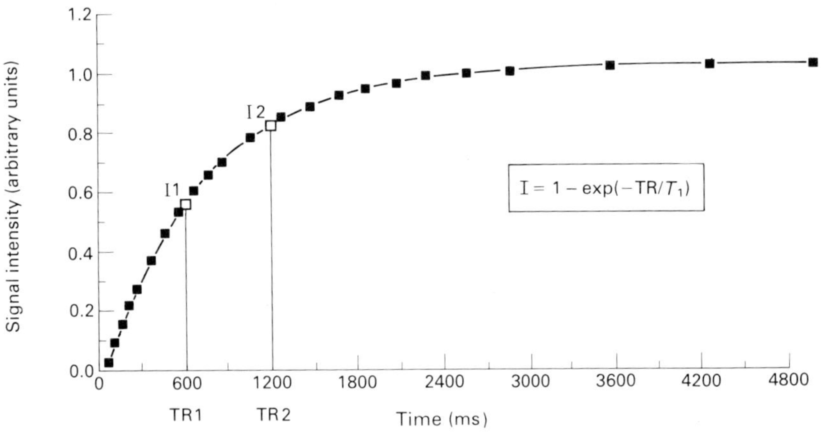

Figure 8.1. Calculation of T_1. Using two different repetition times, TR1 and TR2, two images with different signal intensities are obtained. It is not possible to solve the resulting equations arithmetically and approximations must be used.

8.1.1 The measurement of relaxation times

In vitro determination of relaxation times is usually performed by spectrometric measurements of homogeneous tissue samples. T_1 measurements are obtained using an inversion recovery sequence with additional pulses and T_2 measurements using the Carr–Purcell–Meiboom–Gill sequence, which is a spin echo sequence with multiple 180° pulses, and hence echoes, after the 90° pulse. *In vivo* magnetic resonance imaging offers several methods of measuring T_1 including the saturation–recovery or inversion–recovery sequences. However, the spin echo sequence is commonly used as it allows both T_1 and T_2 to be determined. To measure T_1 using the spin echo technique, two images with different repeat times are acquired (figure 8.1). Since the repeat time is restricted to the R–R interval or multiples thereof, the initial sequence is usually gated to every heart beat and the second sequence to alternate beats. Two echo times are required to measure T_2 (figure 8.2) and this is accomplished by using a spin echo sequence with two echoes. For optimal image quality, echo times should be short and echo times of 30 and 60 ms are often employed. Thus, two acquisitions allow the measurement of both T_1 and T_2 with an imaging time of approximately 20 minutes. Regions of interest are drawn on the images to measure mean myocardial signal intensity in the first and second echo images using the short repeat time and on the first echo image using the longer time. The values are used to solve the equations for T_1 and T_2.

Although the techniques for measuring T_1 and T_2 from images are relatively simple, there are a number of problems which lead to inaccuracies. The most important is that although two measurements are in theory sufficient for the calculation of an exponential decay rate, significant errors can be made in practice. Two point measurements are usually unavoidable because of limitations of imaging time but, in the brain, T_2 measurements have an accuracy of 20%[6] and in the heart it is much less. Other problems are the motion artefact from blood which can overlie the myocardium,[7] variation in R–R interval during the acquisition, variation in the time of the cycle for the two echo images, partial volume effects between normal and ischaemic tissues, and the variation in signal caused by motion and diffusion effects.[8] Additional sources of variation depend upon the scanner used. T_1 varies with field strength although T_2 is relatively in-

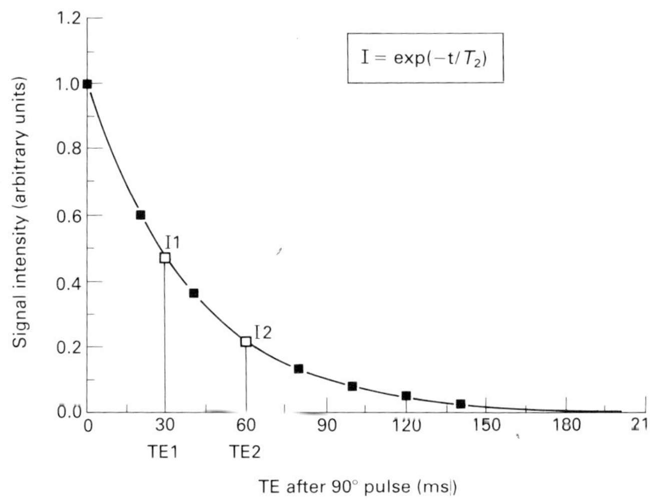

Figure 8.2. Calculation of T_2. Using spin echo sequences with echo times of 30 and 60 ms, two different mean signal intensities can be measured in the myocardial region of interest. T_2 is calculated from these values.

dependent, and errors from inhomogeneities of magnetic and radiofrequency fields will lead to errors. Thus, relaxation time measurements made from images should be considered semi-quantitative at best.

8.1.2 Myocardial ischaemia

Consistent prolongation of T_1 in regions of acute myocardial ischaemia were first observed by spectrometric examination of *ex vivo* animal hearts. Increases are seen as early as 30 minutes after coronary occlusion and become more prominent as the ischaemic time is extended to 60 or 120 minutes.[9] The increases of T_1 largely reflect the increased water content and not the tissue levels of high-energy compounds, lactate, or hydrogen ions. Imaging, however, has been less successful. Partial volume effects adversely affect the accuracy of imaging techniques and probably explain the inability to show differences between T_1 relaxation times of infarcted and normal myocardium in *ex vivo* infarcted dogs' hearts.[10]

T_2 measurements from images show a narrower range of normal values and moderate increases of T_2 compared with normal myocardium have been observed in *ex vivo* infarcts.[10] The increases are linearly related to water content.

In vivo measurements of T_1 using spin echo images at medium and high field have shown too much variability between individuals to be clinically useful,[11,12] although much more success has been achieved at low field (0.08 T) using an inversion recovery sequence with gradient echoes.[13] In this study, maximum prolongation was seen two weeks after infarction at a time when cellular infiltration and repair is greatest, suggesting that factors other than water content can be observed.

Although some investigators question the applicability of magnetic resonance for tissue characterisation in myocardial ischemia,[12] most agree that T_2 is well suited for the purpose.[11,14] Acutely infarcted myocardium shows significantly increased T_2 times as early as 3 hours after coronary occlusion,[11] but difficulties may occur in distinguishing between infarcted myocardium and intracavitary blood, signal from which may be prominent near the infarcted hypokinetic wall (figure 8.3). Differentiation of the two is aided by the phenomenon of even echo rephasing which leads to higher signal for slowly moving blood in the second echo image and an apparently negative T_2 value.[15] In contrast, the signal intensity of infarcted myocardium decreases from the first to the second echo image with a T_2 usually less than 100 ms. Partial volume averaging of intracavitary blood signal with infarcted myocardium results in a T_2 of greater than 100 ms.[16] The problem

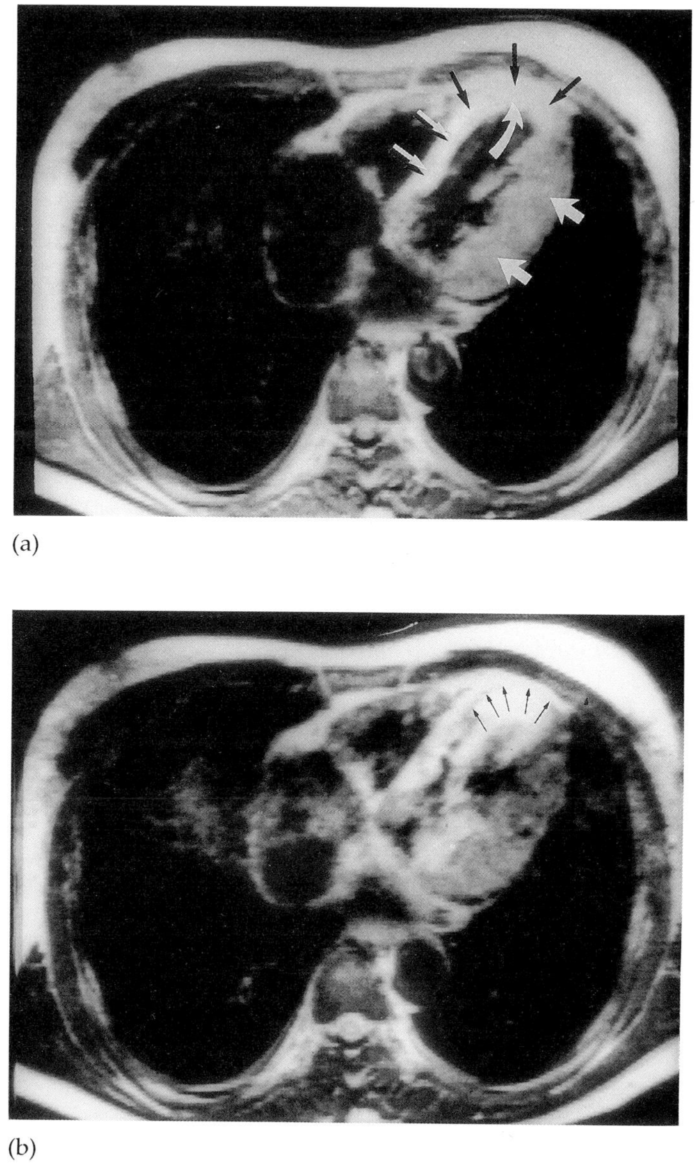

Figure 8.3. (a) Transverse first echo image (TE 30 ms) of a patient with a 7-day-old acute anteroseptal and anterior wall infarct. Intracavitary flow signal adjacent to the infarcted anterior wall (curved arrow) blends with the increased myocardial signal. The infarcted septum and anterior wall have higher signal intensity (black and white arrows) than the normal lateral wall (short arrows). (b) Second echo image (TE 60 ms) of the same patient. Flow signal can now be differentiated from the thinned anterior myocardium and the boundary between intracavitary flow signal and myocardium is marked by small black arrows.

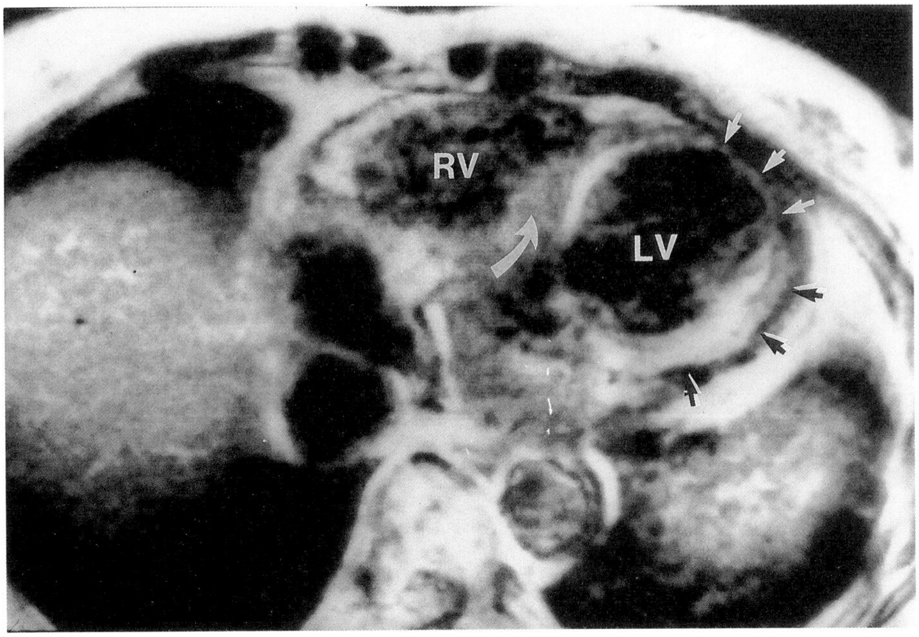

Figure 8.4. Transverse second echo image (TE 60 ms) showing a 9 month old anterior infarct. The infarcted region (black and white arrows) shows lower signal intensity than normal myocardium in the posterior interventricular septum (curved arrow). Left ventricle (LV), right ventricle (RV).

can be further reduced by using a single echo, long echo time image or a third (odd) echo image.

Although there may be difficulties in measuring relaxation time changes accurately, an alternative approach is to compare the signal intensity of a region of interest with normal myocardium. In this way it has been demonstrated that acutely infarcted myocardium has an increased signal intensity on *in vitro* and *in vivo* images without the need for contrast media.[7,15–18] Within 1 hour after coronary occlusion, a significant increase of signal intensity appears in spin echo images in the infarcted region.[19] Differences in signal intensity are most obvious in images with long repeat and echo times which are T_2 weighted. T_1 weighted inversion recovery images do not consistently show areas of high signal[17] because of the relatively small increases and the large standard deviation of T_1 in areas of normal myocardium.

Increased signal intensity of infarcted myocardium can be observed up to 20 days after the acute event.[11,19] The initial increase becomes more pronounced up to 14 days after infarction, and the signal then decreases to values below that of normal myocardium as a fibrous scar is formed.[19]

In patients with chronic infarction, focal myocardial thinning is the most prominent feature,[20,21] and relaxation time measurements are only possible if sufficient myocardium remains. In the majority of patients, myocardial scar has slightly lower signal intensity and shorter T_2 than adjacent normal myocardium (figure 8.4).[21] This finding is consistent with replacement by fibrous scar with low water content and magnetic resonance imaging may be useful for monitoring the healing process and for studying the effects of interventions aimed at modifying the course of infarction.

Many factors influence signal intensity of the acutely infarcted myocardium. The loss of integrity of the myocytes decreases the distinction between extracellular and intracellular water. Intramyocardial haemorrhage, which is a common finding after reperfusion, also causes a substantial increase in signal intensity and T_2. It is possible that myocardial hypokinesis also increases signal intensity.

Unfortunately, areas of increased signal intensity are not confined to infarcted myocardium[7,16,18] and they are observed in a substantial number of normal subjects. Possible explanations include respiratory motion and cardiac motion, and misplaced signal from slowly moving blood in adjacent cardiac chambers.

When compared with other noninvasive imaging techniques for the identification of myocardial infarction, magnetic resonance shows changes earlier than infarct-avid scintigraphy using technetium-99m pyrophosphate and also contrast enhanced computed X-ray tomography, both of which show alterations at 24 hours.[22] Thallium-201 imaging however shows perfusion abnormalities immediately after coronary occlusion.

8.1.3 Reperfusion

Early spectrometric studies of the effects of reperfusion demonstrated large increases of water content and T_1 in the myocardium of animals subjected to relatively long occlusion periods of 1 or 2 hours, with myocardial infarction despite the reperfusion. In contrast, shorter occlusion periods of 40 minutes did not cause changes in water content or T_1. A comparison of reperfusion and nonreperfusion in animals with left anterior descending occlusion for 2 or 3 hours showed that reperfusion produced higher T_1 and T_2 values and water content,[23] which can be explained by the oedema and haemorrhage caused by the reperfusion itself.[24] Relaxation time measurements may however reflect the severity of an ischaemic insult and the degree of reperfusion, as has been shown by *in vitro* spectrometric measurements compared with microsphere measurements of residual flow.[25]

In vivo, magnetic resonance imaging can detect reperfused acute infarction as early as 30 minutes after reperfusion or 90 minutes after the initial coronary occlusion (figure 8.5). The jeopardised myocardium demonstrates high signal intensity caused by prolonged T_2 compared with normal myocardium. Compared with occlusive myocardial infarcts, increases in signal intensity and T_2 are larger and earlier than when reperfusion is established.[26,27] Imaging might therefore be helpful in the identification of patients with successful reperfusion after intravenous thrombolysis.

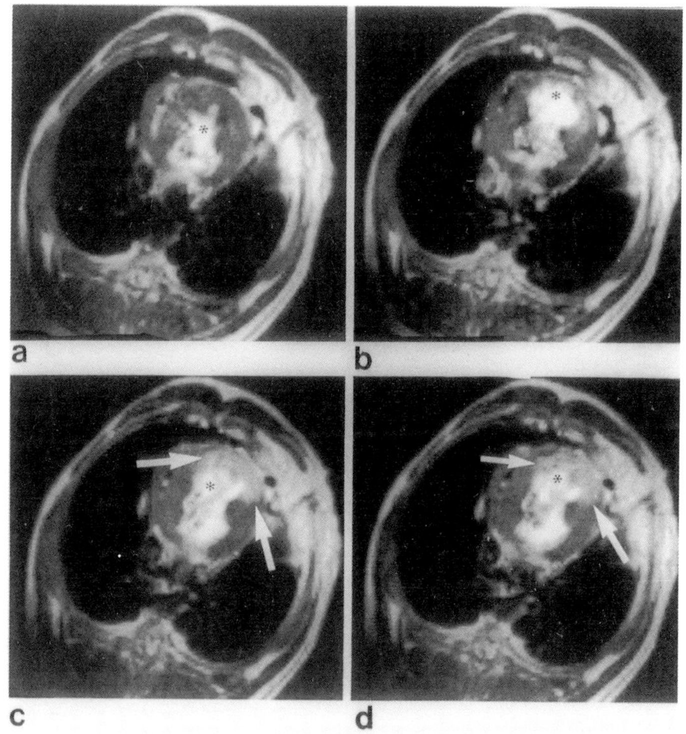

Figure 8.5. Transverse images in a dog following ligation of the left anterior descending coronary artery. The images were gated to alternate heart beats to prolong the R–R interval. Echo time 60 ms. (a) Preocclusion image. (b) Thirty min after ligation of the vessel. Note the thinning of the ischaemic anterior myocardium. (c) Thirty min after reperfusion, signal increase of the ischaemic region can be observed (arrowed). (d) Sixty min after reperfusion, the ischaemic anterior myocardium continues to exhibit high signal intensity and wall thickness has increased above preocclusion values. Intracavitary flow signal (*). (Reproduced with permission from *Am J Roentgenol* 1986; **146**: 925–30.)

8.1.4 Infarct sizing

The T_2 information inherent in first and second echo images can be used to construct a T_2 map of the heart. Such maps allow measurement of the extent of myocardial injury since they provide more consistent differentiation between normal and infarcted tissue compared with the native spin echo images (figure 8.6).

Magnetic resonance sizing of infarcts between 6 hours and 21 days after acute coronary occlusion has shown a good correlation with anatomical estimates in both in vitro and *in vivo* animal studies.[28,29] However, in vivo studies are subject to artefacts introduced by cardiac and respiratory motion which influence the calculation of T_2 and the accuracy of the measurements.

8.1.5 Doxorubicin cardiotoxicity

Present noninvasive techniques for the detection of doxorubicin cardiotoxicity rely on the assessment of myocardial function rather than on the direct measurement of altered tissue properties. Because relaxation times depend on water, lipid, and macromolecular content, and on interactions and exchange processes, magnetic resonance spectrometry has been used in rat models to evaluate the effect of doxorubicin cardiotoxicity on myocardial relaxation times.[30,31] In excised rat hearts with histological evidence of chronic cardiotoxicity, T_1 values have been shown to be significantly elevated compared with controls, and the difference was more pronounced in rats with clinical evidence of toxicity or heart failure.[30] In the study, there were no changes in T_2 or tissue water content and the alterations in T_1 were explained by membrane dysfunction leading

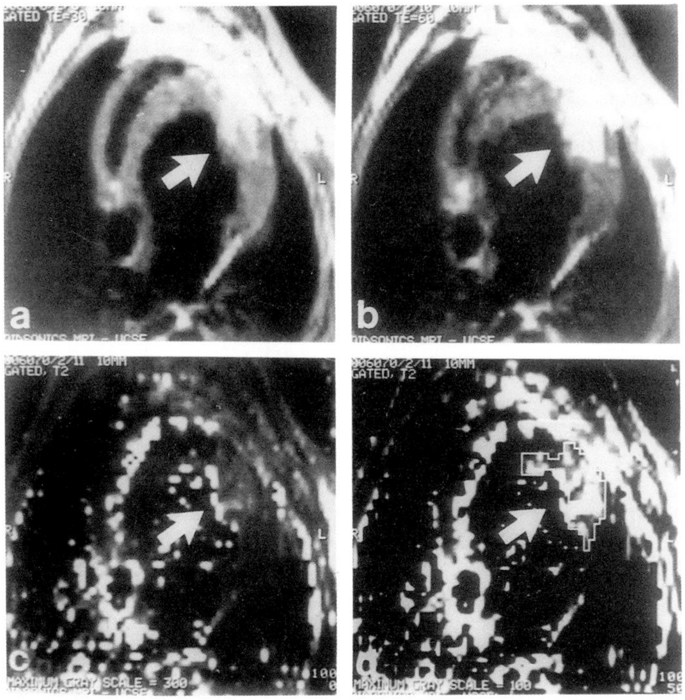

Figure 8.6. Transverse image in a dog with 3-day-old ligation of the left anterior descending artery. Prominent increase in signal intensity is seen in the infarcted anterolateral wall (arrows) on first (a) and second (b) echo images (TE 30 and 60 ms respectively). (c) The T_2 calculated image does not improve contrast between infarct (arrow) and normal myocardium without further manipulation. (d) When an upper level of the display window of 100 ms is used and a lower level of 50 ms, the infarcted region with prolonged T_2 is highlighted (outlined region). Note that the infarct extends into the anterior wall, which is difficult to appreciate from the native images alone. (Reproduced with permission from *Am J Roentgenol* 1987; **149**: 237–43.)

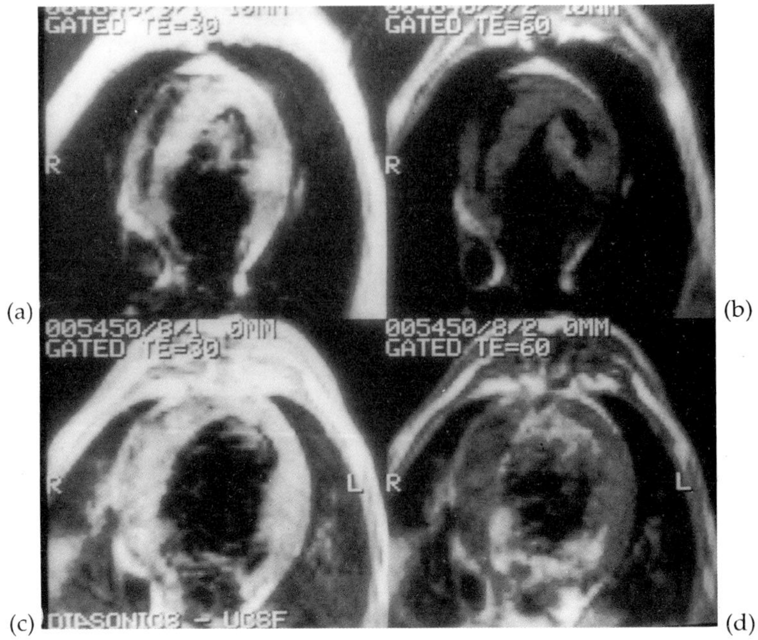

Figure 8.7. Transverse spin echo image in a dog with doxorubicin cardiotoxicity. (a) First echo image before treatment. (b) Second echo image before treatment. (c) First echo image after the development of heart failure. Note the dilatation of the left ventricle. At autopsy, there was histological evidence of severe toxicity. (d) Second echo image after the development of heart failure.

to changes in calcium and sodium content of the myocardium. However, the observed changes in T_1 were small and there was overlap between the two groups.

In our experience using a dog model of doxorubicin cardiotoxicity, it is possible to show the progressive dilatation of cardiac chambers associated with increasing toxicity (figure 8.7) but it has not proved possible to distinguish between normal hearts and those with mild, moderate or severe toxicity by measuring relaxation times. This is probably due to the difficulties of *in vivo* measurements and the absence of changes in water content between groups. *Post mortem* imaging has also failed to reveal differences of statistical significance.

8.1.6 Transplant rejection

Another form of cardiomyopathy is found in cardiac allografts suffering from rejection. It is common practice to perform regular endomyocardial biopsy to detect the histological changes of rejection and although noninvasive tests such as electrocardiography, echocardiography and radionuclide ventriculography are used, they cannot reliably detect rejection before irreversible damage is done. There is therefore an urgent need for a noninvasive technique that can identify the subtle changes of myocardial tissue composition that indicate graft rejection. These changes include inflammation and oedema: processes for which magnetic resonance is known to be sensitive.[17,23] Initial work in a dog model of heterotopic transplantation demonstrated a significant increase in T_2 and signal intensity from 3 days to 14 weeks after surgery.[32] Mean T_1 of native and transplanted hearts showed no significant difference *in vivo*, but *post mortem* it was longer in the transplanted hearts. Extending these experiments, it has been shown that immunosuppression prevents the prolongation of T_2 and that the magnitude of increase correlates well with the intensity of rejection in untreated animals.[33] Typical changes of rejection include an increase in wall thickness and in signal intensity compared with normal controls.

A recent study in humans found increases in T_1 and T_2 more than 25 days after surgery and 14 of 15 patients with late rejection were correctly identified on the basis of the relaxation times.[34] In this study a repeat time approximately equal to myocardial T_1 was used in order to improve the accuracy of the T_1 measurements.[5] Widespread clinical application is however limited by a low specificity because nonrejecting grafts also showed increases in T_1 and T_2 when imaged within 24 days of implantation. This is possibly caused by a prolonged period of cold anoxic arrest and subsequent oedema which seems to subside after 3–4 weeks.

Other groups have reported less optimistic results in human recipients of cardiac transplants: Revel and colleagues have demonstrated that T_2 is increased in transplant patients compared with normal subjects but that it is not related to the presence of biopsy evidence of rejection.[35]

8.1.7 Other applications of relaxation measurements

Relaxation times are a convenient method of incorporating the information from signal intensities and imaging parameters into a single number. However, because of the difficulties of measuring relaxation times accurately, some investigators prefer to use relative signal intensities on first and/or second echo images for tissue characterisation. The approach has been successfully applied in patients with lipomatous hypertrophy of the interatrial septum[36] and in contrast with echocardiography which depicts the anatomical features of the mass, magnetic resonance imaging can identify the adipose nature of the tissue by its characteristic high signal intensity. Normal myocardium and subcutaneous fat serve as an internal reference. However it is important to remember that such findings are not specific and that other pathological processes such as subacute haemorrhage and proteinaceous fluid may exhibit similar high signal.

Another promising field of myocardial tissue characterisation is the assessment of myocardial iron in patients with iron overload using the relative signal intensities of cardiac and skeletal muscle.[37] Although

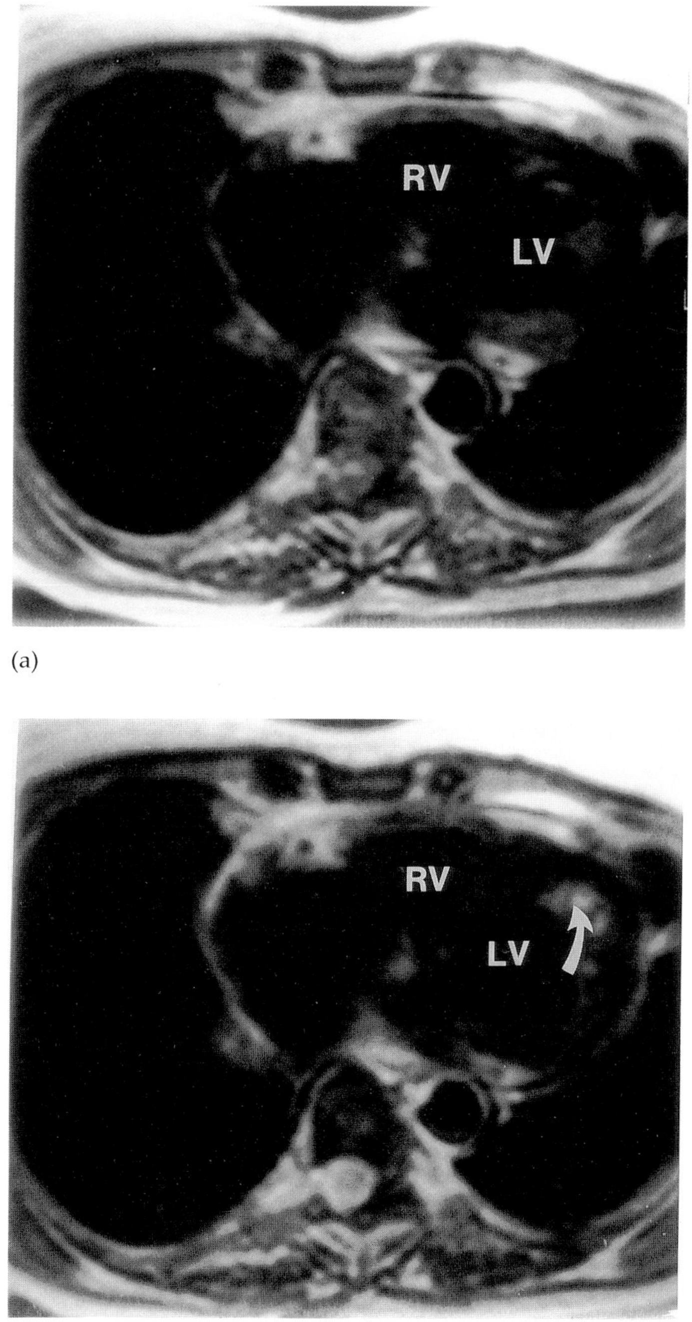

(a)

(b)

Figure 8.8. (a) Transverse first spin echo image (TE 30 ms) in a patient with severe iron overload due to repeated blood transfusion. The myocardium has very low signal intensity because of the T_2 shortening caused by myocardial iron deposition. (b) The second echo image (TE 60 ms) still shows low myocardial signal intensity consistent with T_2 shortening and there is some flow related adjacent next to the anterior wall (curved arrow). Left ventricle (LV), right ventricle (RV).

iron deposition in the myocardium is a late event in patients requiring multiple blood transfusions, the technique may be valuable for the follow-up of patients treated with erythropoetin (figure 8.8).

8.2 Contrast media

Although current magnetic resonance techniques usually provide excellent contrast between different soft tissues, alterations in signal intensity may be too small to allow the visualisation of some abnormalities. In such cases, magnetic resonance contrast media may be helpful. The major objectives in the use of contrast media for the myocardium are:

1 Delineation of the area at risk after acute coronary occlusion.

2 Improved demarcation of normal and infarcted myocardium, and hence an increase in the sensitivity and specificity of magnetic resonance for the detection of infarction.

3 The differentiation of occlusive and reperfused myocardial infarction.

4 An assessment of myocardial perfusion.

8.2.1 Physical properties and pharmacokinetics

Magnetic resonance contrast agents are paramagnetic compounds that influence the relaxation times of tissues with which they have close contact, by virtue of unpaired electrons in the outer shell of a central atom or ion.[38] Gadolinium (Gd) is a rare earth transition metal belonging to the lanthanide series, and it is a particularly powerful paramagnetic substance because of the seven unpaired electrons in its outer shell. Uncomplexed lanthanide ions are highly toxic. They antagonise the effects of calcium upon cells and, amongst other things, have a negative inotropic effect on the myocardium and inhibit the clotting system. They do not form covalent bonds with organic molecules but they can be complexed with ligands such as diethylenetriaminepentaacetic acid (DTPA), when they are no longer toxic.[39] At the time of writing (1990) Gd-DTPA is the only magnetic resonance contrast agent approved for human use although other complexes of gadolinium and other metal ions have been used experimentally.

Another paramagnetic metal that has been evaluated in models of myocardial ischaemia is the transition metal manganese (Mn). This is also toxic but it has been chelated with etylenediaminetetraphosphonate (Mn-TP) and with bis-pyridoxal ethylenediamine-diacetate (Mn-DPDP) which lack important cardiovascular side effects in rats.[40,41] Manganese is less paramagnetic than gadolinium because it has only five unpaired electrons.

The effect of paramagnetic molecules upon the relaxation of neighbouring nuclei arises from the motion of their strong magnetic moments (approximately 700 times that of a proton) and the resulting fluctuating electromagnetic field. Components of this field fluctuating at the same frequency as the precession of neighbouring hydrogen nuclei lead to transitions between energy levels of the hydrogen and reduce its longitudinal relaxation time, T_1. The same fluctuations also produce random variations of the precession frequency, leading to a loss of phase coherence and a decrease of transverse relaxation time, T_2.

The effectiveness of a paramagnetic substance in inducing relaxation is proportional to its concentration and to the square of its magnetic moment. Other factors include the number of water molecules associated with it, the rate of exchange of associated water with free water, and the distance between the paramagnetic ion and the relaxing protons.[42] The effect of paramagnetic contrast on signal intensity is complex and depends upon the sequence used. In a T_1-weighted image signal will increase and in a T_2-weighted image it will decrease. The concentration of the contrast agent is also important and in the low concentrations used clinically, the predominant shortening of T_1 compared with T_2 causes an increase in signal intensity, but with increasing concentrations, T_1 shortening becomes less important because the protons are able to relax completely between 90° pulses and there is a decrease in signal because of T_2 shortening.

To understand the complex effects of Gd-DTPA on myocardial images, a knowledge of its pharmacokinetics is important. After intravenous injection, there is rapid distribution throughout the tissues in proportion to blood flow and tissue perfusion. It is confined to the extracellular compartment and is not taken up by cells because of its hydrophilia, its charge and its relatively high molecular weight. In normally perfused tissues, the effects of the contrast agent are most pronounced within the first minutes after injection but in areas of necrosis later imaging may give optimum contrast. Gd-DTPA is mainly excreted through the kidneys and its plasma half-life is approximately 20 minutes. More than 90% of the injected dose is excreted in 24 hours.[39]

Contrast materials with large magnetic susceptibilities create inhomogeneities in the applied magnetic field which accelerate proton dephasing and decrease T_2. When given following coronary occlusion, the ischaemic zone is highlighted because of the shortened T_2 and reduced signal in the normally perfused myocardium. Dysprosium-DTPA is a recently developed contrast agent which exerts such a magnetic susceptibility effect for approximately 60 minutes and it is under evaluation in animal models of acute myocardial infarction.[43]

8.2.2 Applications in ischaemic heart disease

Although myocardial infarction can be detected after several hours of coronary occlusion by magnetic resonance imaging without contrast agents, the detection of ischaemia of short duration is more difficult. Some of the problems have already been discussed and they include the differentiation between signal from slowly moving blood in the cavity and the myocardium, and the areas of high signal in the myocardium caused by motion artefact. Contrast agents have therefore been used for some time to exploit the flow dependent alteration of myocardial signal intensity associated with ischaemia.

Injection of Gd-DTPA in a high dose of 0.5 mmol/kg into dogs with acute coronary occlusion leads to relative enhancement of the ischaemic region as early as two minutes after the occlusion because of the shortened T_2 in the normal myocardium.[44] T_1 and T_2 within the ischaemic segment may also be slightly reduced suggesting that residual flow to the jeopardised myocardium through collateral arteries can be observed. At 5 minutes after injection, differential washout of the contrast material results in shorter T_1 and T_2 of the infarcted zone when compared with normal myocardium.[45] The slow appearance of contrast material in the infarcted region is accompanied by impaired clearance, resulting in a net accumulation of Gd-DTPA at 5 minutes. The consequent increase in signal is most marked in T_1-weighted images. Improved visualisation of infarcts due to T_1 effects can also be seen 24 hours–5 days after infarction and for up to 120 minutes after administration of 0.34 mmol/kg of Gd-DTPA.[46]

The effects of reperfusion have also been studied in animal experiments. Two groups of dogs underwent left anterior descending coronary arterial occlusion for either 15 minutes (reversible injury) or for 60 minutes (irreversible injury), followed by reperfusion for 24 hours.[47] Intravenous administration of 0.5 mmol/kg of Gd-DTPA resulted in significant T_1 shortening of a well demarcated area of injured myocardium producing high signal intensity on T_1-weighted images 5 minutes after the injection of contrast. In this experimental setting of irreversible injury followed by reperfusion, a greater wash-in and a diminished washout of Gd-DTPA when compared with occlusive infarcts might be expected because of the patency of the ischaemia related vessel and compression of the draining veins by oedema. In the animals with short lived occlusion and reversible injury no differences in relaxation times or signal intensity were observed.

In another experiment, enhancement of irreversibly damaged myocardium was seen 55 minutes after 0.35 mmol/kg of Gd-DTPA.[48] Thus, although reperfused infarcts already show an increased signal intensity without contrast administration, Gd-DTPA produces further increases suggesting that it may be useful as a marker of reperfusion.

Although contrast enhanced magnetic resonance imaging is able to identify severe ischaemia and infarction, more subtle alterations in myocardial perfusion are not detected.[49] It has been possible, however, to identify the myocardium at risk in an *ex vivo* dog model of coronary occlusion and reperfusion by virtue of the hyperaemic response.[50] Hyperaemia of both ischaemic and infarcted tissue led to an increased delivery of Gd-DTPA and an increased signal of the reperfused myocardium. The area demonstrated was larger than the infarcted area and it agreed well with the myocardium at risk defined by a dual isotope technique. The use of Gd-DTPA for the definition of myocardium at risk after thrombolytic therapy depends upon further validation *in vivo*.

Several studies have investigated Gd-DTPA in human myocardial infarction.[51–53] Patients imaged 7 days after infarction have shown significant enhancement of the infarcted region after intravenous injection of 0.1 mmol/kg of Gd-DTPA and the mean intensity ratio between infarcted and normal myocardium increased from 1.1 to 1.6.[51] Although there was no such increase in the second echo images, Gd-DTPA is likely to be helpful because first echo images offer a better signal-to-noise ratio and shorter imaging times. Gd-DTPA may also be helpful to discriminate between infarction and spurious high intensity artefacts caused by motion. The effect of Gd-DTPA in chronic infarction is unclear. No signal changes were observed in one study[52] but

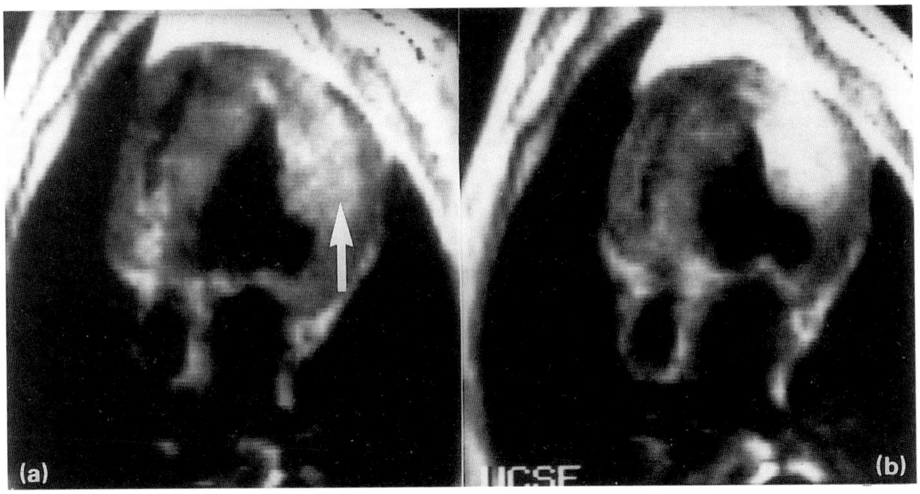

Figure 8.9. Transverse spin echo images of a dog with acute anterior infarction after ligation of the left anterior descending artery. (a) Second echo (TE 60 ms) image without contrast medium. The infarct zone (arrow) has slightly higher signal intensity than the surrounding normal myocardium. (b) First echo image (TE 30 ms) 5 minutes after administration of albumin bound Gd-DTPA. Signal intensity of the infarcted region has clearly increased and the effect persisted for more than 30 minutes.

Table 8.1. The effects of contrast agents on normal myocardium

Contrast agent	Dose (mmol/kg)	Type of study	Reference	Time between injection and imaging (min)	T_1	T_2
Gd-DTPA	0.5	*ex vivo*	45	1	↓↓	↓↓
Gd-DTPA	0.35	*ex vivo*	46	1½	↓	↓
Gd-DTPA	0.35	*ex vivo*	46	5	↓	↔
Gd-DTPA	0.5	*ex vivo*	48	5	↓	↓
Mn-TP	0.05	*in vivo*	41	5	↓↓	↔

↓↓ Pronounced decrease, ↓ slight decrease, ↔ no change.

Table 8.2. The effects of contrast agents on ischaemic myocardium

Contrast agent	Dose (mmol/kg)	Type of study	Reference	Time between occlusion and imaging	Time between injection and imaging (min)	T_1	T_2	TR/TE for best contrast
Gd-DTPA	0.5	*ex vivo*	33	2 min	1	↓	↓	2000/56
Gd-DTPA	0.35	*ex vivo*	46	24 hr	1½	↓	↔	500/56
Gd-DTPA	0.35	*ex vivo*	46	24 hr	5	↓↓	↓	500/56
Gd-DTPA	0.34	*ex vivo*	48	1 hr/reperf 24 hr	5	↓↓	↓	500/28
Gd-DTPA	0.34	*in vivo*	47	1–5 days	15			RR/30
Gd-DTPA	0.2	*ex vivo*	50	3½ min	1	↓	↓	300/15
Gd-DTPA	0.1	*in vivo*	49	<7 days	10			RR/30
Gd-DTPA	0.05	*in vivo*	41	1–2 hr	15–16	↓	↔	RR/20*

* Heart rate 260/min, no other echo time investigaed.
↓↓ Pronounced decrease, ↓ slight decrease, ↔ no change, RR : TR equal to R–R interval.

infarcted myocardium showed a 26% increase in signal intensity in another study.[53] Any lack of enhancement in chronic infarction may be due to opposing concentration dependent effects on T_1 and T_2.

To avoid the rapid extravascular distribution and renal excretion of Gd-DTPA, further complexing with human serum albumin (HSA) has been employed.[54] Gd-DTPA-HSA remains within the blood pool and significant shortening of T_1 of normal myocardium persists for 30 minutes (figure 8.9). However, the problems of differential delivery and retention in normal and ischaemic myocardium and the dose dependent shortening of relaxation times leave many problems to be solved.

To conclude, Gd-DTPA is useful for outlining regional myocardial blood distribution in experimental coronary occlusion, but the short time course of enhancement and the concentration and flow dependency of relaxation rates make quantitative analysis impossible. Since Gd-DTPA is an extracellular marker of myocardial perfusion, it is not extracted by viable myocardium which would be desirable for an ideal contrast agent. A summary of the effects of Gd-DTPA on normal and infarcted myocardium is given in tables 8.1 and 8.2.

8.2.3 Other contrast agents

Early studies demonstrated the potential of intravenous manganous ions (Mn^{2+}) to depict regions of ischaemia in excised dogs' hearts.[55,56] To reduce toxicity manganese has been chelated with ethylene-diamine-tetraphosphonate (Mn-TP). In T_1-weighted spin echo images, signal intensity of normal myocardium increases dramatically after injection of Mn-TP and it remains almost unchanged 1 hour after injection.[40] In contrast, the signal intensity of ischaemic myocardium rises only moderately (figure 8.10). Surprisingly, myocardial T_2 is unaltered by Mn-TP. Mn-TP is excreted by the liver and it remains in the blood pool for a longer time than Gd-DTPA. It also remains in the heart after plasma clearance. Whether this indicates intracellular uptake of Mn-TP and possible redistribution is unknown. If the ligand is not completely stable and ionic manganese is released, use of the agent will be impossible in man.

Another manganese contrast agent is Mn-DPDP.[41] This has shown promise for the differentiation between occlusive and reperfused infarction and for the delineation of the site and extent of tissue salvaged by reperfusion. Signal is increased in reperfused myocardium at least two fold which is substantially higher than that achieved with Gd-DTPA.[48]

8.2.4 Conclusion

Gd-DTPA improves the visibility of acutely infarcted myocardium almost immediately after occlusion. It

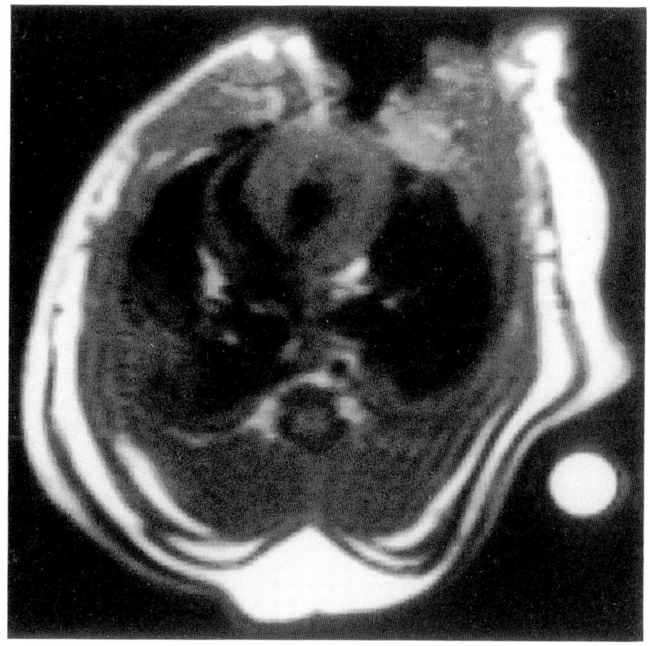

(a)

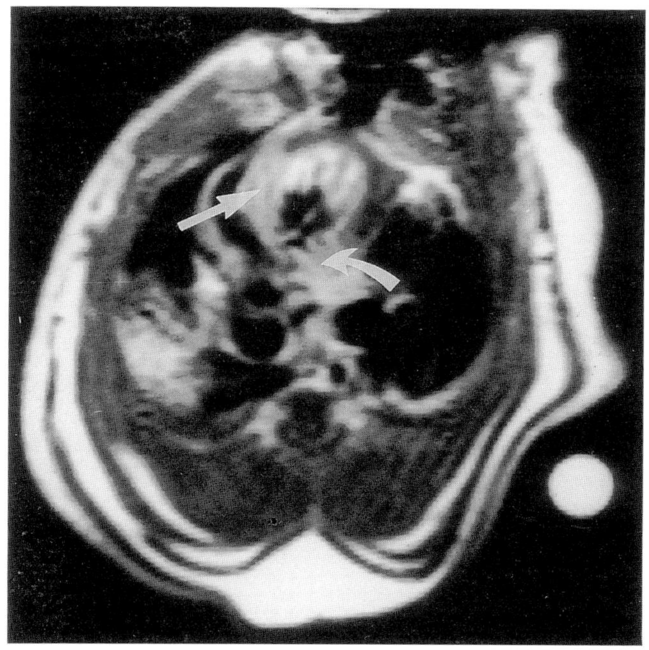

(b)

Figure 8.10. Transverse spin echo image (TE 20 ms) in a rat after occlusion of the left anterior descending artery. (a) Precontrast image. Normal and infarcted myocardium cannot be differentiated. (b) Fifteen minutes after injection of Mn-TP. Normally perfused myocardium in the interventricular septum (arrow) and posterolateral wall (curved arrow) shows higher signal intensity than the infarcted anterior region. Differential enhancement persisted for more than 60 minutes. (Reproduced with permission from *Radiology* 1988; **167**: 129–133.)

aids the identification and delineation of ischaemic myocardium in experimental animals and in man by increasing the signal intensity of ischaemic regions, particularly in spin-echo images with short echo times. An important limitation is the inability to assess myocardial perfusion because of its extracellular distribution. The use of echo planar techniques which permit real-time imaging and the measurement of time-intensity curves may overcome this limitation.

Recently developed manganese compounds have the advantage of slower excretion from the blood pool and more time for imaging. It is not yet clear whether they are retained in the myocardial cells and further elucidation of their toxicity and metabolism will be required before they contrast agents can be safely applied in patients.

References

1 Crooks LE, Hylton NM, Ortendahl DA, Posin JP, Kaufman L. The value of relaxation times and density measurements in clinical MRI. *Invest Radiol* 1987; **22**: 158–69.

2 Herfkens RJ, Sievers R, Kaufman L, *et al.* Nuclear magnetic resonance imaging of the infarcted muscle: a rat model. *Radiology* 1983; **147**: 761–4.

3 Bottomley PA, Hardy CJ, Argersinger RE, Allen-Moore G. A review of 1H magnetic resonance relaxation in pathology: are T_1 and T_2 diagnostic? *Med Phys* 1987; **14**: 1–37.

4 Raaphorst GP, Kruw J, Pintar MM. Nuclear magnetic resonance study of mammalian cell water. *Biophys J* 1964; **15**: 391–402.

5 Prato FS, Drost DJ, King M, *et al.* Cardiac T_1 calculations from MR spin-echo images. *Magn Reson Med* 1987; **4**: 227–43.

6 Johnson G, Ormerod IEC, Barnes D, Tofts PS, MacManus D. Accuracy and precision in the measurement of relaxation times from nuclear magnetic resonance images. *Br J Radiol* 1987; **60**: 143–53.

7 Filipchuk NG, Peshock RM, Malloy CR, *et al.* Detection and localization of recent myocardial infarction by magnetic resonance imaging. *Am J Cardiol* 1986; **58**: 214–9.

8 Majumdar S, Orphanoudakis SC, Gmitro A, O'Donnell M, Gore JC. Errors in the measurements of T_2 using multiple-echo MRI techniques. I: Effects of radio-frequency pulse imperfections. *Magn Reson Med* 1986; **3**: 397–417.

9 Williams ES, Kaplan JI, Thatcher F, Zimmerman G, Knobel SB. Prolongation of proton spin lattice relaxation times in regionally ischaemic tissue from dog hearts. *J Nucl Med* 1980; **21**: 449–53.

10 Higgins CB, Herfkens R, Lipton MJ, *et al.* Nuclear magnetic resonance imaging of acute myocardial infarction in dogs: alteration in magnetic relaxation times. *Am J Cardiol* 1983; **52**: 184–8.

11 Tscholakoff D, Higgins CB, McNamara, Derugin N. Early-phase myocardial infarction: evaluation by MR imaging. *Radiology* 1986; **159**: 667–72.

12 Dilworth LR, Aisen AM, Mancini GBJ, Buda AJ. Serial nuclear magnetic resonance imaging in acute myocardial infarction. *Am J Cardiol* 1987; **59**: 1203–5.

13 Been M, Smith MA, Ridgway MP, *et al.* Serial changes in the T_1 magnetic relaxation parameter after myocardial infarction in man. *Br Heart J* 1988; **59**: 1–8.

14 Wesbey G, Higgins CB, Lanzer P, Botvinick E, Lipton MJ. Imaging and characterization of acute myocardial infarction in vivo by gated nuclear magnetic resonance. *Circulation* 1984; **69**: 125–130.

15 McNamara MT, Higgins CB, Schechtmann N, *et al.* Detection and characterization of acute myocardial infarction in man with use of gated magnetic resonance. *Circulation* 1985; **71**: 717–24.

16 Fisher MR, McNamara MT, Higgins CB. Acute myocardial infarction: MR evaluation in 29 patients. *Am J Roentgenol* 1987; **148**: 247–51.

17 Pflugfelder PW, Wisenberg G, Prato FS, Carroll SE, Turner KL. Early detection of canine myocardial infarction by magnetic resonance imaging in vivo. *Circulation* 1985; **71**: 587–94.

18 Johnston DL, Thompson RC, Liu P, *et al.* Magnetic resonance imaging during acute myocardial infarction. *Am J Cardiol* 1986; **57**: 1059–65.

19 Pflugfelder PW, Wisenberg G, Prato FS, Turner KL, Carroll SE. Serial imaging of canine myocardial infarction by in vivo nuclear magnetic resonance. *J Am Coll Cardiol* 1986; **7**: 843–9.

20 Higgins CB, Lanzer P, Stark D, *et al.* Imaging by nuclear magnetic resonance in patients with chronic ischemic heart disease. *Circulation* 1984; **69**: 523–31.

21 McNamara MT, Higgins CB. Magnetic resonance imaging of chronic myocardial infarcts in man. *Am J Roentgenol* 1986; **146**: 315–20.

22 Higgins CB, Siemers PT, Schmidt W, Newell JD. Evaluation of myocardial ischemic damage of various ages by computerized transmission tomography. *Circulation* 1979; **60**: 284–91.

23 Johnston DL, Brady TJ, Ratner AV, *et al.* Assessment of myocardial ischemia with proton magnetic resonance: effects of a three hour coronary occlusion with and without reperfusion. *Circulation* 1985; **71**: 595–601.

24 Nayler WG, Elz JS. Reperfusion injury: laboratory artifact or clinical dilemma? *Circulation* 1988; **74**: 215–21.

25 Ratner AV, Okada RD, Newell JB, Pohost GM. The relationship between nuclear magnetic relaxation parameters and myocardial perfusion with acute coronary arterial occlusion and reperfusion. *Circulation* 1985; **71**: 823–8.

26 Tscholakoff D, Higgins CB, Sechtem U, Caputo G, Derugin N. MRI of reperfused myocardial infarcts in dogs. *Am J Roentgenol* 1986; **146**: 925–30.

27 Johnston DL, Liu P, Rosen BR, Levine RA, Beaulieu PA, Brady TJ, Okada RD. In vivo detection of reperfused myocardium by nuclear magnetic resonance imaging. *J Am Coll Cardiol* 1987; **9**: 127–35.

28 Rokey R, Verani MS, Bolli R, *et al.* Myocardial infarct size quantification by MR imaging early after coronary artery occlusion in dogs. *Radiology* 1986; **158**: 771–4.

29 Caputo GR, Sechtem U, Tscholakoff D, Higgins CB. Measurement of myocardial infarct size at early and late time intervals using MR imaging: an experimental study in dogs. *Am J Roentgenol* 1987; **149**: 237–43.

30 Thompson RC, Canby RC, Lojeski EW, Ratner AV, Fallon JT, Pohost GM. Adriamycin cardiotoxicity and proton nuclear magnetic resonance relaxation properties. *Am Heart J* 1987; **113**: 1144–9.

31 Ng TC, Daugherty JP, Evanochko WT, Digerness SB, Durant JR, Glickson JD. Detection of antineoplastic agent induced cardiotoxicity by P–31 NMR of perfused rat hearts. *Biochem Biophys Res Commun* 1983; **110**: 339–47.

32 Tscholakoff D, Aherne T, Yee ES, Derugin N, Higgins CB. Cardiac transplantation in dogs: evaluation with MR. *Radiology* 1985; **157**: 697–702.

33 Aherne T, Tscholakoff D, Finkbeiner W, *et al*. Magnetic resonance imaging of cardiac transplants: the evaluation of rejection of cardiac allografts with and without immunosuppression. *Circulation* 1986; **74**: 145–156.

34 Wisenberg G, Pflugfelder PW, Kostuk WJ, McKenzie FN, Prato FS. Diagnostic applicability of magnetic resonance imaging in assessing human cardiac allograft rejection. *Am J Cardiol* 1987; 60: 130–6.

35 Revel D, Mathieu D, Helenon O, *et al*. Heart transplantation: follow-up with MR imaging (Abstract). *Radiology* 1987; **165(P)**: 27.

36 Levine RA, Weyman AE, Dinsmore RE, *et al*. Noninvasive tissue characterization: diagnosis of lipomatous hypertrophy. *J Am Coll Cardiol* 1986; **7**: 688–92.

37 Johnston DL, Rice L, Vick W, Roberts R, Rokey R. Assessment of myocardial iron by nuclear magnetic resonance imaging. *J Am Coll Cardiol* 1988; **11**: 226A.

38 Saini S, Frankel RB, Stark DD, Ferruci JT. Magnetism: a primer and review. *Am J Roentgenol* 1988; **150**: 735–43.

39 Weinmann HJ, Brasch RC, Press WR, Wesbey GE. Characteristics of Gadolinium-DTPA complex: a potential NMR contrast agent. *Am J Roentgenol* 1984; **142**: 619–24.

40 Pflugfelder PW, Wendland MF, Holt WW, *et al*. Acute myocardial ischemia: MR imaging with Mn-TP. *Radiology* 1988; **167**: 129–33.

41 Saeed M, Wagner S, Wendland M, Derugin N, Higgins CB. In vivo differentiation between occlusive and reperfused myocardial infarctions with myocardial persistent NMR contrast media (Abstract). *Circulation* 1988; **78** (Suppl II): II–539.

42 Koutcher JA, Burt CT, Lauffer RB, Brady TJ. Contrast agents and spectroscopic probes in NMR. *J Nucl Med* 1984; **25**: 506–513.

43 Brown JJ, Higgins CB. Myocardial paramagnetic contrast agents for MR imaging. *Am J Roentgenol* 1988; **151**: 865–72.

44 McNamara MT, Higgins CB, Ehman RL, Revel D, Sievers R, Brasch RC. Acute myocardial ischaemia: magnetic resonance contrast enhancement with Gadolinium-DTPA. *Radiology* 1984; **153**: 157–63.

45 Wesbey GE, Higgins CB, McNamara MT, *et al*. Effect of Gadolinium-DTPA on the magnetic relaxation times of normal and infarcted myocardium. *Radiology* 1984; **153**: 165–9.

46 Rehr RB, Peshock RM, Malloy CR, *et al*. Improved in vivo magnetic resonance imaging of acute myocardial infarction after intravenous paramagnetic contrast agent administration. *Am J Cardiol* 1986; **57**: 864–8.

47 McNamara MT, Tscholakoff D, Revel D, *et al*. Differentiation of reversible and irreversible myocardial injury by MR imaging with and without Gadolinium-DTPA. *Radiology* 1986; **158**: 765–9.

48 Peshock RM, Malloy CR, Buja LM, Nunnally RL, Parkey RW, Willerson JT. Magnetic resonance imaging of acute myocardial infarction: gadolinium diethylenetriamine pentaacetic acid as a marker of reperfusion. *Circulation* 1986; **74**: 1434–40.

49 Johnston DL, Liu P, Lauffer RB, *et al*. Use of Gadolinium-DTPA as a myocardial perfusion agent: potential applications and limitations for magnetic resonance imaging. *J Nucl Med* 1987; **28**: 871–7.

50 Schaefer S, Malloy CR, Katz J, *et al*. Gadolinium-DTPA-enhanced nuclear magnetic resonance imaging of reperfused myocardium: identification of the myocardial bed at risk. *J Am Coll Cardiol* 1988; **12**: 1064–72.

51 De Roos A, Doornbos J, van der Wall EE, van Voorthuisen AE. MR imaging of acute myocardial infarction: value of Gd-DTPA. *Am J Roentgenol* 1988; **150**: 531–4.

52 Eichstaedt HW, Felix R, Dougherty FC, Langer M, Rutsch W, Schmutzler H. Magnetic resonance imaging in different stages of myocardial infarction using the contrast agent Gadolinium-DTPA. *Clin Cardiol* 1986; **9**: 527–35.

53 Seiderer M, von Arnim T, Moser E, Rienmueller R, Hahn D. Gd-DTPA in der kernspintomographischen Diagnostik chronischer Myokardinfarkte. *Fortschr Röntgenstr* 1986; **145**: 666–73.

54 Schmiedl U, Ogan M, Paajanen H, *et al*. Albumin labeled with Gd-DTPA as an intravascular, blood pool-enhancing agent for MR imaging: biodistribution and imaging studies. *Radiology* 1987; **162**: 205–10.

55 Brady TJ, Goldman MR, Pykett IL, *et al*. Proton nuclear magnetic resonance imaging of regionally ischemic canine hearts: effect of paramagnetic proton signal enhancement. *Radiology* 1982; **144**: 343–7.

56 Goldman MR, Brady TJ, Pykett IL, *et al*. Quantification of experimental myocardial infarction using nuclear magnetic resonance imaging and paramagnetic ion contrast enhancement in excised canine hearts. *Circulation* 1982; **66**: 1012–6.

Chapter 9
Magnetic Resonance Angiography

DAVID FIRMIN

Because signal from flowing blood can be manipulated almost at will, there has been considerable interest in magnetic resonance angiography in which images of blood vessels are produced without detail from surrounding stationary tissue. The aim is to produce angiograms that avoid the need for invasive arteriography and, although important progress is being made, the task is not easy. Tomographic imaging is not an ideal method of demonstrating tortuous vessels and three dimensional imaging becomes important despite the problem of coping with large amounts of data. A further problem is to ensure that blood in the vascular lumen always gives signal because an area of signal loss caused by turbulence could be interpreted as a stenosis. At the time of writing (1990) magnetic resonance angiography is still developing and workers in the field are searching for a robust technique. Large clinical trials comparing magnetic resonance with X-ray angiography have not been performed. Nonetheless, very promising images can be obtained from static vessels such as those in the head and the periphery. X-ray angiography may still be needed if surgery is contemplated, but magnetic resonance angiography is a valuable addition to conventional imaging.

All the angiographic imaging techniques make use of one or more of the factors that affect the signal from flowing blood and these are described in detail in chapter 10. The potential of magnetic resonance to produce angiograms was realised at least 2 years before any clinical results were presented.[1] Nishimura and colleagues have reviewed the technical aspects of angiography[2] and Alfidi and colleagues have reviewed the more clinical aspects.[3] The techniques fall into two categories: phase shift and time of flight methods.

9.1 Phase shift angiography

Wedeen and colleagues[4] were the first group to describe a method of producing a subtraction angiogram showing a projection image of arterial blood. They used a spin echo sequence but without slice selection gradients during the 90 and 180° pulses so that signal was obtained from all tissue within the receiving coil. Two images were acquired, one in systole during the phase of rapid arterial flow, and the other in diastole during slow flow. In the systolic image, the rapid flow causes loss of signal from flowing blood but there is little or no loss in the diastolic image. The signal from static material outside the arteries is identical in the two images and subtraction leaves only the signal from arterial blood. Because venous flow is much less pulsatile and signal is preserved in both images, the veins are not seen in the subtracted image. Meuli and colleagues[5] used this method in a number of normal subjects and four selected patients. The images showed the same features as conventional X-ray angiography.

The main disadvantage of this method is that the two images are not acquired synchronously and any change of shape or position of the vessels between systole and diastole will produce artefacts on the subtraction image. Methods were therefore developed that used alterations in the pulse sequence to change the signal from blood depending upon its rate of flow.[6,7] Velocity sensitive gradient profiles were used in one sequence and velocity insensitive profiles in the other, with all other sequence parameters being identical. The velocity sensitive sequence causes loss of signal from flowing material but there is no loss in the velocity insensitive sequence, and stationary material gives the same signal in both sequences. Reasonable subtraction angiograms can be produced (figure 9.1), but problems still exist because complete dephasing of the flow signal in one acquisition and rephasing in the other rarely occurs, particularly in tortuous or bifurcating vessels. A second problem arises from the effects of eddy currents on the static tissue signal which differ slightly in the two sequences and lead to incomplete cancellation of stationary tissue.

These methods use the fact that flow in the direction of a magnetic field gradient introduces phase shifts and loss of signal. Dumoulin and Hart[8] also used phase shifts but in a more controlled way. They imaged during diastole or used even echo rephasing (see chapter 10) to ensure that signal from flowing blood was not lost. Data was collected twice using slightly different sequences (figure 9.2). In the first, a bipolar gradient was introduced which had no effect on stationary material but which imparted a phase shift to material with a component of flow in the direction of the gradient. In the second, the polarity of the bipolar gradient was reversed and so the flow-related phase shift was also reversed. Complex subtraction of the data sets acquired in this way results in signal only from flowing material, and the amplitude of the signal is proportional to velocity. The relationship between velocity and signal amplitude is linear only for phase shifts in the range of ± 1 radian, but the bipolar gradients can be adjusted to keep the phase shifts within this range.

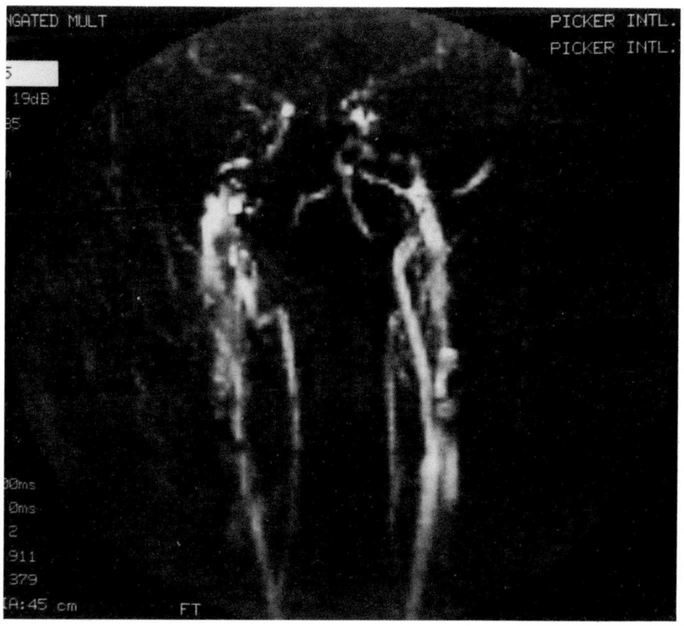

Figure 9.1. Magnetic resonance angiogram produced by the subtraction of images produced with velocity-sensitive and velocity-insensitive sequences. Multiple contiguous coronal slices were acquired of the neck of a normal subject without cardiac triggering. After image subtraction, the images were combined to produce a projection angiogram through the neck.

Although the method only detects vessels with a component of flow in a single direction, additional acquisitions can be made to show tortuous vessels, at the expense of imaging time. More recently it has been adapted for three-dimensional acquisition so that projection images can be reconstructed from any region of interest and can be viewed at any angle. Excellent angiograms have been produced, particularly of the intracranial and peripheral arteries, but the main disadvantages are imaging time and the requirement for an extremely stable imaging system.

9.2 Time of flight methods

9.2.1 Magnetic tagging

Dixon and colleagues[9] developed a method of angiography in 1986 using magnetic tagging. An important advantage of tagging is that it has very little effect upon the later part of the sequence in which data is collected, and this allows very good subtraction of stationary tissue. They used a special form of radiofrequency pulse in a small localised transmitter coil, which was designed to affect only flowing spins. This transmitter coil was positioned on the subject's neck

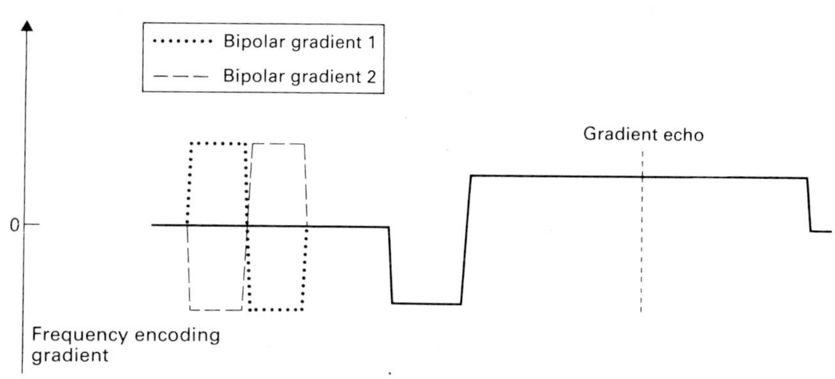

Figure 9.2. Typical frequency encoding gradient profile with added bipolar gradient sections of opposite polarity similar to those used by Dumoulin and Hart in their form of phase contrast angiography.[8]

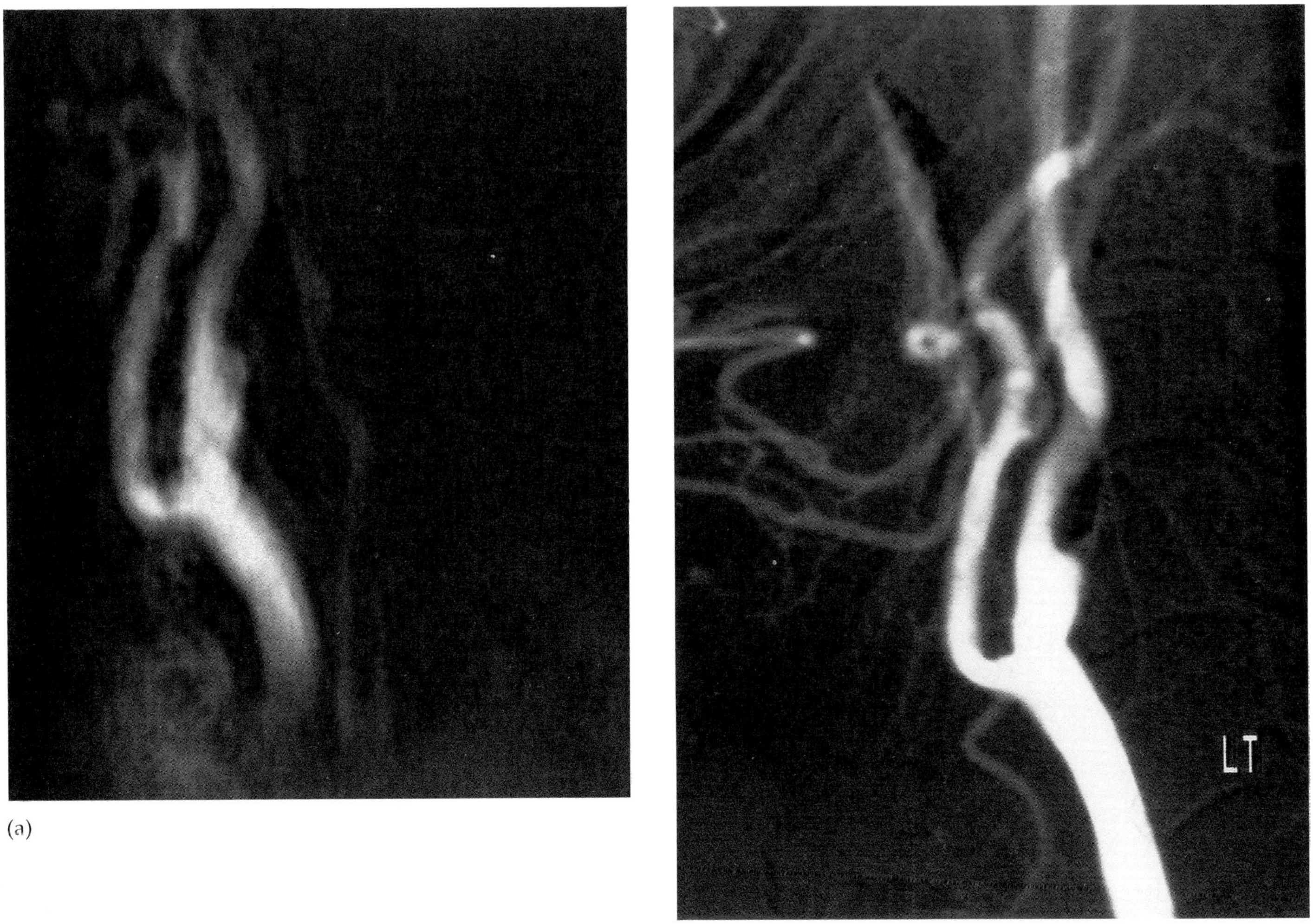

Figure 9.3. A comparison between a magnetic resonance subtraction angiogram (a) and a conventional contrast X-ray angiogram (b) of a stenotic lesion causing a 50% narrowing of the internal carotid artery. The magnetic resonance angiogram was acquired in approximately 4 min and has a spatial resolution of 0.5 mm (horizontal) by 0.7 mm (vertical).[11] (Reproduced with permission from Dr D.G. Nishimura.)

such that the magnetisation of blood flowing through the underlying carotid artery was inverted. The duration of the pulse was chosen so that a reasonable length of the carotid artery contained inverted spins, and two different methods were used to separate flowing blood from the surrounding stationary tissue. In the first method, the inversion was applied on alternate pulses so that flowing blood was given an extra phase encoding term and mispositioned into an empty area of the image. In the second method, two acquisitions were averaged, one with the special radio-frequency pulse and the other without. Subtraction of the two acquisitions cancelled stationary material as its phase was the same for both, but added signal from flowing material which was 180° out of phase in each acquisition.

Any slight difference in the acquistions of the two data sets to be subtracted may result in poor subtraction of signals from stationary tissue and a 'ghost' appearance on the subtraction image. Dixon has described a useful method of reducing remaining signal from stationary tissue without affecting the signal from smaller structures such as blood vessels.[9] A low amplitude short duration 'twister' gradient is applied through the image projection. This gradient causes a phase shift which is dependent on depth through the

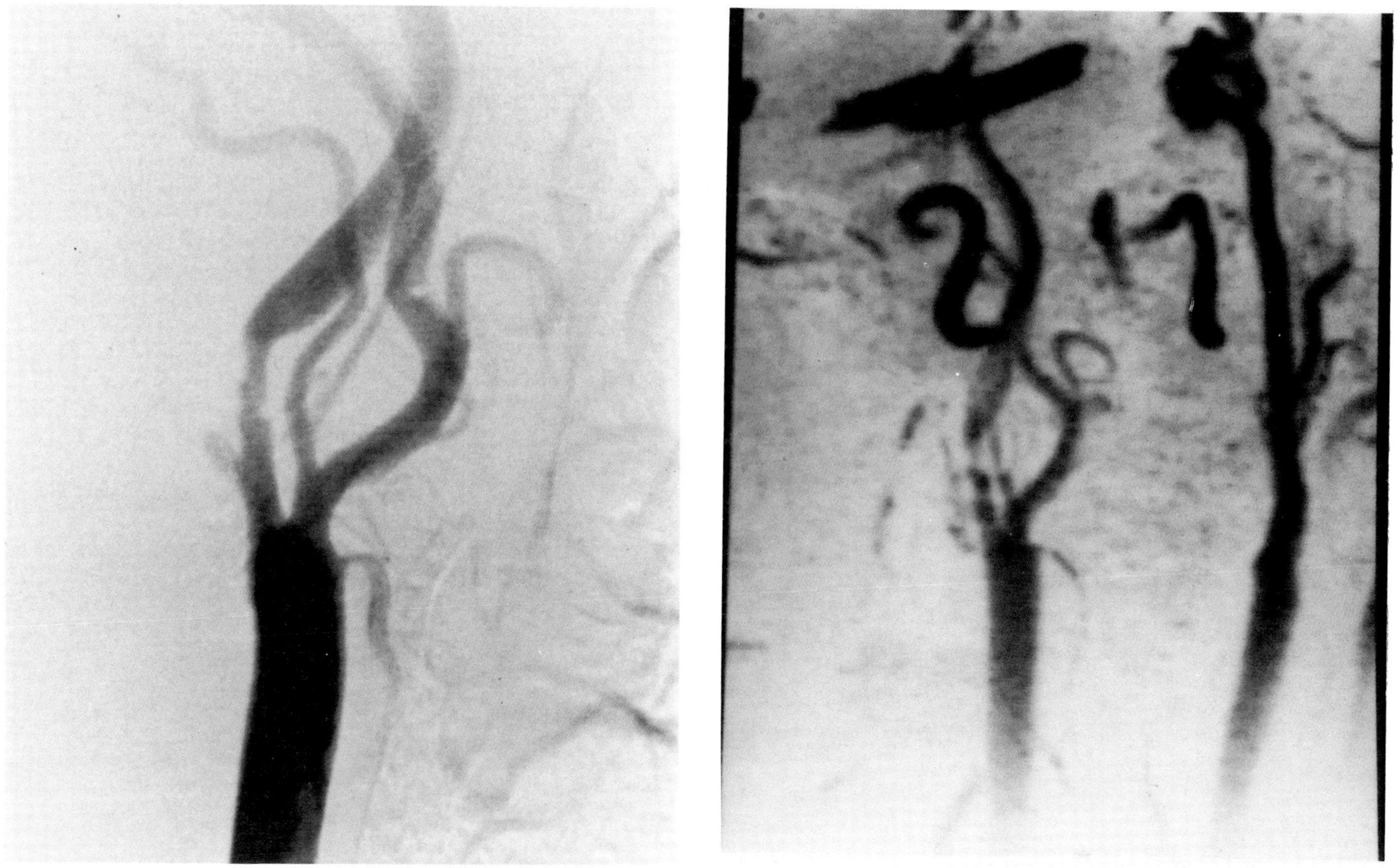

(a) (b)

Figure 9.4. Comparison between an intra-arterial digital subtraction angiogram (a) and a magnetic resonance angiogram (b) of a patient with bilateral carotid stenoses. For the magnetic resonance study both carotid arteries were acquired simultaneously using a 32 mm sagittal slab selection with 16–32 partitions. The data set was post-processed using a maximum intensity projection ray tracing algorithm. (Reproduced with permission from Dr T.J. Masaryk.)

projection. For large objects such as stationary tissue which cover a large range of depths through the projection, signal cancellation will occur, but the signal from small structures will be phase shifted but not cancelled. Although successful, problems can occur when vessels cross in the projection image as the phases of their signals will be unknown and could add or subtract in an unpredictable manner.

Magnetic tagging has also been described by Nishimura and colleagues[10,11] who used two inversion recovery sequences, one with and one without a slice selection gradient during the 180° pulse. Without a slice selective 180° pulse unexcited spins wash into the slice in the period between inversion and reading of the signal and reduce the signal from flowing blood. Subtraction of the two signals leads to good suppression of static material. Figure 9.3 shows examples of this technique, each angiogram being acquired in 4 min with an in-plane resolution of 0.5 × 0.7 mm.

9.2.2 Wash-in effects

A rapid method of high resolution three-dimensional angiography uses the signal enhancement produced by wash-in and wash-out effects. If a gradient echo sequence is repeated rapidly, stationary tissue becomes saturated and produces a low signal, but blood flowing into the excited region is unsaturated and produces a high signal. Three-dimensional acquisition involves the excitation of a thick slab of material followed by phase encoding gradients to resolve the signal in two dimensions and a frequency encoding gradient in the third. Laub and colleagues successfully adapted the technique for angiography.[12,13] This form of spatial encoding has advantages because the phase encoding gradients produce smaller phase shifts and therefore less phase dispersion and signal loss than conventional slice selection. The slab thickness, repeat time and the radio-frequency flip angle have to be optimised for good contrast between the blood and stationary tissue, but one problem is that slowly flowing blood is difficult to image because of saturation. Clinical examples are shown in figure 9.4.

Another approach which uses similar ideas but which is designed to overcome the problem of slow flow, is to use a saturation recovery sequence.[14] A slice of tissue is saturated by a radio-frequency pulse and a dephasing gradient so that its signal contribution to any sequence which follows rapidly is minimal. Very little is seen apart from high signal where fully magnetised blood has washed into the image plane. The sequence is repeated rapidly with phase encoding steps so that an image can be acquired in a matter of seconds. As each image is acquired in only a matter of seconds a large number of very narrow contiguous image slices can easily be obtained and can then be combined into a three-dimensional image.

9.3 Functional angiography

Magnetic resonance velocity mapping (chapter 10) has allowed functional angiograms to be acquired in which arterial flow velocities are displayed as opposed to a purely anatomical image.[15] The technique is particularly suitable for the study of large vessels, and stenoses can be detected and quantified from the increase in velocity which occurs across them. Velocity mapping is particularly useful because moderate variations in signal intensity which occur from wash-in and wash-out or dephasing effects do not reduce its accuracy. The acquisition is normally from a single slice in systole but short echo time sequences with very short repeat times can produce a limited multislice acquisition over a short period of systole when velocity is relatively unchanged. Multislice projection angiograms can then be combined to form a projection image and the technique is illustrated in chapter 11.

References

1 Mackovski A. Selective projection imaging: Applications to radiography and NMR. *IEEE Trans Med Imag* 1982; **MI–1**: 42–7.

2 Nishimura DG, Macovski A, Pauly JM. Magnetic resonance angiography. *IEEE Trans Med Imag* 1986; **MI–1**: 140–51.

3 Alfidi RJ, Haacke EM, Lenz GW, *et al*. MR angiography of peripheral, carotid, and coronary arteries. *Am J Roentgenol* 1987; **149**: 1097–109.

4 Wedeen VJ, Meuli RA, Edelman RR, *et al*. Projective imaging of pulsatile flow with magnetic resonance. *Science* 1985; **230**: 946–8.

5 Meuli RA, Wedeen VJ, Geller SC, *et al*. MR gated subtraction angiography: evaluation of lower extremities. *Radiology* 1986; **159**: 411–8.

6 Axel L, Morton D. MR flow imaging by velocity compensated/uncompensated difference images. *J Comput Assist Tomogr* 1987; **11**: 31–4.

7 Nayler GL, Firmin DN. Multislice MRI Angiography. *Magn Reson Imag* 1986; **4**: 156 (Abstract).

8 Dumoulin CL, Hart HR. Magnetic resonance angiography. *Radiology* 1986; **161**: 717–20.

9 Dixon WT, Du LN, Faul DD, Gado M, Rossnick S. Projection angiograms of blood labeled by adiabatic fast passage. *Magn Reson Med* 1986; **3**: 454–62.

10 Nishimura DG, Macovski A, Pauly JM, Conolly SM. MR angiography by selective inversion recovery. *Magn Reson Med* 1987; **4**: 193–202.

11 Nishimura DG, Macovski A, Pauly JM. Considerations of magnetic resonance angiography. *Magn Reson Med* 1988; **7**: 472–84.

12 Laub G. Magnetization Recovery Angiography. *Proceedings of the Eighth Annual Meeting of the Society of Magnetic Resonance in Medicine*. 1989: **153** (Abstract).

13 Masaryk TJ, Ross JS, Modic MT, Lenz GW, Haacke EM. Carotid bifurcation: MR imaging—work in progress. *Radiology* 1988; **166**: 461–6.

14 Keller PJ, Drayer BP, Fram EK, Williams KD, Dumoulin CL, Souza SP. MR angiography with two-dimensional acquisition and three-dimensional display. *Radiology* 1989; **173**: 527–32.

15 Mohiaddin RH, Sampson C, Firmin DN, Underwood SR, Rees RSO, Longmore DB. MR flow imaging in atherosclerotic vascular disease. *Proceedings of the Eighth Annual Meeting of the Society of Magnetic Resonance in Medicine*, 1989: **204** (Abstract).

Chapter 10
Magnetic Resonance Flow Imaging

DAVID FIRMIN AND
RICHARD UNDERWOOD

The purpose of the heart is to maintain flow in the cardiovascular system and the ability of magnetic resonance to measure flow is one of the reasons why it is such an important imaging technique. The study of the effects of flow and motion on the magnetic resonance signal has a history almost as long as the experimental studies of magnetic resonance itself. In 1948, 2 years after the first description of magnetic resonance,[1,2] Bloembergen and colleagues studied the effect of molecular motion on the line width of the signal.[3] The first to note the effect of coherent motion or flow was Suryan.[4] Applications were soon developed using Suryan's finding that longitudinal relaxation was effectively increased by motion. These were aimed at increasing the signal to noise ratio in high resolution spectroscopy and accurate measurements of T_1 in liquids. Although a number of the studies indicated that flow measurement would be possible, it was not until 1959 that the first work on this was presented.[5,6] Interestingly, these early studies were developed with the measurement of blood flow in mind.

In the following years a wide variety of methods of flow measurement were developed, all of which used one of three different effects:

1 In-flow/out-flow
2 Time of flight
3 Phase shift

After the development of magnetic resonance imaging the way in which flow affected the image was studied and methods of flow measurement were investigated. Again, the same three effects were used and many have now been applied both *in vitro* and *in vivo*.

10.1 Flow effects on the magnetic resonance signal

Most of the early work on flow used continuous wave systems. In these, the absorption of the radiofrequency radiation is measured either by sweeping the frequency through the Larmor frequency, or by altering the magnetic field with a fixed frequency. In continuous wave systems the magnetic resonance signal is proportional to the population difference between the two allowed nuclear energy states. For a stationary sample this difference can be altered by previous exposure to radio-frequency radiation at the Larmor frequency. If the sample is flowing, the population difference can be altered in two further ways. Firstly, by exchange of saturated spins for unsaturated spins as material flows out of the region being examined and, secondly at higher flows, from the wash-in of unpolarised spins from outside the magnetic field. The first of these mechanisms will increase the signal amplitude and the second will decrease it.

The early non-imaging studies have been reviewed by Jones and Child[7] and by Zhernovoi and Latyshev.[8] Bowman and Kudravcev, in 1959,[5] described experimental arrangements and observed the effect of flow on the magnetic resonance signal, and they demonstrated that slight adjustments to the arrangement could alter the relationship. They suggested that this was due to the signal's dependence upon a number of phenomena including relaxation, saturation, radiofrequency absorption coefficients and, in particular, upon the geometrical arrangement of the receiving coil. They concluded that a method of flow measurement might be conceived but they did not suggest a method.

10.2 Flow effects in magnetic resonance imaging

10.2.1 Wash-in/wash-out

The same effects influence the signal in images as in non-imaging experiments. Unless the sequence is re-

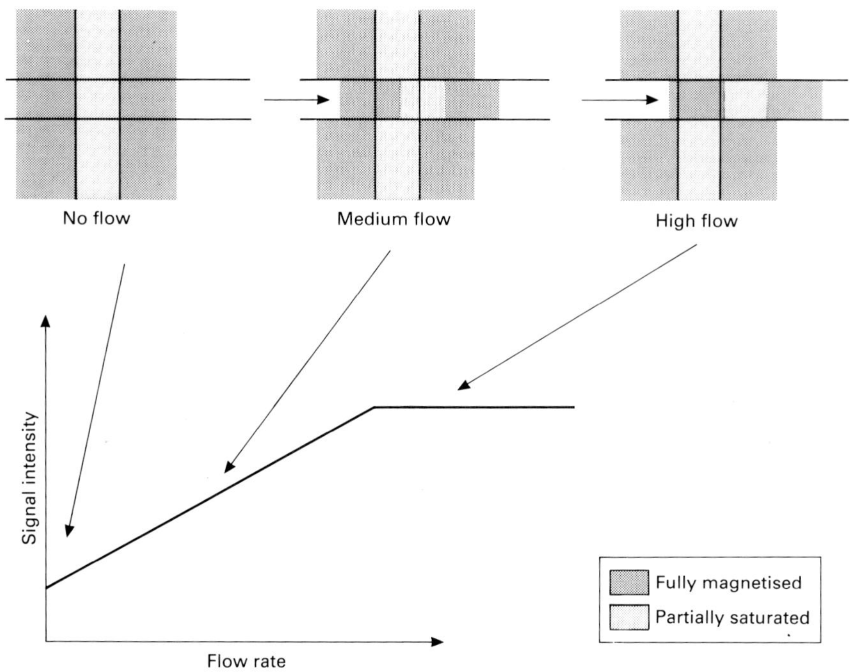

Figure 10.1. Stationary material within the imaging plane is partially saturated and its signal is reduced. Fully magnetised material flowing into the slice refreshes the saturated material and increases the signal. The faster the flow the greater the enhancement until all the material within the slice has been replenished in the time between the pulses.

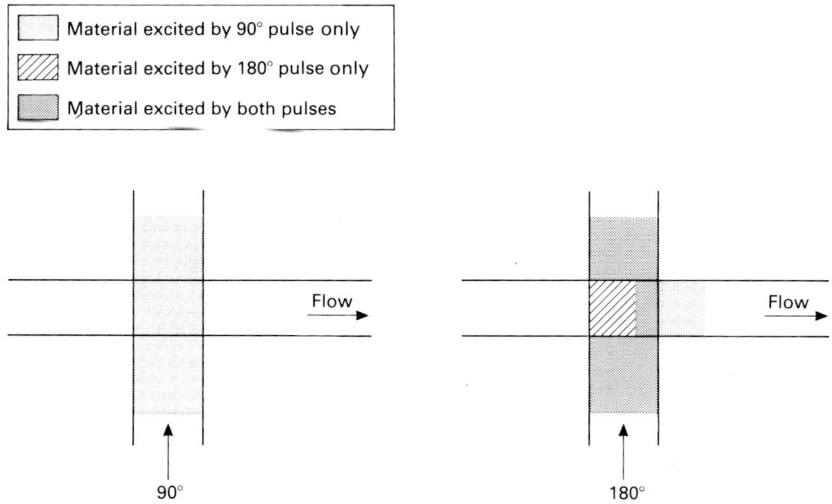

Figure 10.2. A fully selective spin echo sequence requires that material that is in the slice during the 90° pulse is also in the slice for the 180° pulse. When flow is perpendicular to the slice there will be a certain amount of washout between the two pulses and the spin echo signal reduced or lost altogether.

peated very slowly, material in the imaging plane is partially saturated by previous excitations. Flowing material refreshes the saturated material and increases the signal. The faster the flow, the greater the enhancement until all the material within the slice has been replenished in the time between pulses (figure 10.1). Singer and Crooks[9] were among the first to point this out in images and later workers investigated the effect during multislice imaging.[10] The enhancement occurs only in the first few slices in multislice imaging and deeper slices require higher flow for the effect to be observed. With laminar flow, the presence of a small area of higher velocity laminae at the centre of a blood vessel confirms the effect.

Another way in which signal is reduced is by through plane flow. With the spin echo sequence for example, if a slice selection gradient is applied during both the 90 and the 180° pulses, material which flows out of the slice between the two pulses will not contribute to the image (figure 10.2). Grant and Back[11] were the first to

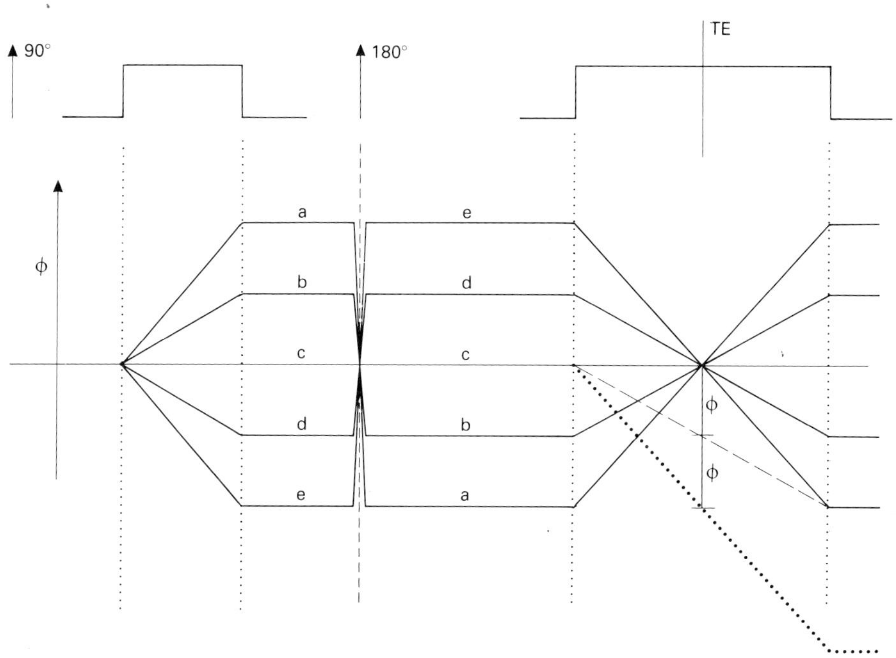

Figure 10.3. The effect of a typical frequency encoding (read) gradient and radio-frequency pulses of a spin echo sequence on the phase of the signal from equally spaced points along the direction of the gradient (a, b, c, d and e). The signal from stationary material is dephased and then rephased by the two gradient portions to form an imaging echo at time TE. If material moves between the times of the two gradient sections then the signals will be phase shifted by different amounts and will not rephase at time TE. The dashed trace is from material which moves from c to d between the gradients, and this results in a phase shift, φ, at time TE. The dotted trace shows material which has moved twice as far, from c to e, and this results in twice the phase shift, 2φ.

investigate this effect, and Bradley and colleagues[12] later described a linear relationship between the signal decrease and the velocity.

10.2.2 Signal dephasing

The effect of a magnetic field gradient on the phase of spins is described in chapter 1, and figure 10.3 shows the frequency encoding gradient of a spin echo sequence and its effect on the phase of signals from different positions (a, b, c, d and e) which dephase and then rephase to form an echo at time TE. If the material at position c moves to position d between the two lobes of the gradient, then the effect of the second gradient is no longer equal to the first and the signal no longer rephases at time TE and it does not contribute fully to the echo. If the material moves twice as far to position e, the resultant phase shift will be twice as large. In fact, if the material moves with a constant velocity the phase does not follow the exact path shown in figure 10.3 but the result is the same. The actual phase paths are shown in figure 10.4. Simplified analysis shows that the phase shift φ caused by motion with velocity v in the direction of a typical frequency encoding gradient profile is:

$$\phi = \gamma G \Delta \delta v$$

where G is the gradient amplitude, δ is the duration of each portion and Δ is the time between the two portions.

If all the material moves at the same velocity (that is, a moves to b, b to c, c to d, and so on) then the phase shifts will be the same and, although the resultant phase will not be zero, the gradient echo will be formed correctly (figure 10.5). Alternatively if the material has a range of velocities then the rephasing will not be complete and the size of the echo will be diminished (figure 10.6). In an image it is necessary to consider the phases within each voxel as opposed to across the whole imaging plane, but the above description still applies and a voxel containing blood moving with a range of velocities will lose signal. Figure 10.7 shows the situation for a tube with a parabolic flow profile. The high shear at the edge of the tube leads to phase dispersion and signal loss but the low shear in the centre results in a large overall phase shift without signal loss. This description applies whether the gradient consists of a positive and a negative lobe or two positive lobes separated by a 180° pulse (figure 10.8). In practice both the slice selection and the frequency encoding gradients of spin echo and gradient echo sequences cause dephasing in voxels containing a range of velocities.

Pulsatile flow and variations in velocity in a single voxel between each phase encoding step result in even greater signal loss and produce image artefacts. These

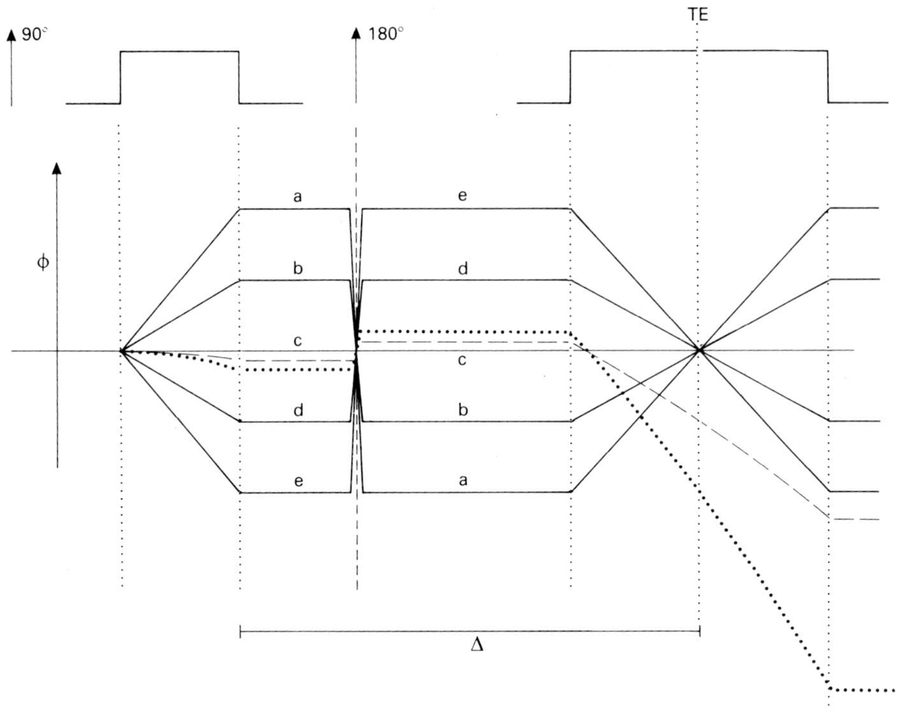

Figure 10.4. The actual phase paths that occur when material is moving continuously. The dashed trace shows material that has flowed from c to d in time Δ, and the dotted trace shows material moving twice as fast producing twice the phase shift. The phase changes are curved rather than linear when flow occurs during the gradient.

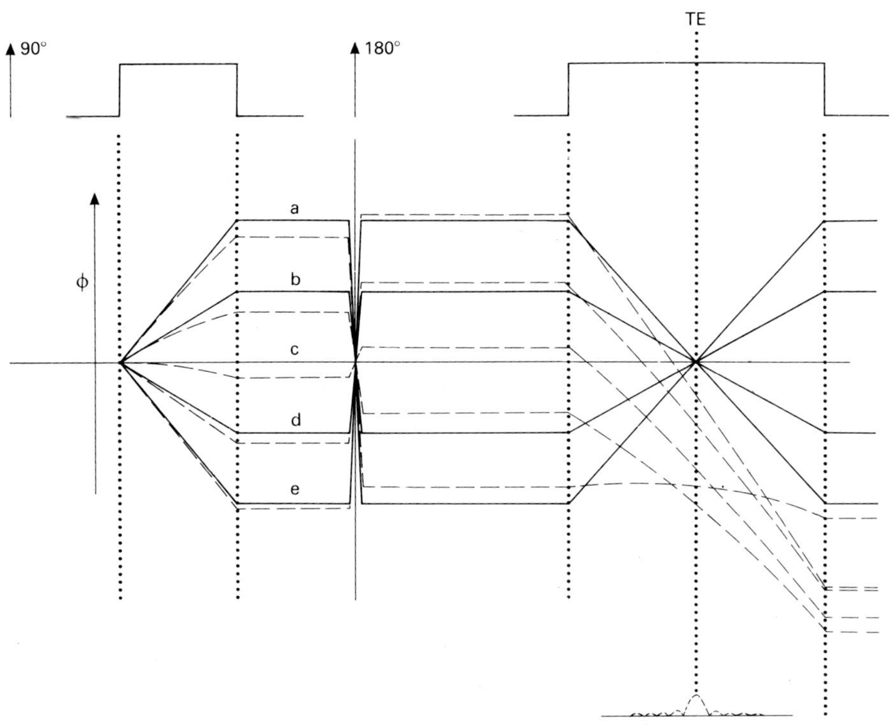

Figure 10.5. Comparison between the phases of stationary material (solid lines) and flowing material (dashed lines) initially at points a, b, c, d and e, all of which have the same velocity in the direction of the frequency encoding gradient. The phases reconverge at time TE to form an imaging echo although the absolute value of the phases is not zero as it is for the stationary material.

velocity related phase shifts are superimposed upon the phase shift of the phase encoding gradient and on reconstruction the signal is incorrectly placed, or smeared across the image as an artefact in the phase encoding direction. Perman and colleagues have investigated these artefacts in detail.[13]

These two effects dominate the appearance of blood in most images of the heart and blood vessels. The

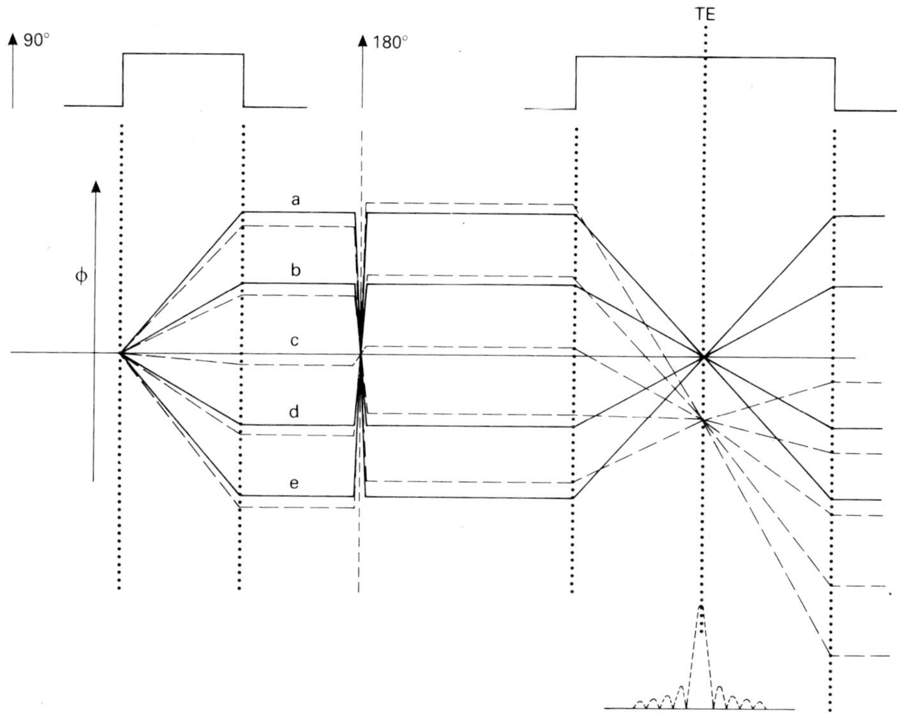

Figure 10.6. Similar to figure 10.5, although for material at points a, b, c, d and e with different velocities in the frequency encoding direction. The phases do not reconverge completely at time TE and the amplitude of the imaging echo is diminished. Signal loss due to dephasing has occurred.

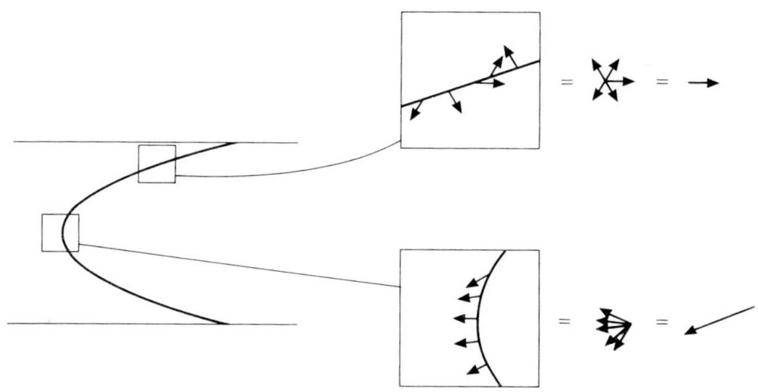

Figure 10.7. The phase shifts and dispersions that result from flow in the direction of the frequency encoding gradient with a parabolic velocity profile. The central voxel contains fast flow with a small range of velocities and its signal is phase shifted but only slightly reduced by phase dispersion. The peripheral voxel contains slower flow with a large range of velocities and the signal is greatly reduced by phase dispersion.

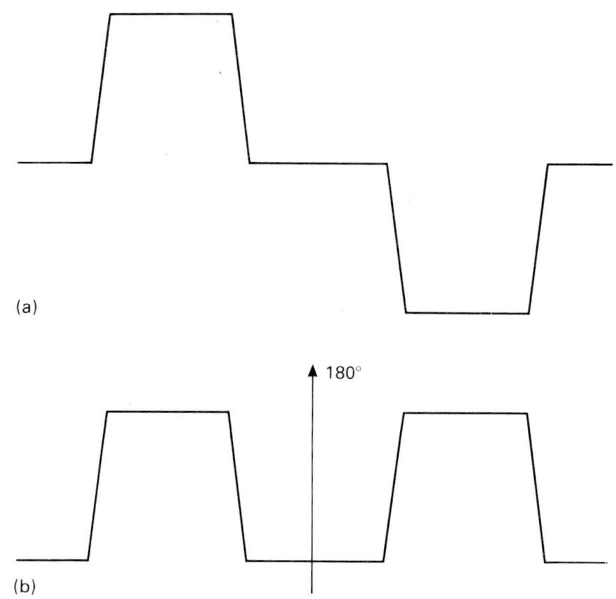

Figure 10.8. Both a positive (a) followed by a negative gradient lobe or two positive lobes (b) separated by a 180° radio-frequency pulse cause the same type of phase shifts for signal from flowing and stationary material.

majority of the signal from blood is lost, but that which remains is smeared across the image as artefact.

10.2.3 Even echo rephasing

The phase shift of the echo formed by motion in the direction of a bipolar gradient is reversed if a second echo is formed. Figure 10.9 shows this effect. The gradient profile can be considered in two halves which are of equal but opposite polarity, producing equal but

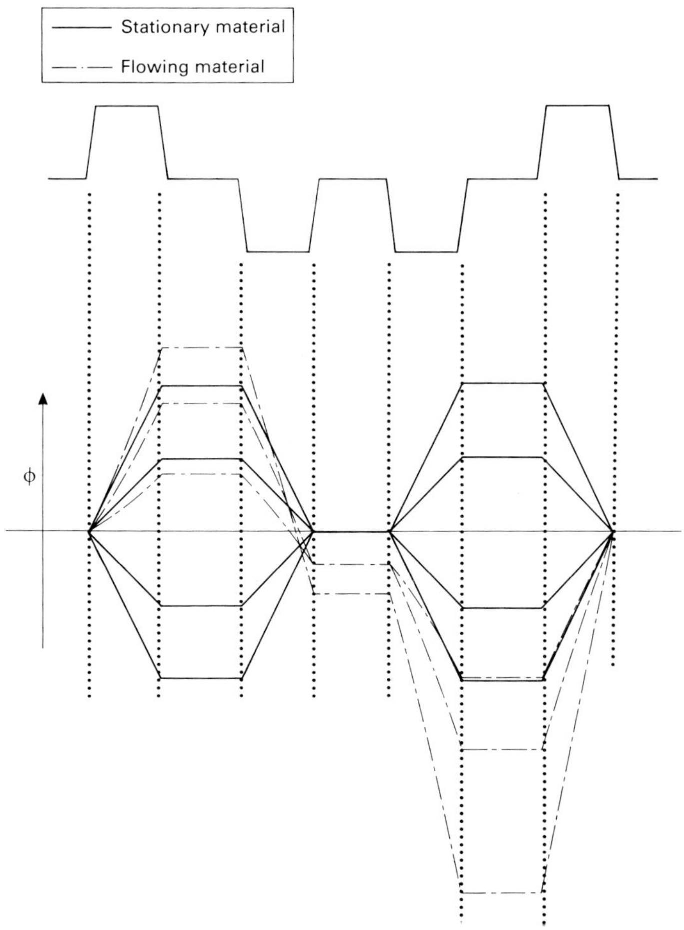

Figure 10.9. The effect on the phase of flowing and stationary material of a bipolar gradient followed by another of opposite polarity. The signal from stationary material rephases after both bipolar gradients to form an echo. The signal from flowing material is phase shifted after the first bipolar gradient but the effects are reversed by the second bipolar gradient and an echo is formed.

opposite phase shifts. For a train of multiple echoes formed in this way, rephasing occurs for each even numbered echo but the odd echoes are dephased.[14] Hence the name: even echo rephasing. Waluch and Bradley[15] were the first to differentiate between the forms of flow-related signal enhancement, namely in-flow/out-flow effects[9] and even echo rephasing.

If material is not flowing with a constant velocity but is accelerating, then the spins are not rephased by even echo rephasing and loss of signal and image artefacts may still occur. Sequences with symmetrical gradients such as those seen in figure 10.12 will rephase all the odd higher order derivatives of position as well as velocity (that is velocity, jerk, etc).[16] Because turbulence and other complex flow types contain a number of higher orders of motion, these areas can be identified as areas of signal loss on an even echo image. Loss of signal is loosely referred to as 'turbulence' although the real situation is more complex. The clinical value of these areas of signal loss is discussed in more detail in chapter 7.

Although gradients can be designed that rephase any number of the derivatives of position longer sequences are required which may introduce fresh problems. The motion artefact suppression technique (MAST) is an example and it has proved particularly useful for reducing or removing artefacts due to eye motion, carotid blood flow, and respiratory motion.[17]

10.2.4 Misregistration effects

If material moves between the times of slice selection, phase encoding and frequency encoding then its signal can be misplaced in the resulting image.[18] For example, the signal from flowing blood may be displaced in its direction of motion so that it appears partly outside the vessel containing it. This effect can be minimised both by keeping echo times as short as possible and by ensuring that the direction of flow is perpendicular to the imaging plane. Since this is not always possible, it is important to be aware of the effect when examining clinical images.

10.3 Flow measurement using wash-in/wash-out effects

10.3.1 Non-imaging methods

In 1959, Singer was the first person to measure blood flow using wash-in/wash-out effects.[6] He studied the absorption curve obtained from a mouse's tail using a tourniquet to alter flow. Absorption was increased by flow and he attributed this effect to unsaturated blood entering the volume of the spectrometer coils. Zhernovoi and Latyshev,[8] later used the method to measure flow in the femoral artery of a dog but they diverted the circulation from the artery to the spectrometer and so their technique was unsuitable for clinical application. Battocletti and colleagues[19] adapted the technique for non-invasive measurement by designing an instrument with a magnetising magnet upstream and a detecting magnet with transmitter and receiver coils downstream. The degree of magnetisation as blood passed through the magnetising magnet, and hence the signal detected downstream, depended on the flow rate. Both *in vitro* and *in vivo* studies produced good results although it was not possible to discriminate between flow in different arteries. In the following decade the group described a number of methods of localising the signal,[20–22] and in 1981 they reviewed their progress.[23–25]

10.3.2 Imaging methods

Garroway described the first imaging technique for the measurement of flow in 1974.[26] He used a sequence with two 90° pulses separated by a time τ and with a gradient applied perpendicular to the direction of flow. The Fourier transform of the signal from the first pulse gave a measure of the spin density across a tube and that of the second pulse gave a velocity profile. The first pulse served two purposes. It enabled an image to be formed but it also saturated the spins in the fluid. As long as τ was greater than T_2^* and much shorter than T_1, then the second pulse would not produce a signal if there was no flow. If however fully magnetised fluid flowed into the active region between the two pulses, a signal would be obtained. The technique was successful and in 1981 Thulborn and colleagues suggested a similar approach but added a gradient pulse between the radio-frequency pulses.[27] This effectively shortened T_2^* and provided greater flexibility in the timing between the two pulses. Two years later, Singer and Crooks adapted these one dimensional techniques to produce two dimensional flow images which were used to measure blood flow through the internal jugular veins of a normal subject's neck.[9]

In 1986 Mueller and colleagues measured flow by using the fact that it appears to modify the transverse relaxation of blood.[28] The apparent relaxation time (T_2') with flow of velocity v perpendicular to the slice of thickness d is given by the equation:

$$\frac{1}{T_2'} = \frac{1}{T_2}+\frac{v}{d}$$

A multi-echo spin echo sequence was used to measure the T_2 decay of signal from any point on the image and the findings agreed with theory for velocities between 0 and 3.5 cm/s. Flow was also measured in the abdominal aorta, although an 8 cm slice was required in order to avoid loss of signal from the wash-out effect.

Wehrli and colleagues demonstrated that the gradient echo sequence was less sensitive to phase dispersion caused by flow than the spin echo sequence.[29] Using this sequence signal loss was reduced and the accuracy of flow measurements was improved. In 1987 Hennig and colleagues showed that by adjusting the radio-frequency pulse flip angle and the sequence timings static material could be saturated and signal from flowing material was enhanced.[30] They measured flow in the jugular vein and also produced an angiogram of a volunteer's hand.

10.4 Flow measurement using time of flight effects

10.4.1 Non-imaging methods

Time of flight methods of measuring flow involve labelling the flowing material magnetically and then detecting the position of the label after a period of time, or measuring the time required for it to move between fixed points. In Singer's famous paper of 1959[6] he not only described the absorption method of measuring flow which is described above, but he also described the possibility of using a receiver coil downstream from a transmitter coil and using a time of flight method.

Zhernovoi and Latyshev proposed similar approaches in 1965[8] although the methods were devised as automated techniques for use in industry. They used a magnetising coil upstream from a detector coil and they either magnetised the upstream coil each time a signal was detected downstream, or they applied a regular magnetising pulse upstream. In the first method the rate of energising the upstream coil was proportional to flow, and in the second the phase shift between the applied and detected pulses was used. Another industrial flowmeter was designed by Genthe and colleagues in 1968[31] and it was used for a number of applications including the monitoring of flow of solvents such as xylene, butanol and naphtha in a paint manufacturing plant, and of concentrated hydrochloric acid in an agricultural chemical plant. The main advantages in these applications were the independence of fluid properties such as conductivity, temperature, viscosity, density, opacity, and gas or solid entrainment, and the fact that there were no moving parts and no mechanical or electrical contact with the fluid.

In 1970 Morse and Singer described their measurement of venous flow in the human arm,[32] although it had been more of a problem than anticipated in 1959 to apply Singer's original suggestions *in vivo*. They used two small surface coils placed over a vein with the forearm between the poles of a 3.6 T magnet. The main problem was a very low signal to noise ratio, and most of the noise was generated within or picked up by the body of the subject.

10.4.2 Imaging methods

Feinberg and colleagues[33] pointed out a limitation in the wash-in/wash-out methods that were suggested by Kaufman and colleagues[34] and by Singer and Crooks[9] which is that they were only suitable for very low velocities in the range between 0 and 10 cm/s. To overcome this they described a variation in the spin echo sequence where two echoes were formed using slice selective 180° pulses but the first slice was offset by 3 mm from the slice of the 90° pulse and the second slice was offset by 9 mm. The first slice overlapped sufficiently with the excited slice to form an anatomical image but with absent signal from flowing blood because of the dephasing effects of the first echo. The second slice did not overlap at all and signal was only seen from material that had flowed between the excited slice and the slice of the second echo in the time between the 90° pulse and image formation. Using the technique, they successfully identified flow in the carotid and vertebral arteries of a volunteer.

In 1986 Shimizu and colleagues described another approach.[35] They applied slice selection and frequency encoding gradients along the same axis and so material that moved in this direction between slice selection and reading was displaced relative to the stationary material. In other words, they made use of a flow artefact to measure flow. With velocity encoded in one direction the other two directions could be spatially encoded using stepped phase encoding gradients. The technique was validated in phantom experiments and was used to measure flow in the abdominal aorta with good agreement with Doppler ultrasound. Matsuda and colleagues used the same technique to measure flow in the descending thoracic aorta in a number of subjects.[36] Again there was good agreement with ultrasound and the main advantage was seen as the ability to measure very high velocities.

Axel and colleagues described a different approach[37] using an 'inner volume' imaging technique similar to that described by Feinberg.[38] The slice selection gradients for the 90 and 180° pulses are applied in orthogonal directions. Static material appeared as a line but moving material was displaced from this zero line in the direction of frequency encoding. The method was tested on a variety of flowing phantoms but only with relatively low flow velocities (maximum 10 cm/s).

10.5 Flow measurement using phase changes

10.5.1 Non-imaging methods

These methods rely upon the phase changes produced in material that is moving along a magnetic field gradient. Although non-imaging techniques are unsuitable for measuring flow in blood vessels because the surrounding static material significantly affects the detected phase, a number of techniques were developed to measure flow in other systems.

In 1960 Hahn described a method of measuring the motion of sea water (approximately 10^{-3} cm/s) using the Earth's magnetic field, and he suggested that a phase shift as small as 0.3 radians could be measured by comparing the acquired signal with a reference signal.[39] Packer later developed a method of studying slow coherent molecular motion.[40] He initially demonstrated the phase shift produced by flow during a spin echo and a Carr–Purcell–Meiboom–Gill sequence,[41] and he designed a sequence with radio-frequency pulses of 90°-τ-180°-τ-180°-τ-180°-τ-etc, where the signal phase change due to coherent motion is maximised whereas the signal attenuation due to diffusion is minimised. Lucas and colleagues also described the measurement of very low flow convection currents.[42] They studied slow bidirectional flow of liquids in a column and a gradient was applied in the direction of flow so that the resulting phase shifts varied the signal measured according to the velocity profile in the column. Water was initially used but later a mixture of helium-3 and helium-4 was driven through the column by thermal convection. They demonstrated that flow could be measured accurately down to 10^{-5} m/s. Borodin used a toroidal coil and tube in the design of a flowmeter using the Earth's magnetic field that was intended for industrial use.[43] The coil was used to magnetise the sample flowing around it and then to detect the resulting signal, the phase of which was proportional to flow.

The year 1977 saw the first of a number of articles by Hemminga and the group at the Agricultural University of the Netherlands where the effects of flow dependent phase shifts on the signal amplitudes from a flowing sample were analysed. They initially measured low to medium velocities from the decay of echoes in a Carr–Purcell–Meiboom–Gill sequence,[44] and they studied flow in plant stems, where only about 2% of the sample is flowing. In 1978 de Jager and colleagues continued this work by designing a sequence with a series of 180° pulses.[45] The sequence had the advantage that stationary material gave no signal, but for flowing material there was a linear relationship between the mean velocity and the reciprocal of the time from the exciting pulse to the maximum signal. Van As and colleagues combined these two techniques with a sensitive line or plane selection, such as was described by Hinshaw.[46] The selection process enabled flow to be localised spatially, and results were presented for spatially resolved real time flow in two capillary tubes, as well as non-spatially resolved flow from a subject's index finger.

In 1986 Altobelli and colleagues described a very simple method of rapid flow measurement.[47] They monitored the phase of the signal throughout the second echo of a Carr–Purcell–Meiboom–Gill sequence and they used this to calculate the mean flow over the period of the echo or, alternatively, the slope of plot of phase against time measured instantaneous flow.

10.5.2 Imaging methods

In 1982 Moran described the theory of velocity phase encoding which has proved to be the most successful technique in clinical application.[48] The only requirements were the addition a simple bipolar gradient pulse along one axis and the ability to reconstruct the real and imaginary parts of the image separately.

10.5.2.1 Fourier flow methods

Redpath and colleagues described a method in which they produced 8 images with sequences differing only in the magnitude of the bipolar gradient.[49] This produced increments in phase which depended upon the velocity of the spins. A three-dimensional reconstruction of the data set produced eight flow images each displaying a different range of velocities. Feinberg and colleagues modified the same type of approach by removing the spatial phase encoding to shorten the acquisition time whilst velocity phase encoding in two directions.[50] They used a double spin echo technique with spatial encoding from a gradient in the x direction during signal acquisition. Stepped velocity phase encoding gradients were applied in the y and z axes in order to encode velocity in the y direction in the first echo and in the z direction in the second echo. The technique was validated in a flow phantom and was also used to produce a velocity profile through the descending aorta of a normal volunteer. Hennig and colleagues developed this approach further in order to overcome the problem of signal from stationary tissue.[51] They used a rapid partial saturation sequence which produced very low signal from stationary material but a high signal from flowing blood. Although venous flow studies could be performed in a matter of seconds, arterial flow required cardiac triggering and took longer.

10.5.2.2 Velocity phase encoding methods

In 1984 both Van Dijk[52] and Bryant and colleagues[53] demonstrated the clinical use of velocity phase encoding. Their methods used the velocity dependent phase shift produced either by two gradient pulses of the same polarity separated by a 180° radio-frequency pulse or by a bipolar gradient without a 180° pulse. In the final image, instead of displaying the signal magnitude, its phase is displayed. Stationary material is normally represented as mid-grey whilst increasing velocities in opposite directions tend towards black and white. Van Dijk used the existing imaging gradients and produced velocity maps showing motion of the left ventricular myocardium. Bryant and colleagues used two additional gradients in the slice selection direction, one before and one after the 180° pulse (figure 10.10). Because phase shifts arise from factors other than motion, such as magnetic inhomogeneity and susceptibility changes in the patient, two images are acquired one with and one without the added gradients. Subtraction of the phase images leaves only the phase shifts caused by motion. The technique was applied to the measurement of flow in the vessels of the neck (figure 10.11).

Wedeen and colleagues described an alternative method and they produced what is known as the 'zebra stripe' image.[54] They moved the time of the echo away from the centre of the data collection period and this had the effect of creating a phase shift of about 10 cycles across the field of view in the read direction. Reconstruction of only the real or imaginary components of the signal, produced an image with equi-

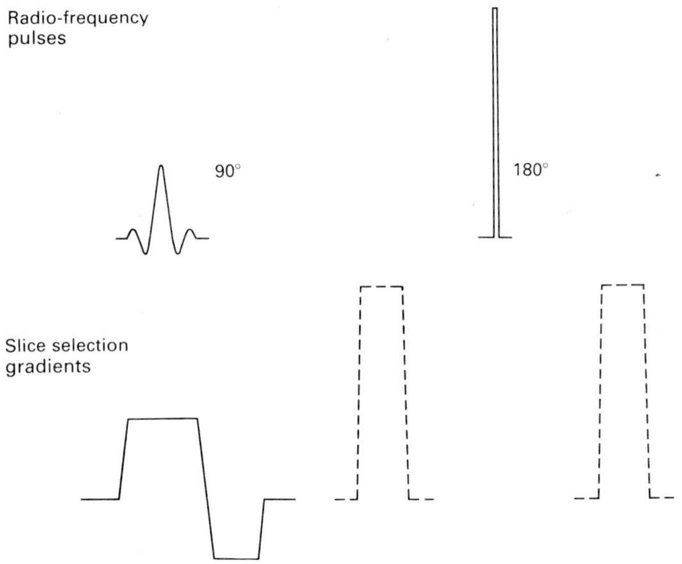

Figure 10.10. The sequence used by Bryant and colleagues for velocity mapping.[53] It is a conventional spin echo sequence with identical gradient pulses either side of the 180° radio-frequency pulse (dashed lines). The signals are acquired with and without the gradient pulses and the phase difference for each pixel is displayed as a velocity map.

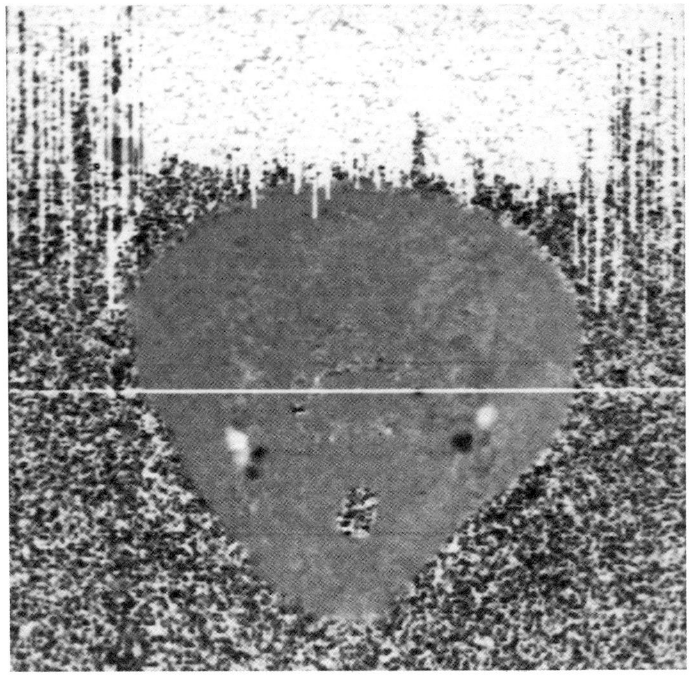

Figure 10.11. A velocity map of a transverse plane through the neck showing flow in the main vessels. Stationary material is displayed as mid grey, cranial velocities in the carotid arteries in darker shades of grey and caudal velocities in the jugular veins in lighter shades of grey.

distant stripes corresponding to the cyclic phase shifts. Moving material had an additional phase shift caused by motion in the slice selection direction and more importantly in the read direction. These additional phase shifts showed as displacement of the regular stripes in the direction of motion and the displacement was proportional to velocity. The technique was applied in a number of phantoms but also in the descending aorta. Dinsmore and colleagues used it to distinguish between slowly moving blood and thrombus in patients with saccular thoracic aortic aneurysms.[55]

10.5.3 The field even echo rephasing sequence

The phase encoding methods described above are extremely sensitive with large phase shifts produced by low velocities. This often led to ambiguity in the velocity measurement when phase shifts of more than one cycle occurred. More importantly, because of signal loss caused by the phase dispersion effects already described, there was often insufficient signal to measure phase. Additional disadvantages were the wash-in/wash-out effects which also caused signal loss and the relatively slow repetition time possible with the spin echo sequence. In order to overcome these problems, Nayler and colleagues developed a gradient echo sequence with even echo rephasing which they called the field even echo rephasing (FEER) sequence.[56]

The sequence uses symmetrically shaped gradient profiles in both the slice selection and frequency encoding directions (figure 10.12), and these result in even echo rephasing with high signal even from moving blood (figure 10.13). With perfect even echo rephasing (that is, complete velocity compensation) there will be no velocity dependent phase shifts, but slight modifications can be made to introduce the phase shifts. These can either take the form of small time shifts (figure 10.14) or changes in the amplitude of the gradient profiles (figure 10.15), and the phase changes can be accurately controlled to measure the velocities typically seen in the cardiovascular system without introducing phase dispersion and signal loss. Velocity can be encoded in any direction with respect to the chosen plane but normally it is either encoded in the slice select direction (perpendicular to the plane) or in the frequency or phase encoding directions within the plane. Because the plane itself can be chosen at will, there is considerable flexibility.

The phase shifts caused by magnet inhomogeneity

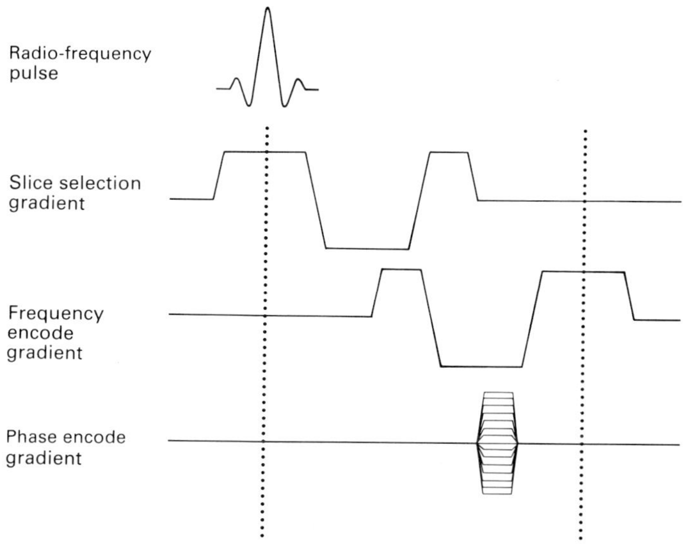

Figure 10.12. The velocity insensitive FEER sequence with symmetrical gradient profiles in the slice selection and frequency encoding directions.

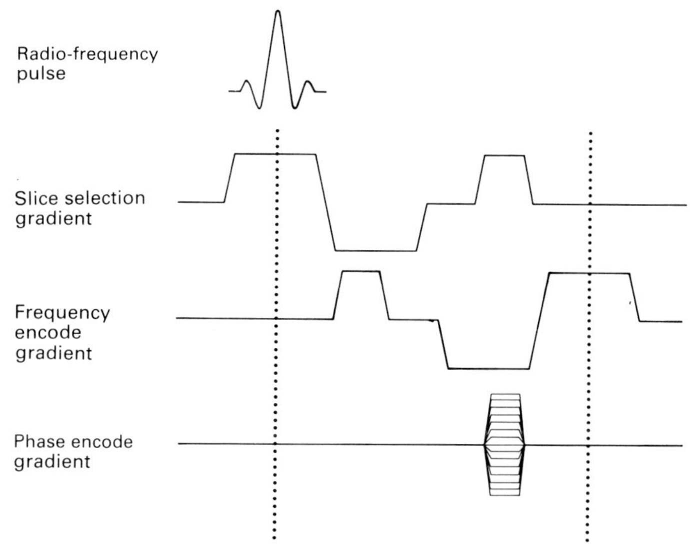

Figure 10.14. The FEER sequence with modifications to encode velocity in the slice selection and frequency encoding directions in the phase of the signal. The modifications involve moving a portion of the gradient in time.

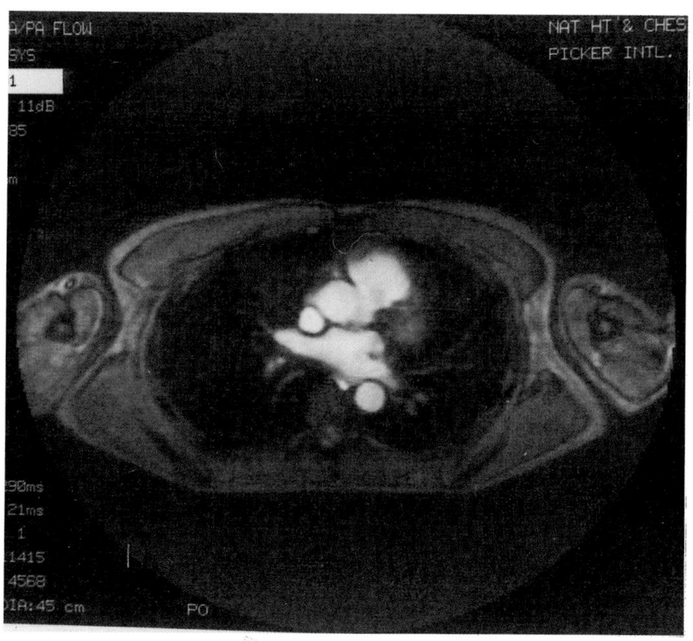

Figure 10.13. A FEER magnitude image of a transverse slice through the major vessels above the heart, showing high signal from the blood in the slice.

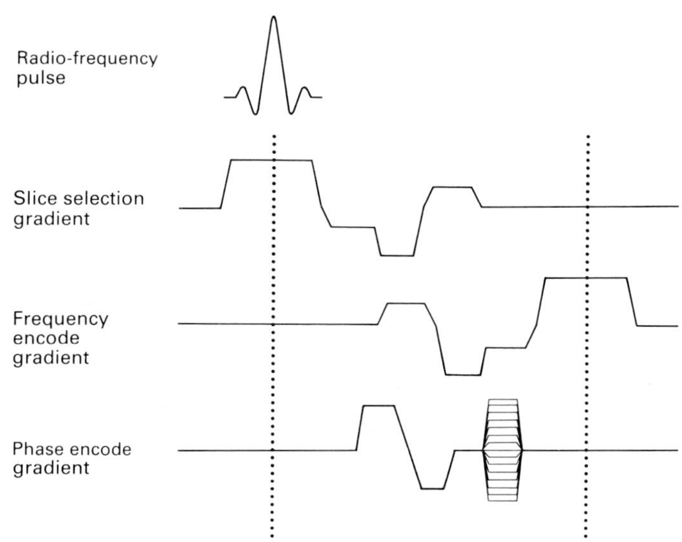

Figure 10.15. The FEER sequence with modifications to encode velocity in all three gradient directions in the phase of the signal. The modifications involve changes to the amplitude of the gradient profiles.

mean that individual phase images are difficult to interpret and so two images are acquired, one with and one without velocity encoding. Subtraction of the two produces an accurate velocity map. An additional correction has to be applied for phase shifts which can arise from non-central sampling of the signal. These appear as a gradient of velocities across the final map, but they can be corrected for by identifying stationary points within the image (either manually or automatically) and setting these points to zero.

10.5.4 Artefacts in velocity mapping

It is important to be aware of factors which can compromise the accuracy of velocity mapping. These include:

1 Aliasing of velocity data
2 Misalignment of flow encoding
3 Partial volume averaging of velocities through the slice
4 Misregistration effects
5 Phase shifts caused by higher orders of motion
6 Signal loss

10.5.4.1 Aliasing

Because phase is cyclic there is a limit of 2π radians that can be measured without ambiguity and this therefore limits the maximum velocity that can be measured. Fortunately, the problem can be overcome both retrospectively and prospectively, unlike the similar phenomenon in Doppler ultrasound. The sensitivity of the velocity encoding of phase is determined by the size of the encoding modifications of the gradient profiles that are used. Thus, before an acquisition it might be decided to use a 2 m/s velocity window and to encode the phase from −1 m/s to +1 m/s. If velocities of +1.3 m/s are encountered then aliasing will occur and this velocity will appear as −0.7 m/s. The same data can be reformatted retrospectively however to show velocities from −0.5 m/s to +1.5 m/s and this would overcome the aliasing in this example. Difficulties occur if the velocity window is moved so far that it no longer encompasses zero velocity, and in these circumstances it would be necessary to repeat the acquisition with a different sensitivity of velocity encoding, for instance with a 4 m/s window from −2 m/s to +2 m/s. The range of velocities that has been measured covers the complete physiological range from 0.1[57] to several m/s.

10.5.4.2 Misalignment of velocity encoding

Because it is only the component of velocity in a chosen direction that is encoded, misalignment between the direction of flow and the direction of encoding will introduce an error proportional to the cosine of the angle between the two (figure 10.16). In practice only small errors are introduced unless the misalignment is severe, with a 6% error for an angle of 20° and less than 1% at 5°. It is, of course, possible to measure velocity in three orthogonal directions and this would provide accurate measurements irrespective of direction. Such an acquisition would require a single reference image and three encoded images and would take twice as long as acquisition of a single direction.

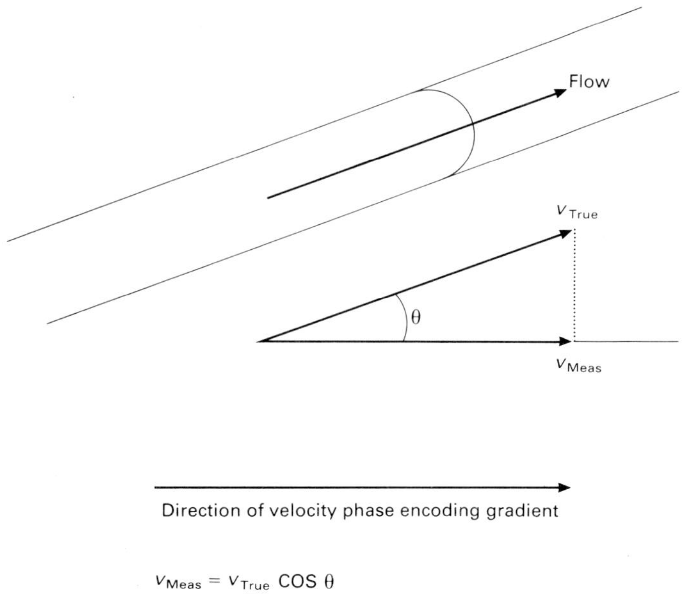

Figure 10.16. The source of misalignment errors and the relationship between the true and the measured velocity.

10.5.4.3 Partial volume averaging

If tissue within a single voxel has a range of velocities then only a mean will be displayed although this mean depends upon the relative amplitudes of the signals with different phases. This partial volume effect will be most important if in-plane velocity is measured in a small vessel using a thick slice and it will be minimised by orienting the slice so that the vessel flows perpendicularly through it. Because the extent of the error depends upon the signal from the surrounding tissue it will depend upon relaxation times and upon the repeat time, echo time, and excitation pulse angle of the sequence used. Figure 10.17 shows the results of a phantom experiment in which a flow with a constant velocity of 0.45 m/s was measured in a 10 mm tube surrounded by air, and by solutions with T_1 of approximately 1 and 100 ms. Velocity maps were acquired with a range of slice thicknesses and the measured velocity can be seen to depend strongly upon slice thickness and surrounding medium. A knowledge of these effects allows acquisitions to be tailored to minimise the error.

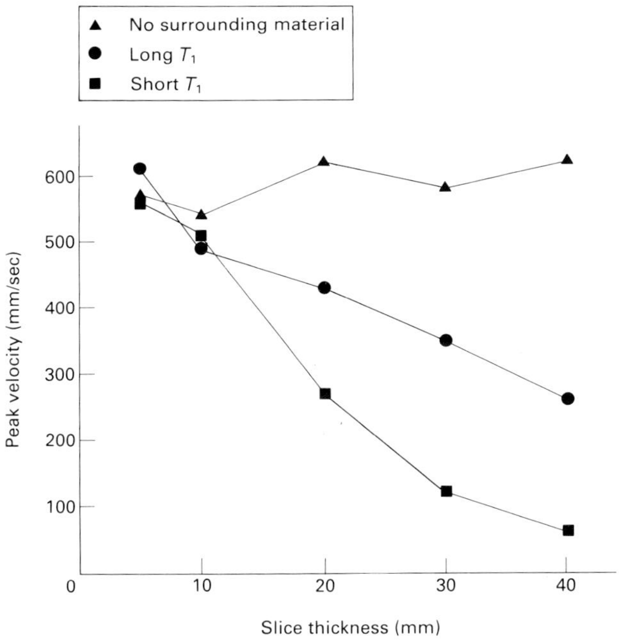

Figure 10.17. The error in velocity measurement caused by the partial volume effect. As the slice thickness is increased signal from surrounding tissue is included in each voxel and the error is increased. Velocity measurements in a tube surrounded by air, by a fluid with a short T_1 (100 ms), and by a fluid with a long T_1 (1000 ms) are shown. In air, the measured velocity is independent of slice thickness because of the absence of signal outside the tube. In the fluids, reduced velocities are measured and the error depends upon the signal from the surrounding stationary fluid: the long T_1 causes saturation and a smaller error than the short T_1. (Reproduced with permission from *Magn Reson Med* 1990; **14**: 230–41.)

10.5.4.4 *Misregistration effects*

Misregistration occurs because of motion between slice selection, phase encoding and frequency encoding and the result is that signal is displaced in the image in the direction of its motion. The effect is most clearly seen in an oblique cine image through the aorta where the signal from the blood in the aorta oscillates between its true anatomical location and a position outside the aorta as its velocity changes throughout the cardiac cycle. If this misregistration results in the signal overlying signal from stationary tissue (as it inevitably will in the example used), a type of partial volume error results and the phases of the stationary and moving material are averaged. The effect can be minimised by using a sequence with very short periods between the different spatial encodings and by arranging the plane to be perpendicular to the direction of flow.

Table 10.1 The error introduced into a velocity measurement of 1 m/s by an acceleration of 10 m/s^2 depends upon echo time

Echo time (ms)	True velocity (m/s)	Measured velocity (m/s)
22	1	1.079
14	1	1.039
6	1	1.017

10.5.4.5 *Phase shifts caused by higher orders of motion*

The equation describing the phase of the signal from a small volume of spins undergoing the same motion (spin isochromat) is:

$$\phi = \int G(t).x(t).dt$$

where $G(t)$ and $x(t)$ are functions describing the variation of the gradient amplitude and the position of the spin isochromat with time. Assuming that x is continuously differentiable over the interval $[0,t]$:

$$x(t) = x(0) + x'(0).t + x''(0).\frac{t^2}{2!} + \ldots + x^{[n]}(0).\frac{t^n}{n!} + \ldots .$$

The equation has a series of terms beginning with displacement and continuing with increasing orders of motion such as velocity, acceleration, jerk, etc. If a velocity measurement is required and a significant acceleration is present, then the final phase shift will have contributions from both orders of motion. The subtraction of velocity sensitive and velocity insensitive phase images removes most of this error but a small error remains, the degree of which depends to a large extent upon the duration of the gradient profile. Table 10.1 shows typical examples.

10.5.4.6 *Signal loss*

Flow related signal loss is probably the most important factor affecting accuracy. Although the FEER sequence is designed to overcome this problem, higher orders of motion can still cause phase dispersion and where there is no signal, phase is of course meaningless. Partial signal loss does not affect accuracy however although only mean phase will be detected.

Two approaches have been suggested for the design of gradients which will minimise signal loss and the success of each depends upon the type of flow. Complex gradient waveforms can be derived that nullify phase shifts caused by the first few derivatives of position[17] but these have the disadvantage of extending the sequence length and so introducing fresh problems. An alternative method that is particularly suitable for turbulent flow with many higher orders of position, is to use the symmetrical gradient profiles of the FEER sequence which nullify phase shifts caused by all the odd order derivatives of position (that is velocity and jerk but not acceleration) and to shorten the sequence as much as possible to reduce the effects of the even order derivatives.

It is thought that a range of values of higher order components of motion in a single voxel is the most important cause of signal loss, not simply its presence. The following analysis emphasises the importance of shortening the sequence in order to avoid this effect. The phase shift caused by the nth order of motion, $x^{[n]}$, is:

$$\phi = S_n . x^{[n]}$$

where S_n is the sensitivity of the signal phase to the nth term and is in turn given by:

$$S_n = G_f . c_n . \tau^{(n+1)}$$

where G_f is a gradient factor related to the gradient shape and amplitude, c_n is a constant of proportionality relevant to the nth motion term and τ is the duration of the gradient waveform. In imaging there is normally a constraint such that:

$$G_f . \tau = C$$

where C is a constant because a higher gradient strength is required to produce the same effect in a shorter time. It follows that:

$$S_n = C . c_n . \tau^n$$

which demonstrates that the sensitivity of the phase of the signal to higher orders of motion becomes increasingly important with long gradient profiles.

Because imaging voxels are normally long and thin, slice orientation can also be important and it might be possible to orientate the slice such that the variation of a higher order motion term within the voxel is reduced. For example, in a vessel which is narrowing because of a stenosis, blood will accelerate along the axis of the vessel as it passes into the narrowing but the acceleration will be uniform across the diameter of the vessel. An in-plane velocity measurement would be less susceptible to signal loss than a through-plane measurement.

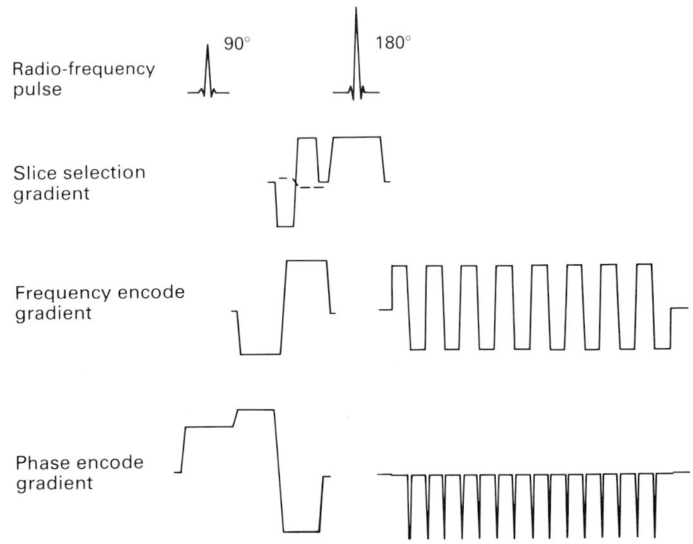

Figure 10.18. Echo planar sequence with gradient profiles designed to zero the velocity dependent phase shifts at the time of the eighth echo. The modification to the slice selection profile (broken line) encodes velocity in that direction in the phase of the signal. (Reproduced with permission from *Magn Reson Med* 1989; **12**: 316–27.)

10.6 Echo planar velocity mapping

Conventional methods of flow imaging acquire information over a period of minutes and so rapid alterations cannot be followed. It is possible to acquire information much more quickly by combining echo planar imaging with velocity mapping. Echo planar imaging has been more fully described in chapter 1 and, although it is difficult to implement, a method has been described using a near standard scanner.[58] Zonal echo planar imaging is used in which a spin echo sequence has a slice selection gradient during the 90° pulse and a perpendicular strip selection gradient during the 180° pulse.[59] Good resolution can be maintained with as few as 16 echoes. The gradients used for echo planar imaging produce large phase shifts from flowing material and hence considerable signal loss. It is possible to rephase these shifts in the centre of the train of echoes (figure 10.18), however, and this overcomes the problem for simple flow although signal is still lost from complex flow patterns.

Figure 10.19 shows echo planar velocity maps with a data acquisition time of 40 ms. Figure 10.20 shows a comparison of echo planar velocity mapping with conventional FEER velocity mapping. The two techniques agree well although it should be remembered that one is an average over time and the other is not.

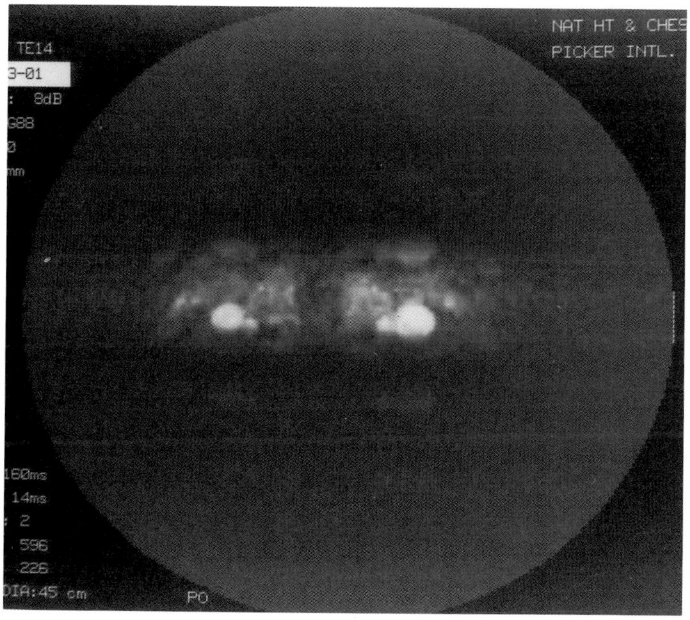

(a)

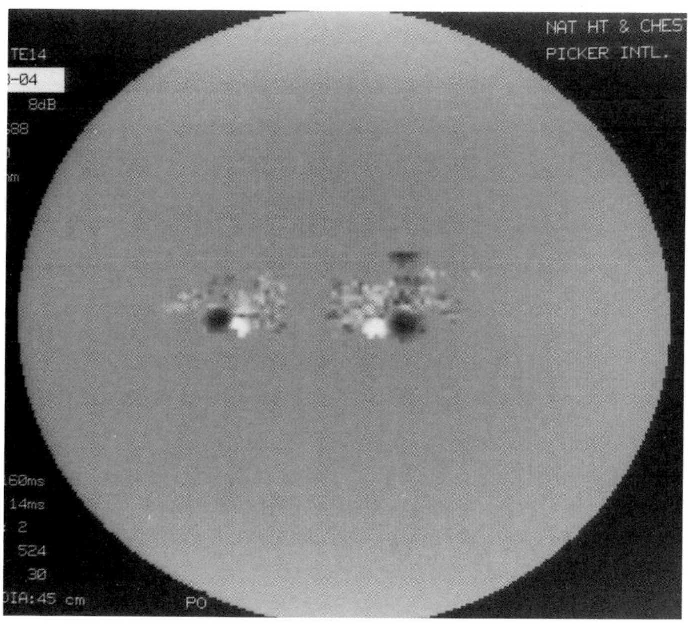

(b)

Figure 10.19. (a) Echo planar magnitude image through the neck acquired with a single excitation. High signal from blood in the carotid arteries and jugular veins is seen. (b) Echo planar velocity map of the same slice reconstructed from a single excitation of each of the velocity encoded and velocity insensitive sequences illustrated in figure 10.18. Velocities in the carotid arteries are shown in white, and in the jugular veins as black. (Reproduced with permission from *Magn Reson Med* 1989; **12**: 316–27.)

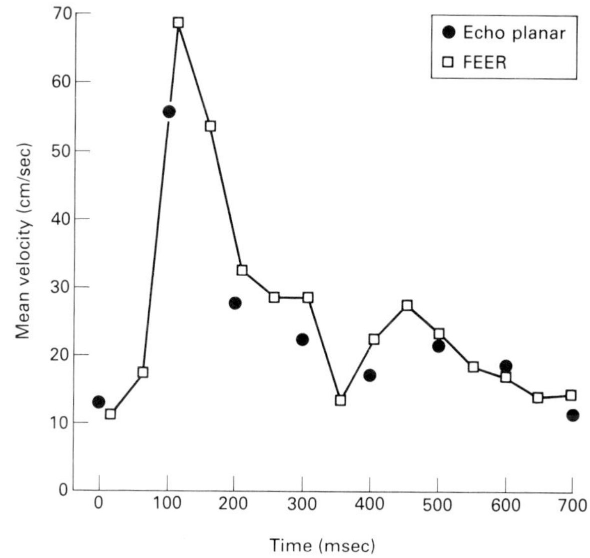

Figure 10.20. Comparison of flow in the right carotid artery of a normal subject obtained by echo planar and by FEER velocity mapping. There is good agreement although the FEER velocity maps show average flow over the period of acquisition and the echo planar maps show measurements from individual cycles. (Reproduced with permission from *Magn Reson Med* 1989; **12**: 316–27.)

10.7 Clinical applications

Although there are many methods of measuring flow using magnetic resonance, the most promising technique is velocity mapping. It is relatively simple to use, it is accurate, and it can be implemented on standard scanners. Its clinical application has depended to some extent on imaging companies recognising its importance and making the technique available for widespread use, but at the time of writing several centres are using the technique successfully.

10.7.1 Validation

As with any technique, it is important to be sure that the measurements are accurate and to be aware of the limitations as well as the strengths of the method. Potential artefacts have already been discussed and providing that these can be avoided or minimised, the measurements of flow are both accurate and reproducible. Validation has been achieved in phantom experiments and by comparison with other methods such as Doppler ultrasound.[56,60] Figure 10.21 shows a rotating disk phantom that has been used and figure 10.22 shows the accuracy of the velocities measured from it.[61]

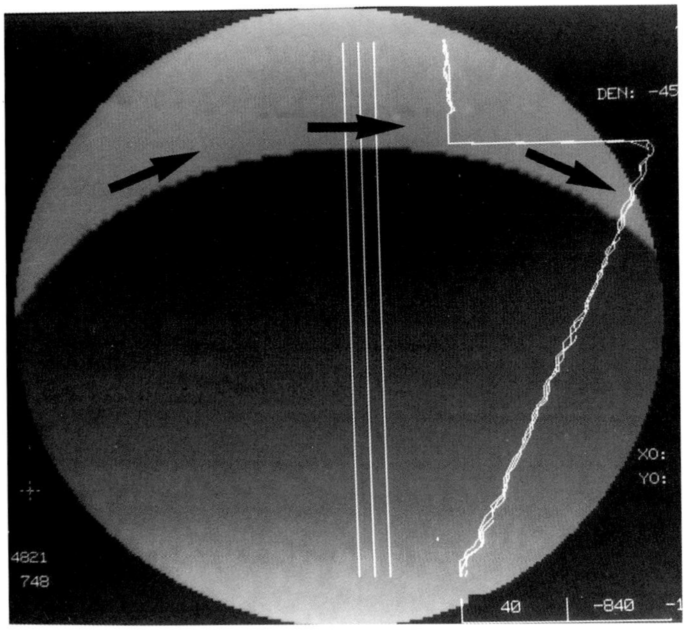

Figure 10.21. Validation of velocity mapping in a phantom consisting of a rotating disk (the centre of rotation is at the bottom of the image). Velocity is encoded from left to right and so a linear gradation would be expected from bottom to top of the image. Three linear profiles are displayed, rising to a maximum of 0.85 m/s. The true velocity profile would be a straight line rising to a maximum of 0.84 m/s.

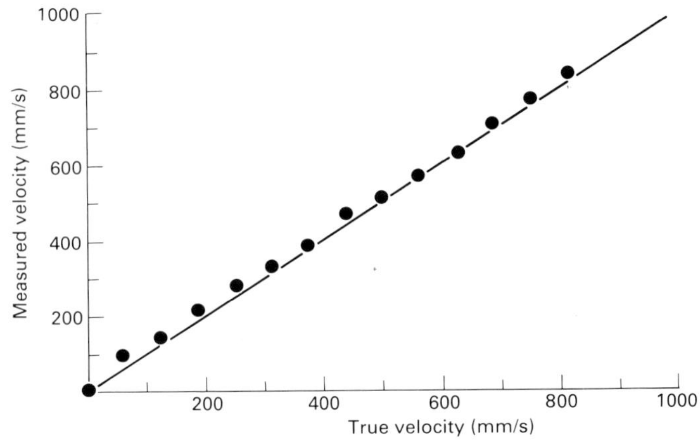

Figure 10.22. Correlation of measured and true velocities measured from the phantom demonstrated in figure 10.21. The line of identity is indicated and the regression equation is $y = 0.999x + 18$, ($r = 0.998$).

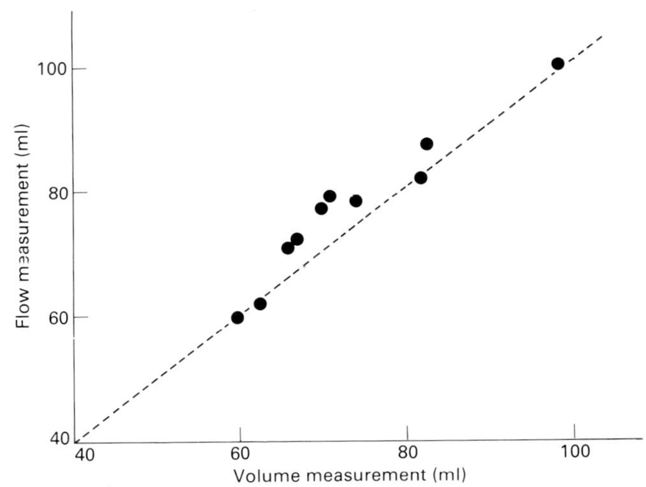

Figure 10.23. The correlation of left ventricular stroke volume measured from the aortic flow with that measured from ventricular volume measurements. The standard error of the estimate is 3.3 ml.

The most convincing validation has been performed *in vivo* and has used the fact that left ventricular stroke volume can be measured by summing areas in multiple contiguous images with an accuracy of 5%.[62] The stroke volume measured in this way should be the same as the flow measured in the aorta using velocity mapping and a comparison has shown a similar accuracy for both techniques.[63] Figure 10.23 shows this comparison in 10 normal subjects. A similar method of validation is to compare flow measured in the aorta and the pulmonary artery since these should also be the same in normal subjects.[64,65]

10.7.2 Congenital heart disease

The most successful clinical application of velocity mapping has been in patients with congenital heart disease.[66,67] This has been discussed in detail in chapter 6 and only brief reference need be made here. Intracardiac shunting can be measured in a number of ways. In an atrial septal defect the shunting can be assessed from the right and left ventricular stroke volumes but this method is not applicable in complex lesions or in ventricular shunts. Flow through atrial and ventricular defects can be visualised directly (figure 10.24), but it is difficult to quantify the flow accurately from such images and it is better to measure aortic and pulmonary flow. This method is particularly helpful in complex lesions and figure 10.25 illustrates an example of a patient with truncus arteriosus. In such patients, the success of surgery depends partly upon pulmonary flow and this can be difficult to measure by any other technique.

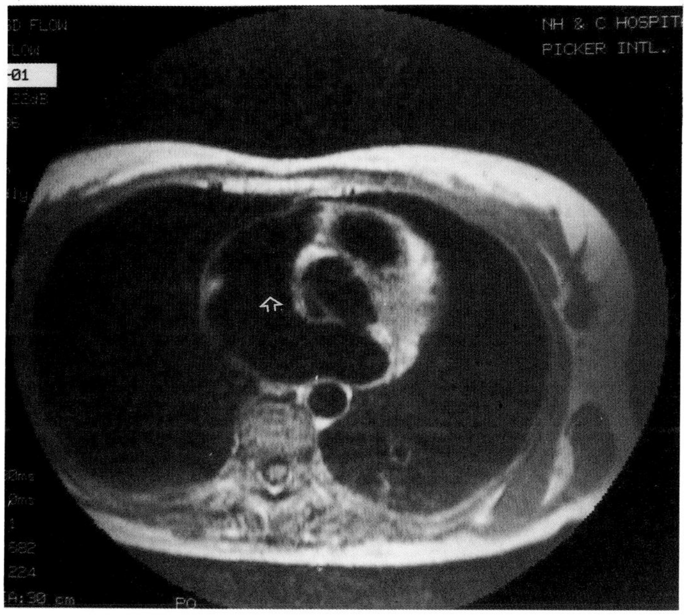

(a)

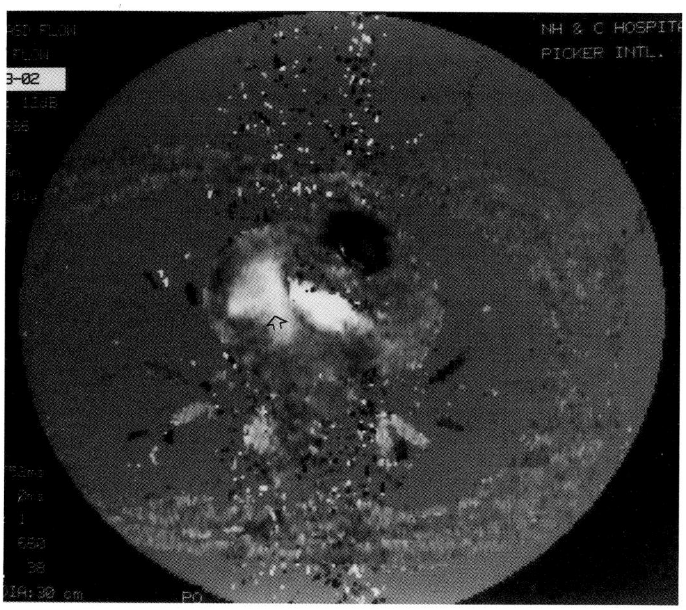

(b)

Figure 10.24. (a) Transverse spin echo image showing a large atrial septal defect. (b) The corresponding velocity map encoded from bottom to top of the image. Flow through the defect is seen as well as flow in the great vessels.

As well as studying natural shunts, the follow-up of flow in surgically created shunts is important. Figure 10.26 shows a patient with transposition of the great arteries, pulmonary stenosis and a ventricular septal defect who had bilateral Blalock shunts created previously. Clinically, it was felt that the left-sided shunt was patent since a murmur could be heard and Doppler echocardiography demonstrated flow within it, but the right sided shunt was though to be occluded because neither a murmur nor Doppler flow could be demonstrated. Magnetic resonance imaging clearly showed the patent right Blalock shunt and flow within it could be measured by velocity mapping.

10.7.3 The assessment of stenoses

The modified Bernoulli equation allows the pressure gradient across a stenosis to be calculated from the peak velocity within it:

$$\Delta P = 4v^2$$

where ΔP is the pressure gradient in mm of mercury and v is the maximum velocity in the orifice in m/s. The equation makes certain assumptions, the most important of which is that the velocity of blood before and after the orifice is small compared with the velocity within the orifice. The method is widely used for assessing stenoses using Doppler ultrasound and it appears to be sufficiently accurate for clinical use.[68,69]

Magnetic resonance velocity mapping should be able to provide the same measurements, but one potential problem is that velocities of up to 6 m/s with severe turbulence can be encountered. Under these conditions, signal is lost from blood with many sequences and if there is no signal then it is impossible to encode velocity. The answer has been to use sequences with very short echo times and using a FEER sequence with an echo time of 3.6 ms aortic valve gradients as high as 120 mmHg have been measured. Figure 10.27 shows an experiment in which the jet through a stenosis in a tube was imaged with different flow rates and different echo times. Although there is significant signal loss with an echo time of 22 ms, velocities up to 6 m/s were measured accurately with an echo time of 3.6 ms. Figures 10.28 and 10.29 show clinical examples in patients with mitral and aortic stenosis respectively. Figure 10.30 shows the correlation between magnetic resonance velocity mapping and either continuous wave Doppler or cardiac catheterisation for the measurement of pressure gradients in a variety of patients with stenosed conduits, valves, or great vessels.

10.7.4 Aortic and pulmonary flow

The size of the great vessels means that they are particularly suitable for velocity mapping and this has

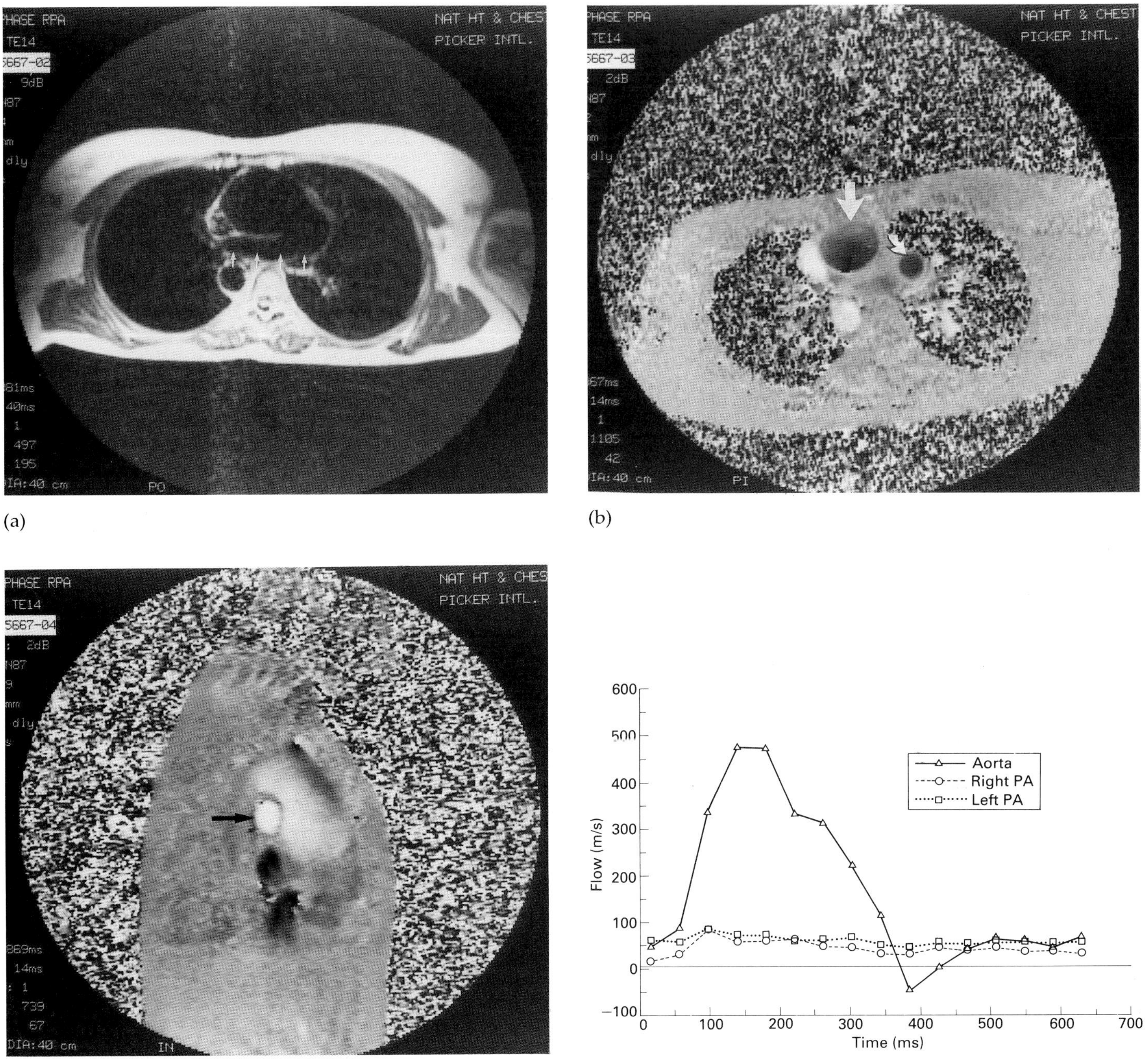

Figure 10.25. (a) Transverse spin echo image in a patient with truncus arteriosus, showing the main and right pulmonary arteries arising posteriorly from the common arterial trunk (arrows). (b) Velocity map in a transverse plane slightly cranial to that of (a) showing flow in the aorta (arrow) and the left pulmonary artery (curved arrow). (c) Sagittal velocity map showing flow in the right pulmonary artery (arrow). (d) Flow profiles in each of the vessels demonstrating the low pulmonary to systemic flow ratio.

provided new insights into their function. Normal systolic flow in the ascending aorta does not have the parabolic flow profile that is so commonly encountered in the laboratory. Instead, it is plug flow and it has a skewed velocity profile with higher velocities around the inside of the arch. In diastole the blood is not static but it continues to move with simultaneous antegrade and retrograde channels (figure 10.31).[64,70] This

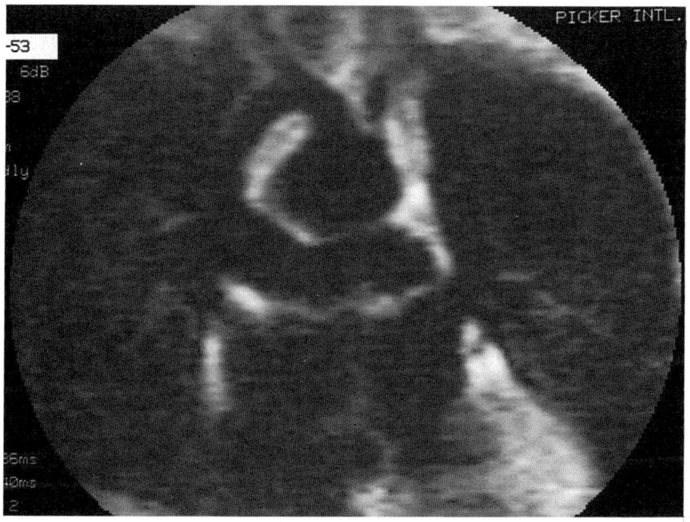

Figure 10.26. Coronal spin echo image showing a right sided Blalock shunt connecting the right subclavian artery to the right pulmonary artery in a patient with transposition of the great arteries, pulmonary stenosis and a ventricular septal defect. The shunt was thought to be occluded because there was no right sided murmur and Doppler echocardiography was unable to demonstrate flow within it. The magnetic resonance image shows it to be widely patent and velocity mapping was able to measure the flow within it.

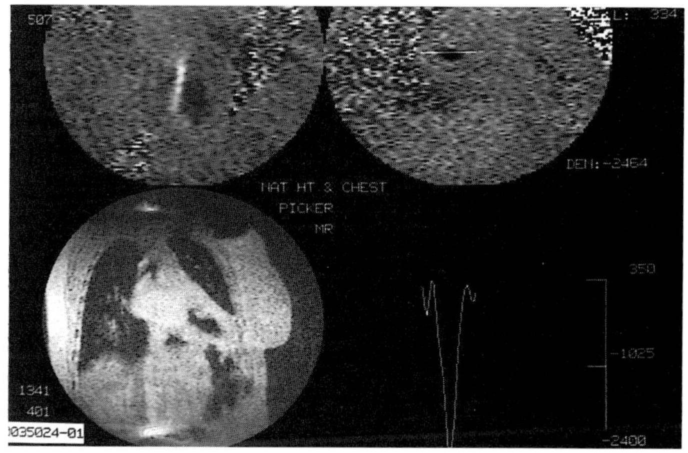

Figure 10.28. Velocity mapping in a patient with rheumatic mitral stenosis. The bottom left image shows a diastolic frame in the vertical long axis plane from a cine gradient echo sequence using an echo time of 14 ms. There is loss of signal in the left ventricle because of the turbulent jet through the mitral valve. Top left is an in-plane diastolic velocity map of the same slice but rotated so that the jet is from top to bottom of the image (acquired using an echo time of 3.6 ms). The jet is clearly seen (white) with reversed flow in the parajet region (black). Top right is a velocity map perpendicular to this and encoded through the plane of the image. The profile through the jet has a peak velocity of 2.4 m/s corresponding to a pressure gradient of 23 mmHg.

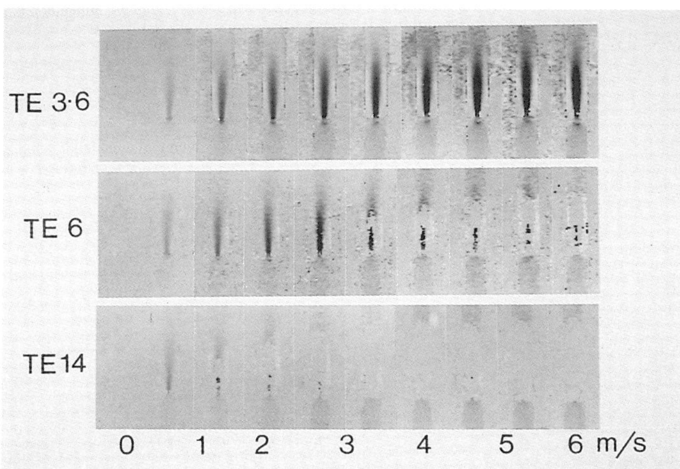

Figure 10.27. Velocity maps of a jet through a 6 mm stenosis in a 20 mm diameter tube. The flow rate increases from left to right and FEER sequences with echo times (TE) of 14, 6 and 3.6 ms were used. Significant signal loss occurs at higher flow rates with the longer echo times, but velocities up to 6 m/s can be measured with TE 3.6 ms.

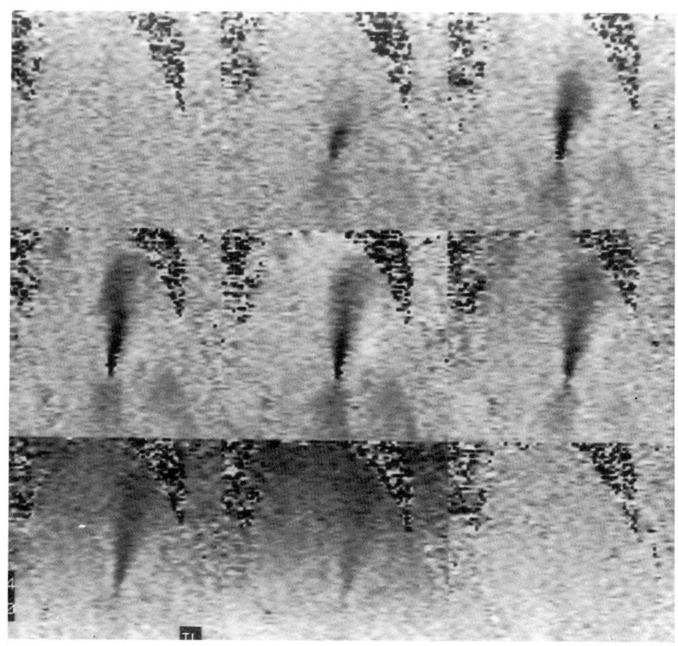

Figure 10.29. Cine velocity mapping in a patient with aortic stenosis. The plane is a tilted coronal plane to include the jet and encoding is from bottom to top of the image. Peak velocity in the jet is 5.6 m/s which corresponds to a pressure gradient of 125 mm of mercury. A gradient of 105 mm was measured at cardiac catheterisation.

complex pattern in diastole is probably the result of the skewed systolic velocity profile. When the aortic valve closes the net momentum of the blood in the ascending

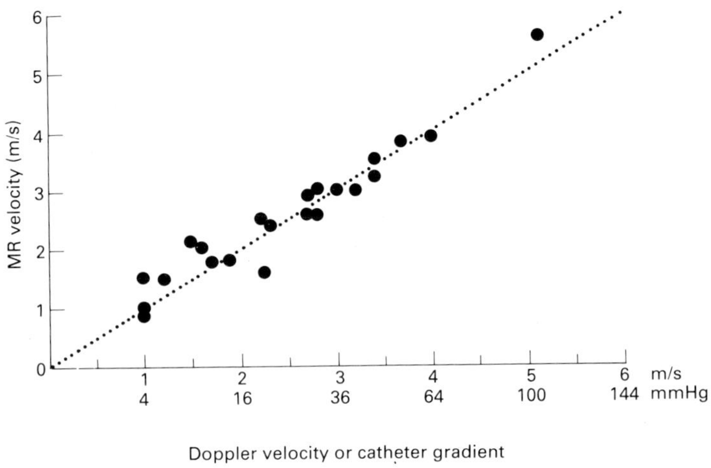

Figure 10.30. Correlation between magnetic resonance peak jet velocity and either continuous wave Doppler measurement or pressure gradient measured by cardiac catheterisation and converted using the modified Bernoulli equation. Twenty two patients are shown with a variety of stenoses in right or left sided valves, surgically created conduits, and great vessels.

aorta must be zero (ignoring the relatively small amount of retrograde flow into the coronary arteries). The differential velocity across the aorta must be maintained however, and so the more rapidly moving blood continues to move forwards at the expense of the rest of the blood which moves backwards.

The reason for this complex pattern is unknown, but in normal subjects the retrograde channel is closely associated with the left coronary sinus and it is tempting to speculate that it augments flow in the left coronary artery by imparting momentum to the blood which is destined to enter it. In patients with coronary artery disease this normal pattern is disturbed.[71] The retrograde channel is smaller and it can be abnormally placed, entering any of the coronary sinuses. There is also a close link between the pattern of flow in the aorta and its compliance (see chapter 11), and in patients with arterial disease and reduced compliance the backflow channel is reduced.

Pulmonary flow profiles have been less well studied but magnetic resonance velocity mapping has confirmed the early systolic peak in patients with pulmonary hypertension;[65] a finding that was already well known from invasive and Doppler flow studies. The early peak is caused by the reflected waves from the distal vasculature which has a high impedance. Detailed analysis of the curve can provide an estimate of characteristic impedance of the pulmonary artery and also, in theory, the impedance of the peripheral vasculature. Such analyses have been touched on using magnetic resonance velocity mapping[72] but detailed studies remain to be performed.

It has also been possible to measure aortic flow wave velocity. Cine velocity mapping is performed with high temporal resolution (8 ms) in a transverse plane through the ascending and descending aorta. The flow wave velocity is calculated from the delay between the appearance of the flow wave in both limbs of the aorta. This parameter is closely related to compliance and it may prove to be useful for the detection and monitoring of arterial disease. The technique is discussed in more detail in chapter 11.

10.7.5 Caval flow

The caval veins are also relatively large, and reliable velocity maps and flow measurements can be obtained.[73] The inferior caval vein is more difficult than the superior caval vein because the hepatic vein often joins very close to the right atrium. The normal pattern of flow has peaks of roughly equal sizes in systole and diastole but this pattern is disturbed by disease.[74] Any condition that causes impaired filling of the right ventricle reduces the diastolic peak, and this pattern is seen in constrictive and restrictive disease, in pulmonary stenosis and in pulmonary hypertension (presumably caused by diastolic right ventricular dysfunction). Magnetic resonance imaging is now commonly requested for the assessment of pericardial disease and so the ability to measure caval flow is an important adjunct, providing an estimate of the functional significance of the disease.

Tricuspid regurgitation attenuates the systolic peak of caval flow, sometimes to the extent that reverse flow occurs. This is perhaps less helpful, because the severity of regurgitation can be assessed by cine imaging or from a comparison of right and left ventricular stroke volumes. Nevertheless, a normal systolic flow peak suggests that tricuspid regurgitation, if it is seen, is not significant.

10.7.6 Coronary flow measurements

Flow has been measured in coronary artery bypass grafts using velocity mapping although the small size of the vessels makes it difficult to obtain reliable results

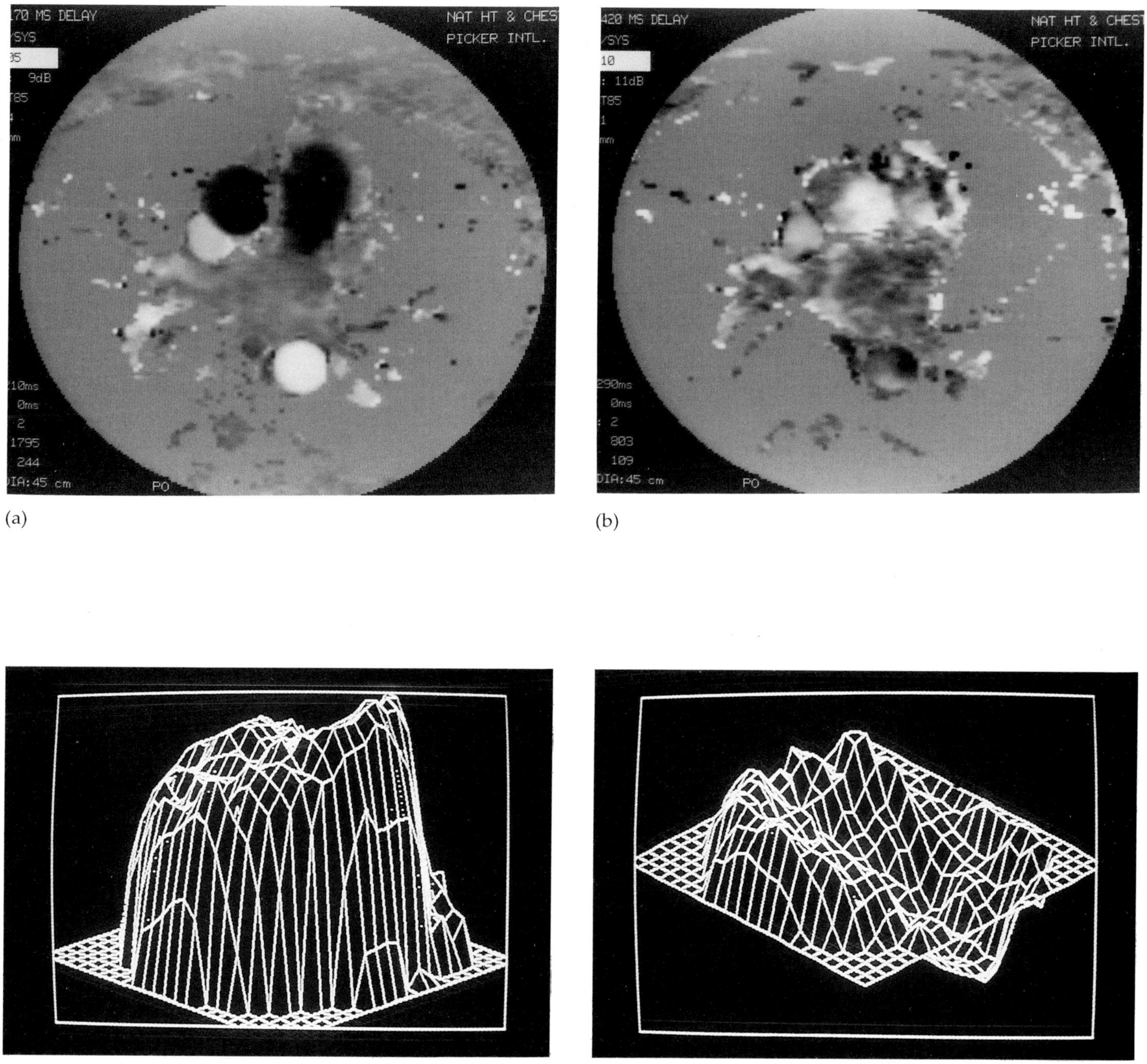

Figure 10.31. (a) Systolic and (b) diastolic velocity maps showing flow in the ascending aorta. The skewed plug flow in systole alters to simultaneous antegrade and retrograde channels in diastole. (c) and (d) show the same information although the aorta is selected out and a pseudo three-dimensional computer display has been used with antegrade velocities above the plane of the section and retrograde velocities below it.

in all cases. Examples have been shown in chapter 5 and peak velocities under 0.1 m/s suggest inadequate flow. Coronary artery flow measurements are more difficult because of the smaller size and the rapid movement but velocity maps showing coronary artery flow can be acquired in favourable circumstance. Figure

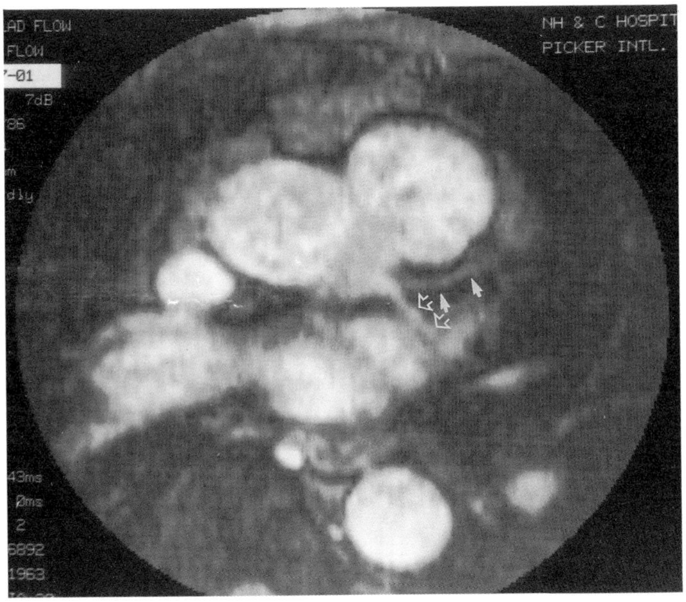

(a)

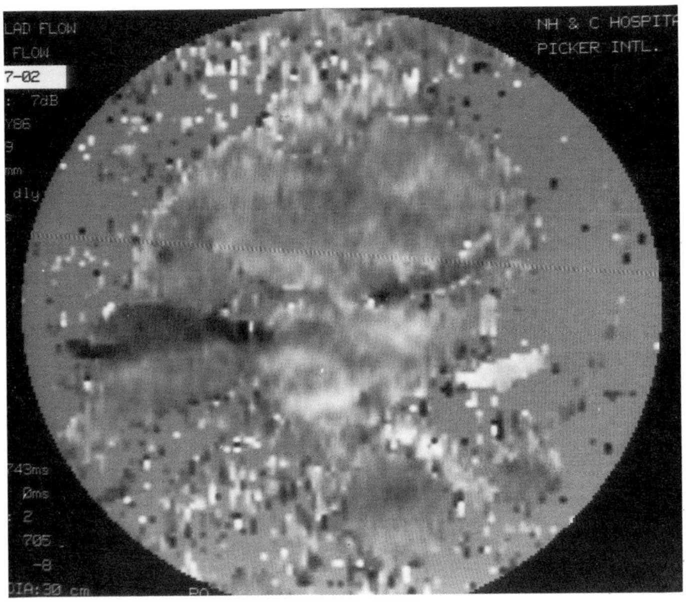

(b)

Figure 10.32. (a) Field echo image showing the left anterior descending (closed arrows) and left circumflex coronary arteries (open arrows). (b) The equivalent velocity map (encoded from right to left) shows flow in the left anterior descending artery.

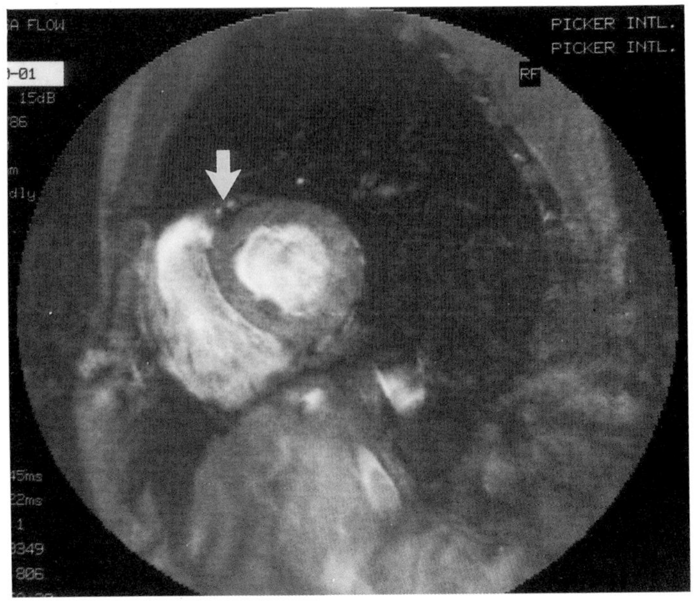

(a)

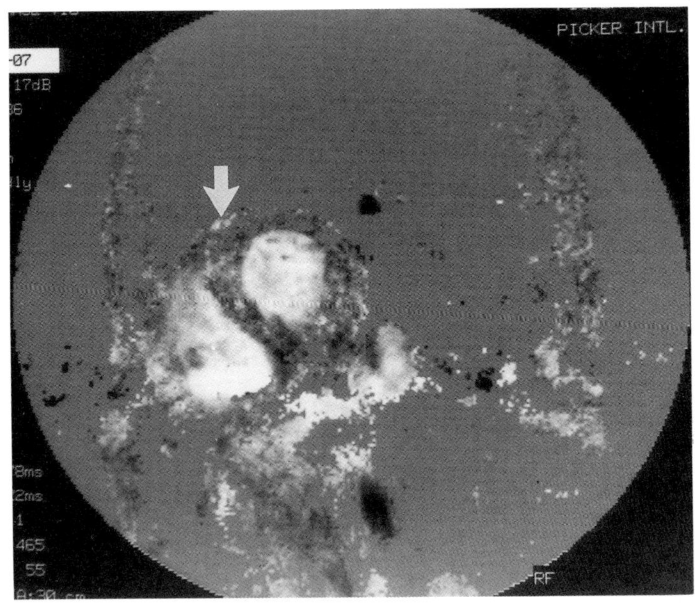

(b)

Figure 10.33. (a) Short axis field echo image showing coronary vessels in the anterior interventricular groove (arrow). (b) Diastolic velocity map encoded through the plane of the image shows flow in coronary vessels and also in the ventricular cavities.

10.32 shows an in-plane velocity map with flow in the left anterior descending artery. Although it is less difficult to acquire an in-plane map, partial volume effects mean that through-plane maps are more accurate (figure 10.33). It is possible that echo planar velocity mapping may overcome some of the problems of imaging such rapidly moving structures.

References

1 Purcell EM, Torrey HC, Pound RV. Resonance absorption by nuclear magnetic moments in a solid. *Phys Rev* 1946; **69**: 37–8.

2 Bloch F, Hansen WW, Packard M. *Phys Rev* 1946; **69**: 127.

3 Bloembergen N, Purcell EM, Pound RV. Relaxation effects in nuclear magnetic resonance absorption. *Phys Rev* 1948; **73**: 679–712.

4 Suryan G. Nuclear resonance in flowing liquids. *Proc Ind Acad Sci (A)* 1951; **33**: 107–11.

5 Bowman RL, Kudravcev V. Blood flowmeter utilizing nuclear magnetic resonance. *IRE Trans Med Elec* 1959; **6**: 267–9.

6 Singer JR. Blood flow rates by nuclear magnetic resonance measurements. *Science* 1959; **130**: 1652–3.

7 Jones DW, Child TF. NMR in flowing systems. *Adv Magn Reson* 1976; **8**: 123–48.

8 Zhernovoi AI, Latyshev GD. *Nuclear Magnetic Resonance in a Flowing Liquid*. Translated from Russian by Turton CN, Turton TE. New York: Consultants Bureau, 1965.

9 Singer JR, Crooks LE. Nuclear magnetic resonance blood flow measurements in the human brain. *Science* 1983; **221**: 654–6.

10 Bradley WG, Waluch V. Blood flow: magnetic resonance imaging. *Radiology* 1985; **154**: 443–50.

11 Grant JP, Back C. NMR rheotomography: feasibility and clinical potential. *Med Phys* 1982; **9**: 188–93.

12 Bradley WG, Waluch V, Lai KS, Fernandez EJ, Spaiter C. The appearance of rapidly flowing blood on magnetic resonance images. *Am J Roentgenol* 1984; **143**: 1167–74.

13 Perman WH, Moran PR, Moran RA, Bernstein MA. Artifacts from pulsatile flow in MR imaging. *J Comput Assist Tomogr* 1986; **10**: 473–83.

14 Carr HY, Purcell EM. Effects of diffusion on free precession in nuclear magnetic resonance experiments. *Phys Rev* 1954; **94**: 630–8.

15 Waluch V, Bradley WG. NMR even echo rephasing in slow laminar flow. *J Comput Assist Tomogr* 1984; **8**: 594–8.

16 Nayler GL, Firmin DN, Longmore DB. Blood flow imaging by cine magnetic resonance. *J Comput Assist Tomogr* 1986; **10**: 715–22.

17 Pattany PM, Phillips JJ, Chiu LC, *et al*. Motion artefact suppression technique (MAST) for MR Imaging. *J Comput Assist Tomogr* 1987; **11**: 369–77.

18 Von Schulthess GK, Higgins CB. Blood flow imaging with MR: spin phase phenomena. *Radiology* 1985; **157**: 687–95.

19 Battocletti JH, Linehan JH, Larson SJ, *et al*. Analysis of a nuclear magnetic resonance blood flowmeter for pulsatile flow. *IEEE Trans Biomed Eng* 1972; **BME–19**: 403–7.

20 Battocletti JH, Sances A, Larson SJ, *et al*. Clinical applications and theoretical analysis of NMR blood flowmeter. *Biomed Eng* 1975; **10**: 12–5.

21 Halbach RE, Battocletti JH, Sances A, Larson SJ, Bowman RL, Kudravcev V. Blood flow detection using the flat crossed-coil nuclear magnetic resonance flowmeter. *IEEE Trans Biomed Eng* 1981; **BME–28**: 40–2.

22 Battocletti JH, Halbach RE, Salles-Cunha SX, Sances A. Nuclear magnetic resonance and transcutaneous electromagnetic blood flow measurement. *J Microwave Power* 1983; **18**: 221–32.

23 Battocletti JH, Halbach RE, Salles-Cunha SX, Sances A. The NMR blood flowmeter-theory and history. *Med Phys* 1981; **8**: 435–43.

24 Halbach RE, Battocletti JH, Salles-Cunha SX, Sances A. The NMR blood flowmeter-design. *Med Phys* 1981; **8**: 444–51.

25 Salles-Cunha SX, Halbach RE, Battocletti JH, Sances A. The NMR blood flowmeter-applications. *Med Phys* 1981; **8**: 452–8.

26 Garroway AN. Velocity measurements in flowing fluids by NMR. *J Phys D: Appl Phys* 1974; **7**: L159–63.

27 Thulborn KR, Waterton JC, Radda GK. Proton imaging for in-vivo blood flow and oxygen consumption measurements. *J Magn Reson* 1981; **45**: 188–91.

28 Mueller E, Deimling M, Reinhardt ER. Quantification of pulsatile flow in MRI by an analysis of T_2 changes in ECG-gated multiecho experiments. *Magn Reson Med* 1986; **3**: 331–5.

29 Wehrli FW, Shimakawa A, Gullberg GT, MacFall JR. Time-of-flight MR flow imaging: Selective saturation recovery with gradient refocusing. *Radiology* 1986; **160**: 781–5.

30 Hennig J, Mueri M, Friedburg H, Brunner P. MR imaging of flow using the steady state selective saturation method. *J Comput Assist Tomogr* 1987; **11**: 872–7.

31 Genthe WK, Vander Heyden WR, Battocletti JH, McCormick WS, Snowball HM. NMR applied to flow measurement. An obstructionless, digital flowmeter. *Instr Tech* 1968; **15**: 53–8.

32 Morse OC, Singer JR. Blood velocity measurements in intact subjects. *Science* 1970; **170**: 440–1.

33 Feinberg DA, Crooks LE, Hoenninger J, Arakawa M, Watts J. Pulsatile blood velocity in human arteries displayed by magnetic resonance imaging. *Radiology* 1984; **153**: 177–80.

34 Kaufman L, Crooks LE, Sheldon PE, Rowan W, Miller T. Evaluation of NMR imaging for detection and quantification of obstructions in vessels. *Invest Radiol* 1982; **17**: 554–60.

35 Shimizu K, Matsuda T, Sakurai T, *et al*. Visualization of moving fluid: quantitative analysis of blood flow velocity using MR imaging. *Radiology* 1986; **159**: 195–9.

36 Matsuda T, Shimizu K, Sakurai T, *et al*. Measurement of aortic blood flow with MR imaging: comparative study with doppler US. *Radiology* 1987; **162**: 857–61.

37 Axel L, Shimakawa A, MacFall J. A time-of-flight method of measuring flow velocity by magnetic resonance imaging. *Magn Reson Imag* 1986; **4**: 199–205.

38 Feinberg DA, Hoenninger J, Crooks LE, Kaufman L, Watts J, Arakawa M. Inner volume MR imaging: technical concepts and their application. *Radiology* 1985; **156**: 743–7.

39 Hahn EL. Detection of sea-water motion by nuclear precession. *Geophys Res* 1960; **65**: 776–7.

40 Packer KJ. The study of slow coherent molecular motion by pulsed nuclear magnetic resonance. *Mol Phys* 1969; **17**: 355–68.

41 Meiboom S, Gill D. Modified spin-echo method for measuring nuclear relaxation times. *Rev Sci Instr* 1958; **29**: 688–91.

42 Lucas PGJ, Penman DA, Tyler A, Vavasour E. Measurement of fluid flow profiles using pulsed NMR. *J Phys E: Sci Instr* 1977; **10**: 1150–2.

43 Borodin PM. Use of free precession of nuclei in the earths magnetic field for the measurement of the velocity and rate of flow of some liquids. *Sov Phys-Tech Phys* 1965; **9**: 1027–32.

44 Hemminga MA, De Jager PA, Sonneveld A. The study of flow by pulsed nuclear magnetic resonance. I. Measurement of flow rates in the presence of a stationary phase using a difference method. *J Magn Reson* 1977; **27**: 359–70.

45 de Jager PA, Hemminga MA, Sonneveld A. Novel method for the determination of flow velocities with pulsed nuclear magnetic resonance. *Rev Sci Instrum* 1978; **49**: 1217–8.

46 Hinshaw WS. Image-formation by the nuclear magnetic resonance sensitive-point method. *J Appl Phys* 1976; **47**: 3709–21.

47 Altobelli SA, Caprihan A, Davis JG, Fukushima E. Rapid average-flow velocity measurement by NMR. *Magn Reson Med* 1986; **3**: 317–20.

48 Moran PR. A flow zeugmatographic interlace for NMR imaging in humans. *Magn Reson Imaging* 1982; **1**: 197–203.

49 Redpath TW, Norris DG, Jones RA, Hutchinson MS. A new method of NMR flow imaging. *Phys Med Biol* 1984; **29**: 891–8.

50 Feinberg DA, Crooks LE, Sheldon P, Hoenninger J, Watts J, Arakawa M. Magnetic resonance imaging and velocity vector components of fluid flow. *Magn Reson Med* 1985; **2**: 555–66.

51 Hennig J, Mueri M, Brunner P, Friedburg H. Quantitative flow measurement with the fast fourier flow technique. *Radiology* 1988; **166**: 237–40.

52 van Dijk P. Direct cardiac NMR imaging of heart wall and blood flow velocity. *J Comput Assist Tomogr* 1984; **8**: 429–36.

53 Bryant DJ, Payne JA, Firmin DN, Longmore DB. Measurement of flow with NMR imaging using a gradient pulse and phase difference technique. *J Comput Assist Tomogr* 1984; **8**: 588–93.

54 Wedeen VJ, Rosen BR, Chesler D, Brady TJ. MR velocity imaging by phase display. *J Comput Assist Tomogr* 1985; **9**: 530–6.

55 Dinsmore RE, Wedeen VJ, Rosen B, Wismer GL, Miller SW, Brady TJ. Phase-offset technique to distinguish slow blood flow and thrombus on MR images. *Am J Roentgenol* 1987; **148**: 634–6.

56 Nayler GL, Firmin DN, Longmore DB. Blood flow imaging by cine magnetic resonance. *J Comput Assist Tomogr* 1986; **10**: 715–22.

57 Young IR, Hall AS, Bryant DJ, *et al*. Assessment of brain perfusion with MR imaging. *J Comput Assist Tomogr* 1988; **12**: 721–7.

58 Firmin DN, Klipstein RH, Hounsfield GN, Paley MP, Longmore DB. Echo-planar high-resolution flow velocity mapping. *Magn Reson Med* 1989; **12**: 316–27.

59 Feinberg DA, Hale JS. Echo planar-inner volume imaging at 0.35 T. *Proceedings of the Fifth Annual Meeting, Society of Magnetic Resonance in Medicine*, 1986: 950.

60 Maier SE, Meier D, Boesiger P, Moser UT, Vieli A. Human abdominal aorta: comparative measurements of blood flow with MR imaging and multigated Doppler US. *Radiology* 1989; **171**: 487–92.

61 Kilner PJ, Firmin DN, Mohiaddin RH, Underwood SR, Rees RSO, Longmore DB. Assessment of valve and great vessel stenosis: trials of a new method using magnetic resonance velocity mapping. *Radiology* (Submitted February 1990).

62 Longmore DB, Klipstein RH, Underwood SR, *et al*. Dimensional accuracy of magnetic resonance in studies of the heart. *Lancet* 1985; **i**: 1360–2.

63 Firmin DN, Nayler GL, Klipstein RH, Underwood SR, Rees RSO, Longmore DB. In vivo validation of MR velocity imaging. *J Comput Assist Tomogr* 1987; **11**: 751–6.

64 Bogren HG, Klipstein RH, Firmin DN, *et al*. Quantitation of antegrade and retrograde blood flow in the human aorta by magnetic resonance. *Am Heart J* 1989; **117**: 1214–22.

65 Bogren HG, Klipstein RH, Mohiaddin RH, *et al*. Pulmonary artery distensibility and blood flow patterns: a magnetic resonance study of normal subjects and of patients with pulmonary arterial hypertension. *Am Heart J* 1989; **118**: 990–9.

66 Underwood SR, Firmin DN, Klipstein RH, Rees RSO, Longmore DB. Magnetic resonance velocity mapping: clinical application of a new technique. *Br Heart J* 1987; **57**: 404–12

67 Rees RSO, Firmin DN, Mohiaddin RH, Underwood SR, Longmore DB. Application of flow measurements by magnetic resonance velocity mapping to congenital heart disease. *Am J Cardiol* 1989; **64**: 953–6.

68 Goldman ME. Real-time two-dimensional doppler flow imaging: a word of caution. *J Am Coll Cardiol* 1986; **7**: 89–90.

69 Come PC. The optimal Doppler examination: pulsed, continuous wave or both? *J Am Coll Cardiol* 1986; **7**: 886–8.

70 Klipstein RH, Firmin DN, Underwood SR, Rees RSO, Longmore DB. Blood flow patterns in the human aorta studied by magnetic resonance. *Br Heart J* 1987; **58**: 316–23.

71 Bogren HG, Mohiaddin RH, Klipstein RH, *et al*. The function of the aorta in ischemic heart disease: a magnetic resonance and angiographic study of aortic compliance and blood flow patterns. *Am Heart J* 1989; **118**: 234–47.

72 Tokuhiro T, Matsuo T. A NMR study of blood flow in aorta. *Proceedings of the Eighth Annual Meeting, Society of Magnetic Resonance in Medicine*, 1989: **202** (Abstract).

73 Mohiaddin RH, Underwood SR, Firmin DN, *et al*. The effect of respiration on caval venous flow determined by cine magnetic resonance velocity mapping. *Proceedings of the Seventh Annual Meeting, Society of Magnetic Resonance in Medicine*, 1988; **182** (Abstract).

74 Mohiaddin RH, Underwood SR, Wann SL, Firmin DN, Rees RSO, Longmore DB. MRI velocity mapping of caval venous flow: clinical study. *Proceedings of the Eighth Annual Meeting, Society of Magnetic Resonance in Medicine* 1989; **206** (Abstract).

Chapter 11
Atherosclerotic Vascular Disease

RAAD MOHIADDIN

Atherosclerotic vascular disease is the most common cause of death and disability in the western world[1] and so the potential contributions of magnetic resonance to its detection and assessment are important. The pathogenesis of the disease is controversial[2] but the hypothesis that it is a response to injury, dating from the pioneering work of Virchow in 1856[3] and recently reviewed by Ross,[4] has gained widespread acceptance. A variety of lesions affects the arterial wall, from non-protruding fatty streaks to more complex lesions consisting of lipid, smooth muscle, fibroblasts, and occasionally calcification. In addition to discrete atherotic lesions a localised and generalised sclerosis occurs. Sclerosis, or stiffness, can be demonstrated both in experimental disease in animals[5] and in man,[6] and regression leads to reduced stiffness.[7]

Magnetic resonance provides techniques which allow all the aspects of atherosclerosis to be studied. Atheroma can be imaged directly, its size can be measured, its shape can be described, its lipid content can be assessed and its effects upon vascular haemodynamics can be studied.[8,9] In addition, arterial compliance, pulse wave velocity, and the pattern of flow within the aorta can be studied.[10,11] It is thus a potential tool not only for the detection of disease but also for studying its natural history, risk factors and the effects of pharmacological or surgical interventions. In this chapter we review these techniques which, although at an early stage of development, promise an important role for magnetic resonance in the assessment of arterial disease.

11.1 The assessment of atherosis

11.1.1 Chemical shift imaging

Because signal is absent from flowing blood, high natural contrast exists between the arterial lumen and the wall, providing ideal circumstances for the demonstration of vascular anatomy and of atherosclerotic plaques. Magnetic resonance angiography has been described in chapter 9 and conventional imaging has been used to study atheromatous lesions in *post mortem* human arteries, in experimental animal models, and in patients with atherosclerosis.[12,13] Most of these studies, however, have relied upon distortion of the arterial lumen and have not involved direct visualisation of the atheroma. Those that have, have used conventional techniques which image hydrogen irrespective of chemical environment, and have not exploited the chemical shift of resonant frequency between the hydrogen in water and fat (3.3 ppm). Imaging nuclei with only a particular resonant frequency rather than the entire spectrum of resonant frequencies is called chemical shift imaging.[14] Several techniques of proton chemical shift imaging have been described.[15] The original method of Dixon[16] results in an image where pure water and pure fat produce no signal and tissues with a mixture of water and fat have higher signal (figure 11.1). The method of Hinks[17] is a true water or fat imaging technique where only signal from water or from fat contributes to the image.

Figures 11.2–11.4 show applications of the Dixon technique. In figure 11.2, a raw egg is imaged. The subtraction image, which shows high signal from tissues with high concentration of lipid, shows high signal from the lipid-rich yolk. Figure 11.3 shows a lipid rich atheromatous plaque in a *post mortem* human aorta. The in-phase image shows both the plaque and an area of extravascular fat without information on lipid concentration, but the subtraction image shows that the plaque has a high lipid content. In contrast, figure 11.4 shows a lipid deficient plaque with very low signal in the subtraction image. Figure 11.5 shows an example of the Hinks technique in a *post mortem* aortic specimen. High signal is seen in the extra-

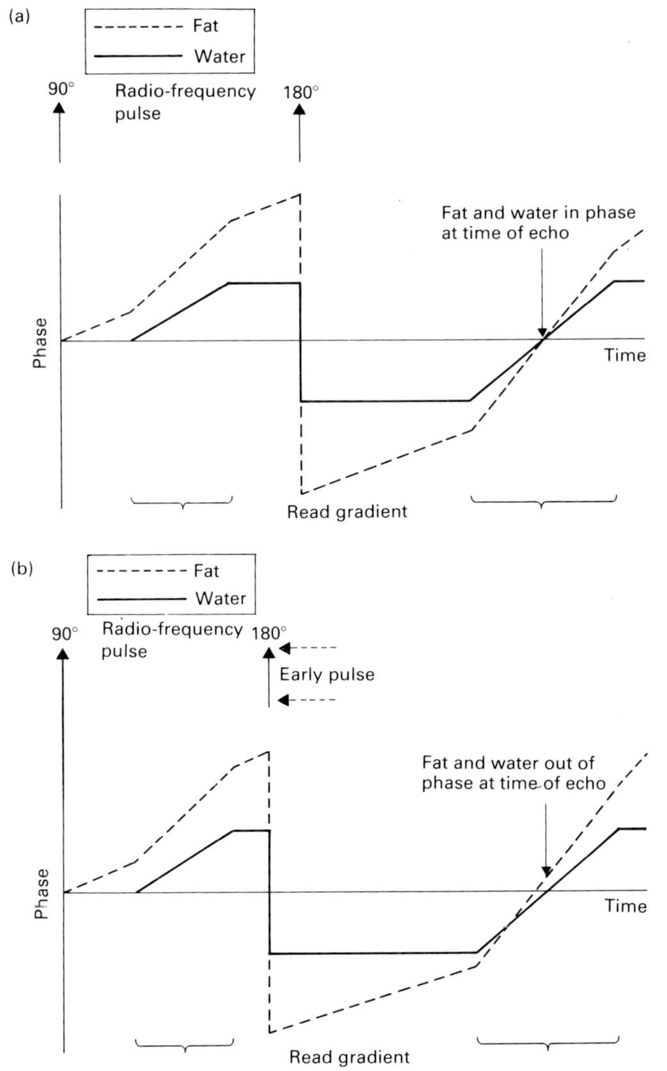

Figure 11.1. Diagram of the Dixon pulse sequences. (a) A conventional spin echo sequence gives an 'in phase' image because fat and water precess with the same phase at the time of the echo and the signal is the sum of that from fat and water. (b) The second sequence is an asymmetrical spin echo sequence in which phase of fat and water differs by 180° at the time of signal acquisition. Subtraction of the 'in phase' and the 'out of phase' images produces an image in which there is only signal in voxels containing both fat and water. (Reproduced with permission from *Br Heart J* 1989; **62**: 81–90.)

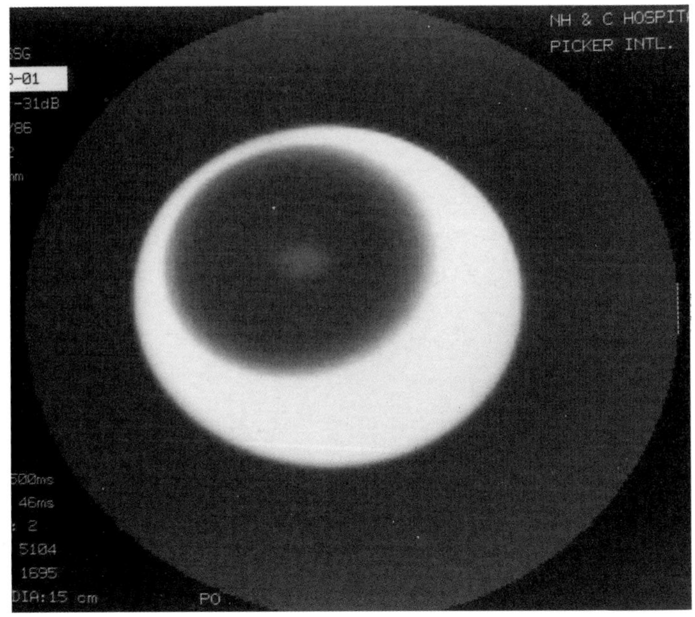

(a)

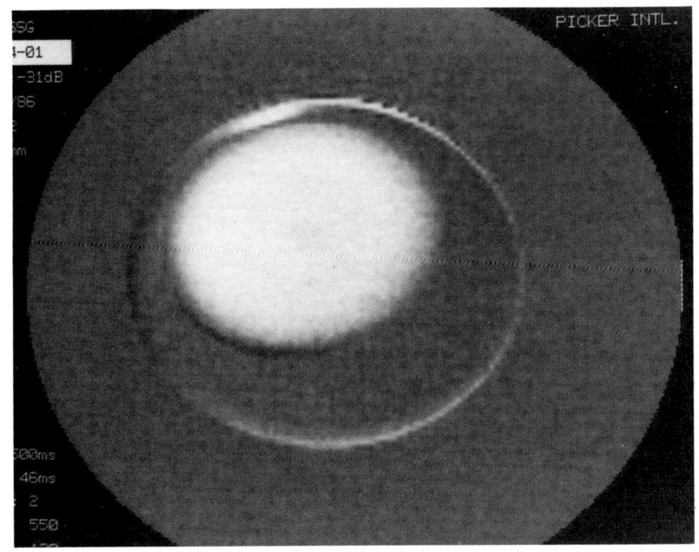

(b)

Figure 11.2. (a) Conventional spin echo image of a raw egg showing high signal from the white (aqueous) and lower signal from the yolk (lipid). (b) The subtraction image shows high signal in the lipid-rich yolk. (Reproduced with permission from *Br Med Bull* 1989; **45**: 968–90.)

vascular fat but the lack of signal in the vessel wall indicates absence of lipid.

Patients with documented peripheral vascular disease have also been studied. Figure 11.6 shows an image of the descending abdominal aorta in which the circular lumen is distorted by thickening of the wall with an atheromatous plaque. The Dixon subtraction image shows that this plaque has low lipid content. Figure 11.7 shows another patient with a high lipid plaque.

The morphology and composition of arterial segments containing atheroma is of considerable importance. Plaques of different morphology (concentric or eccentric for example) have different effects on the

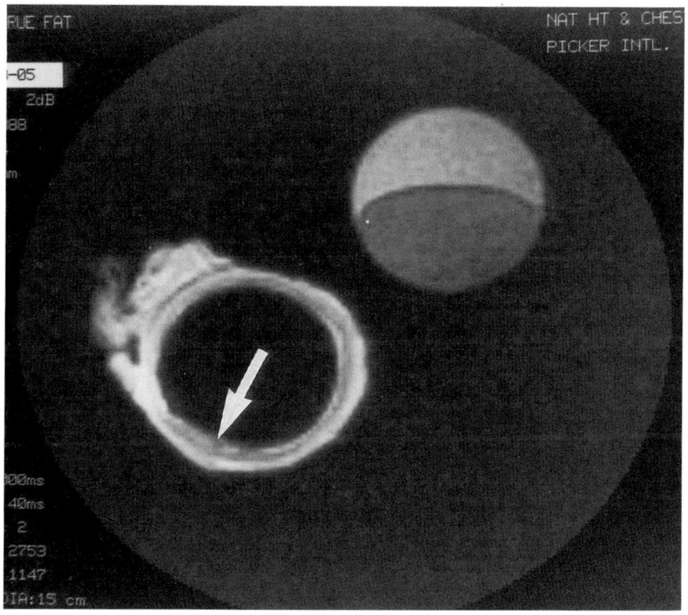

(a)

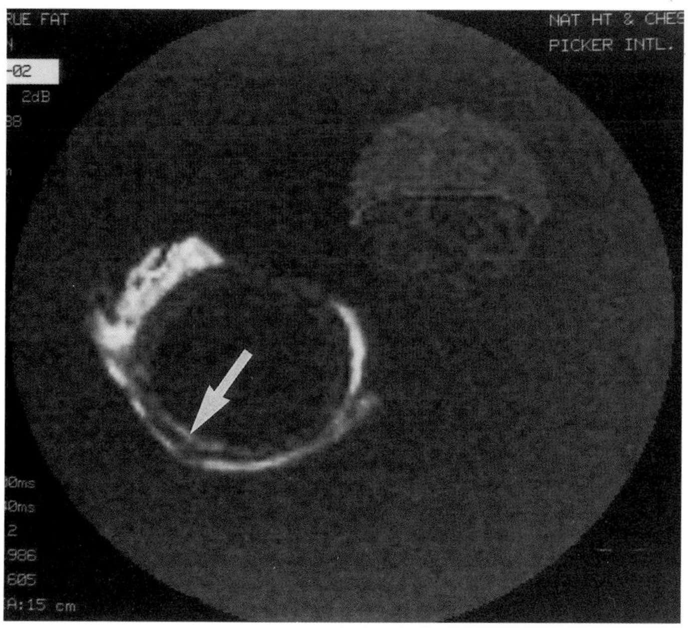

(b)

Figure 11.3. (a) *Post mortem* aortic specimen imaged using a conventional spin echo sequence together with a phantom containing oil floating on water. Atheroma involves approximately half of the circumference of the vessel and the largest accumulation is arrowed. (b) The subtraction image shows high signal in extravascular fat and in the lesion. The ratio of signal intensity compared with extravascular fat is 45%. The oil and water in the phantom give low signal as expected. (c) (See plate 2, facing p. 36) Histology of the same plaque (oil red O stain) showing lipid deposition (red) within the intima. (Reproduced with permission from *Br Heart J* 1989; **62**: 81–90.)

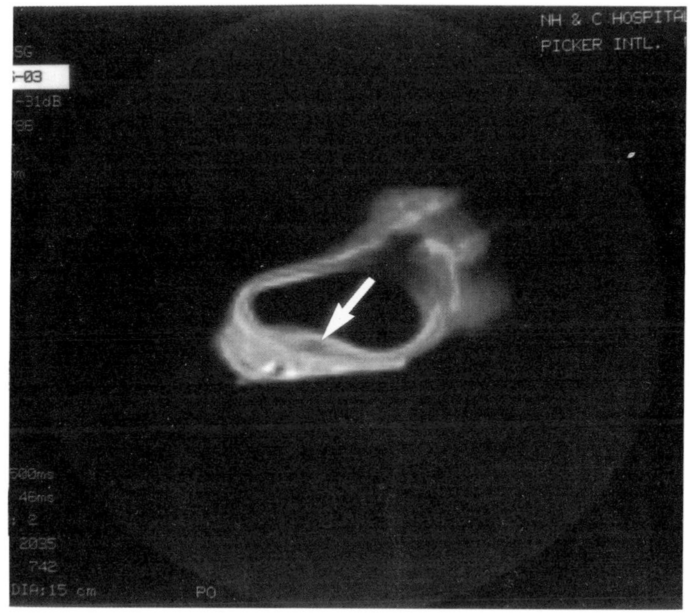

(a)

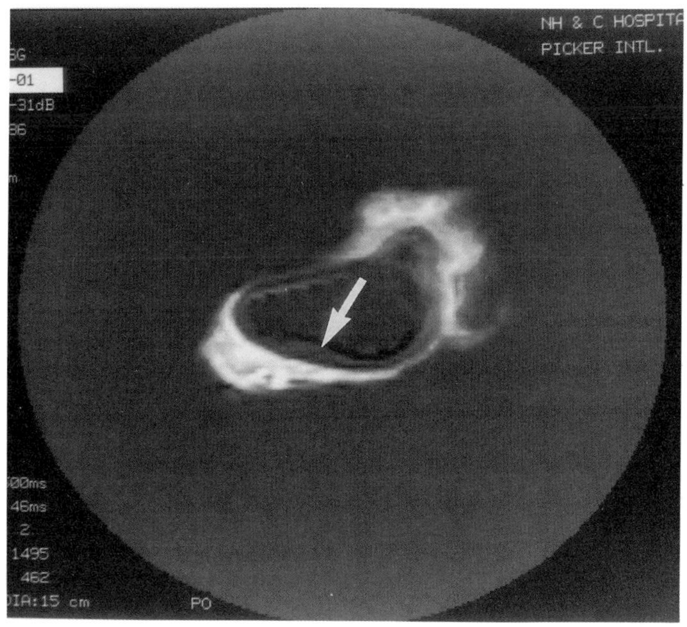

(b)

Figure 11.4. (a) Conventional image of a lipid deficient plaque in a *post mortem* aortic specimen (arrowed). (b) The subtraction image shows very low signal (8%) compared with that from the extravascular fat. (c) (See plate 3, facing p. 36) Elastic Van Gieson stain of the same plaque indicates a predominantly smooth muscle and fibrous plaque. Lipid deposition would appear as vacuoles in this alcohol treated stain, but there are none. (Reproduced with permission from *Br Heart J* 1989; **62**: 81–90.)

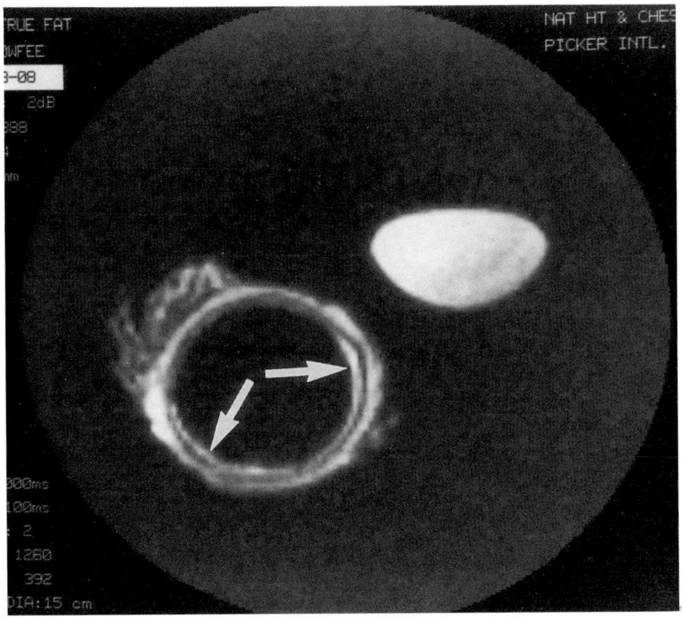

(a)

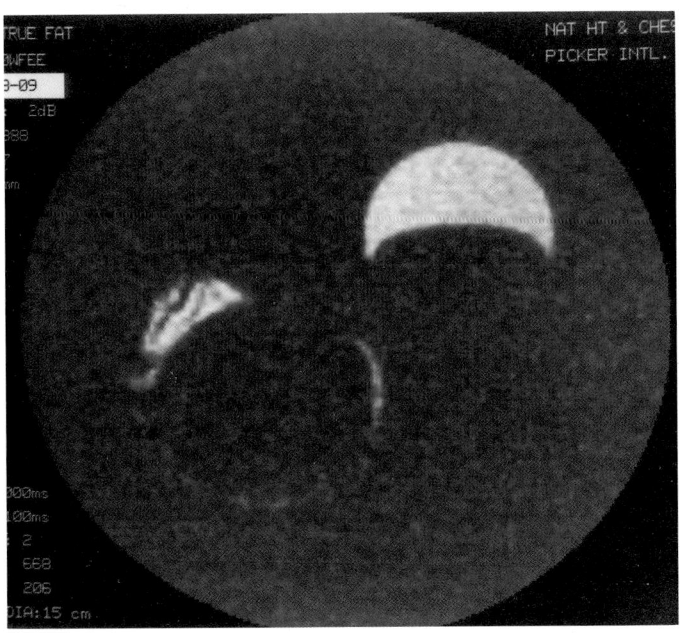

(b)

Figure 11.5. True fat and true water images acquired using the Hinks technique. (a) In the water image, a *post mortem* aortic specimen lies beside a phantom containing oil floating upon water, but only the water is seen. The vessel wall is thickened by atheroma for 60% of its circumference (arrowed). (b) The fat image shows high signal from the extravascular fat, but low signal from the areas of atheroma, and in the phantom only the oil is seen. (Reproduced with permission from *Br Heart J* 1989; **62**: 81–90.)

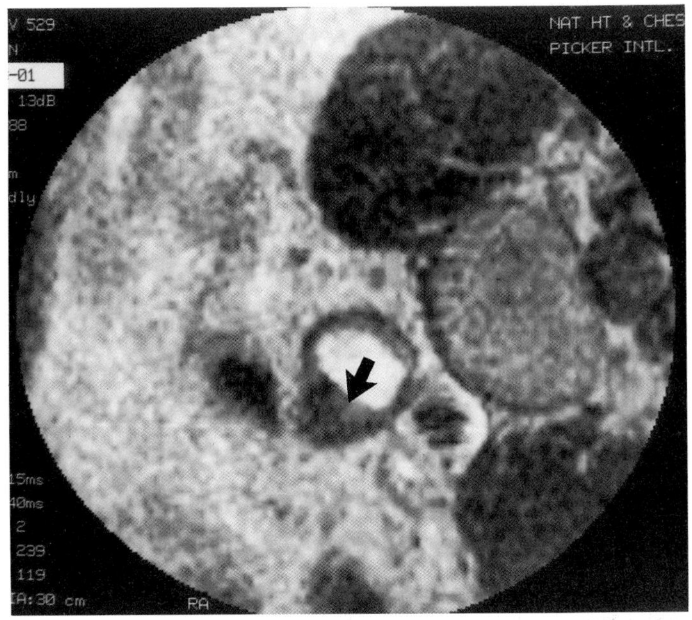

(a)

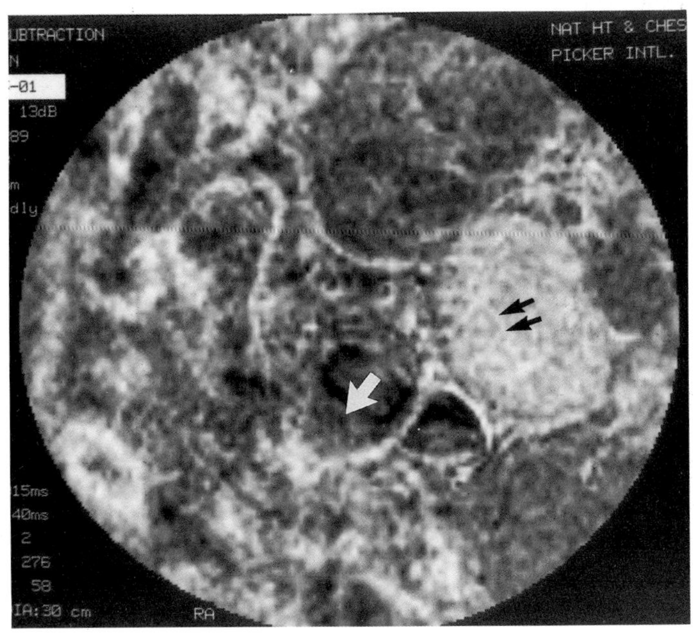

(b)

Figure 11.6. (a) Spin echo image perpendicular to the descending aorta of a 60-year-old man with peripheral vascular disease, showing a large atheromatous plaque expanding the vessel wall (arrowed). (b) The subtraction image shows low signal in the lesion (white arrow) indicating low lipid content. There is high signal from extravascular fat and from the bone marrow in the body of the lumbar vertebra (black arrows). (Reproduced with permission from *Br Heart J* 1989; **62**: 81–90.)

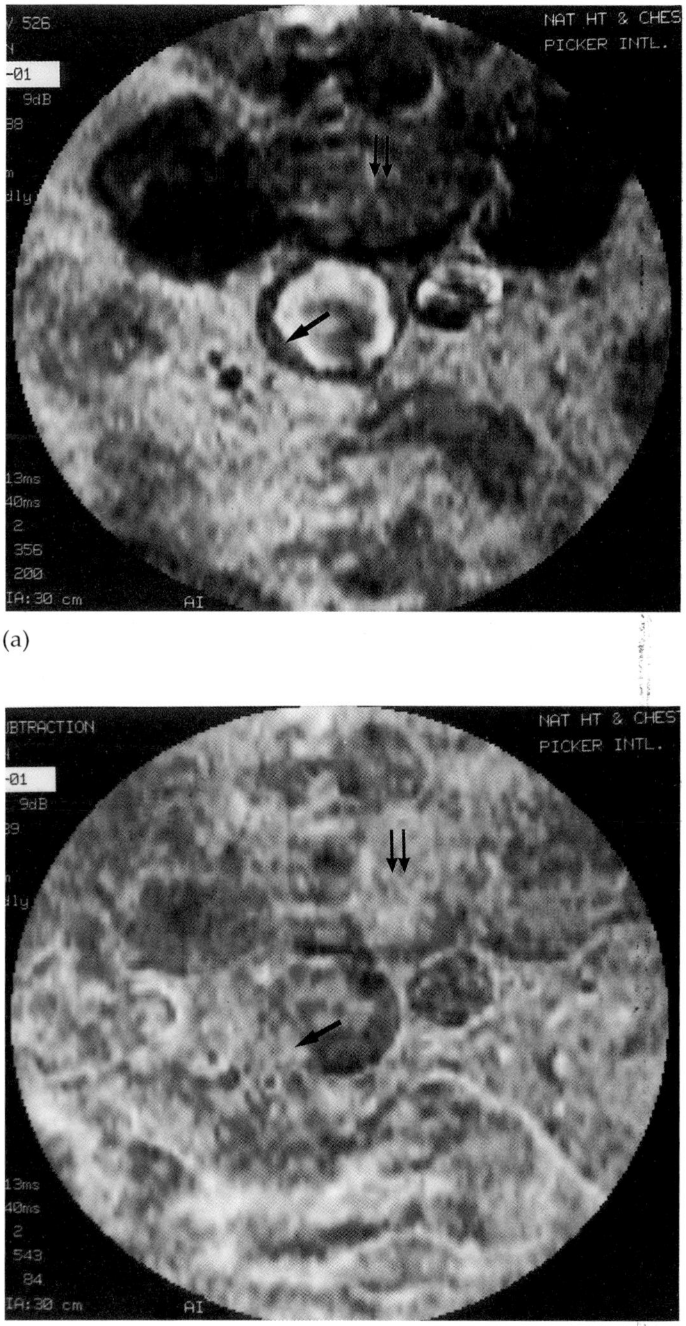

(a)

(b)

Figure 11.7. (a) Spin echo image perpendicular to the descending aorta of a 57-year-old man with peripheral vascular disease. The wall is irregularly thickened with atheroma and the main accumulation is indicated (single arrow). The subtraction image (b) shows high signal within the lesion indicating high lipid content, similar to the marrow in the lumbar vertebral body (double arrow). (Reproduced with permission from *Br Heart J* 1989; **62**: 81–90.)

arterial wall, such as the potential for thrombosis and the effect of arterial spasm.[18] The lipid content may also affect the propensity for fissuring, ulceration and thrombosis.[19] Other properties of atheroma that may be affected by the lipid content are the short and long-term outcome of angioplasty, and the potential for regression.[20] Although little is known of these areas it is possible that there is a link between the composition of atheroma and its susceptibility to chemical or mechanical intervention. There is evidence that regression can occur in experimental animals and that it may be possible to alter the rate of progression in man.[21]

11.1.2 Velocity mapping

The technique of magnetic resonance velocity mapping has been described in chapter 10. Velocity profiles along an atheromatous vessel are particularly useful to localise disease and to measure the degree of stenosis. Blood flowing into a stenosed region must accelerate and the mean velocity increase is proportional to the reduction of cross sectional area.[22] This principle is illustrated in the following figures. Figure 11.8 shows anatomical images and velocity maps of a normal abdominal aorta. The arterial wall is smooth and the velocity profiles through the aorta and iliac vessels are similar. Figure 11.9 shows images in a patient with peripheral vascular disease. The left iliac artery is narrowed and the velocity map shows high velocity past the obstruction. Figure 11.10 shows more extensive atheromatous disease involving the aortic bifurcation and the common iliac arteries.

Magnetic resonance vascular imaging shares with other tomographic techniques the disadvantage of interrupted display of the vessel. This problem has been solved in magnetic resonance angiography by three-dimensional acquisition and display. An alternative approach for velocity mapping is to acquiring information in multiple slices and then to combine these in an image in which only the maximum of each pixel is displayed, irrespective of the slice in which it is seen. Figure 11.11 shows an example in a normal volunteer.

11.2 The assessment of sclerosis

In 1904 Marchand recognised the association between fatty degeneration of the arteries and stiffening of the arterial wall and coined the term atherosclerosis.[23] Since then the fatty component of the disease (atherosis) has been extensively investigated, but less attention has

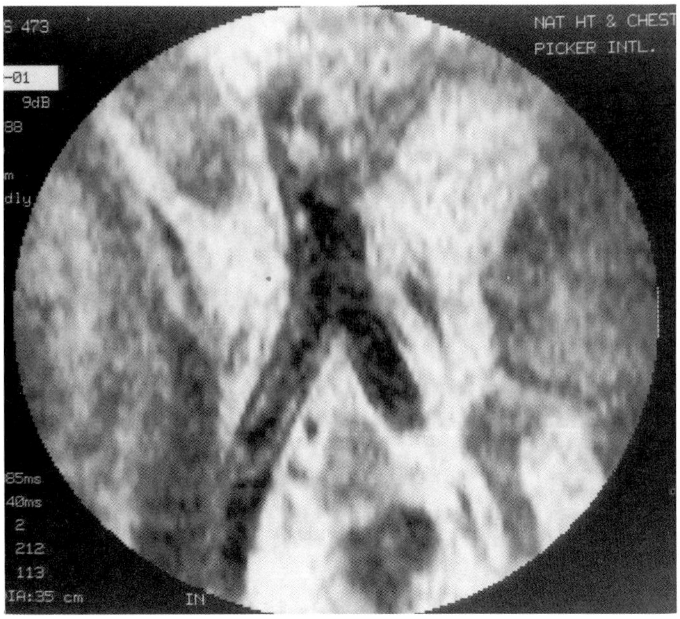

(a)

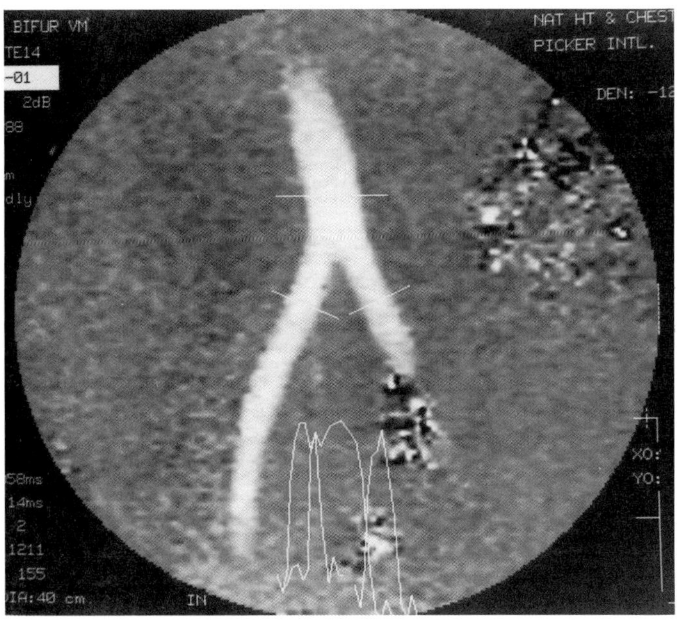

(b)

Figure 11.8. (a) The aortic bifurcation in a normal 43-year-old male. There is some signal from static blood within the lumen. (b) The velocity map encoded from top to bottom of the image shows the same velocity in the aorta and in both iliac arteries (seen from the profiles). This confirms the normal luminal diameter.

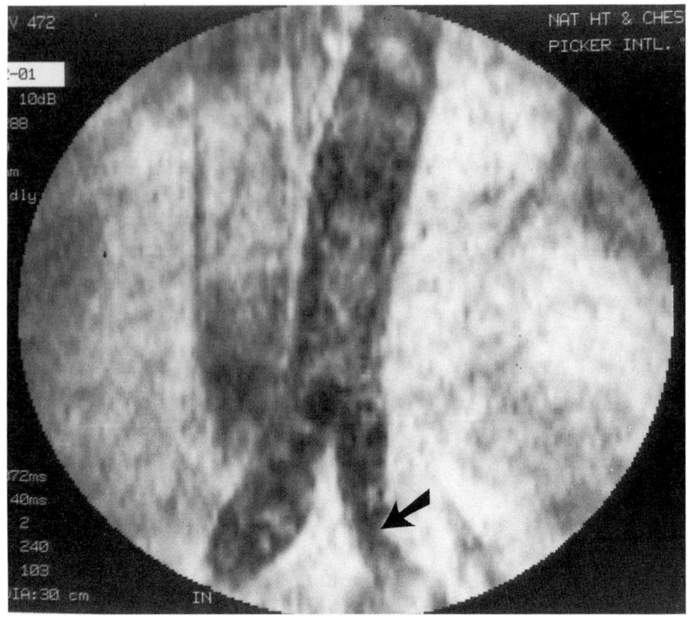

(a)

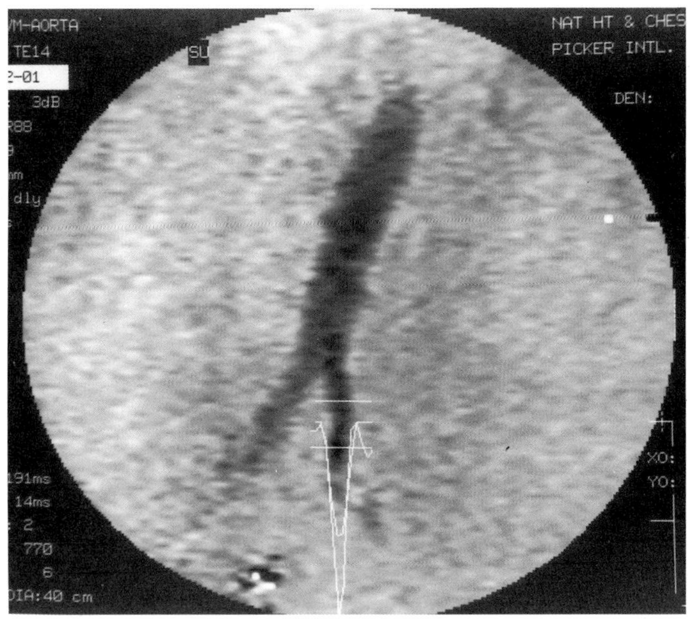

(b)

Figure 11.9. (a) A 57-year-old male with atheromatous disease. The left iliac artery is narrowed (arrow) on the anatomical spin echo image. (b) The velocity map shows high velocities past the obstruction. (Reproduced with permission from *Br Med Bull* 1989; **45**: 968–90.)

been paid to the sclerosis. The elasticity or compliance of an artery is determined by the ratio of elastin, smooth muscle and collagen in the wall, and sclerosis arises from structural changes which include loss of elastin and an increase in collagen.[24] The changes are widespread and they are not necessarily associated with

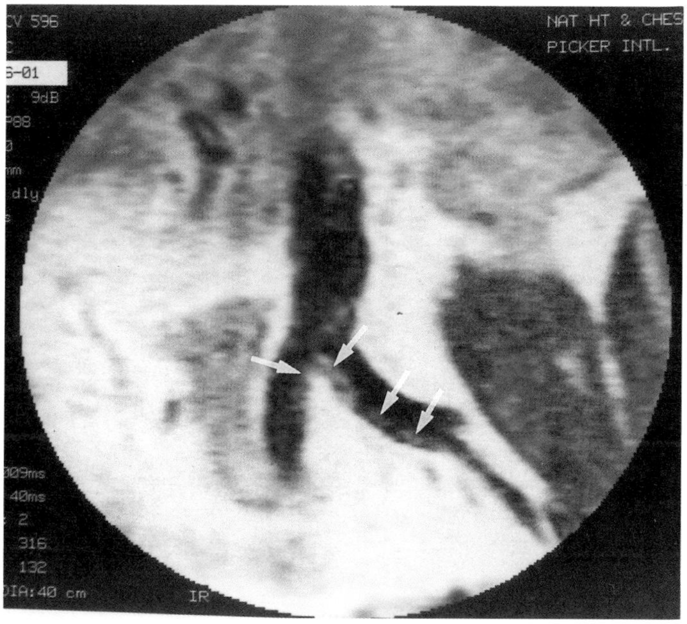

(a)

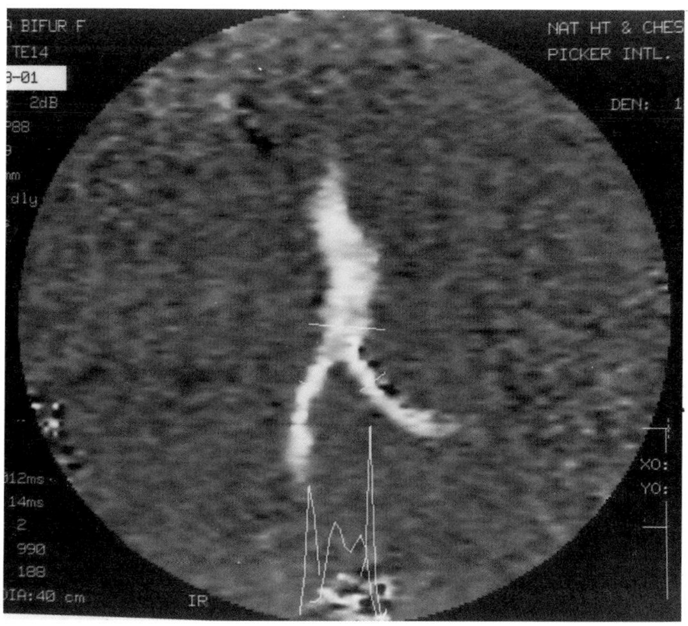

(b)

Figure 11.10. (a) A 61-year-old male with extensive atheroma at the aortic bifurcation (arrows). (b) The velocity map shows high velocity in the obstructed areas. (Reproduced with permission from *Br Med Bull* 1989; **45**: 968–90.)

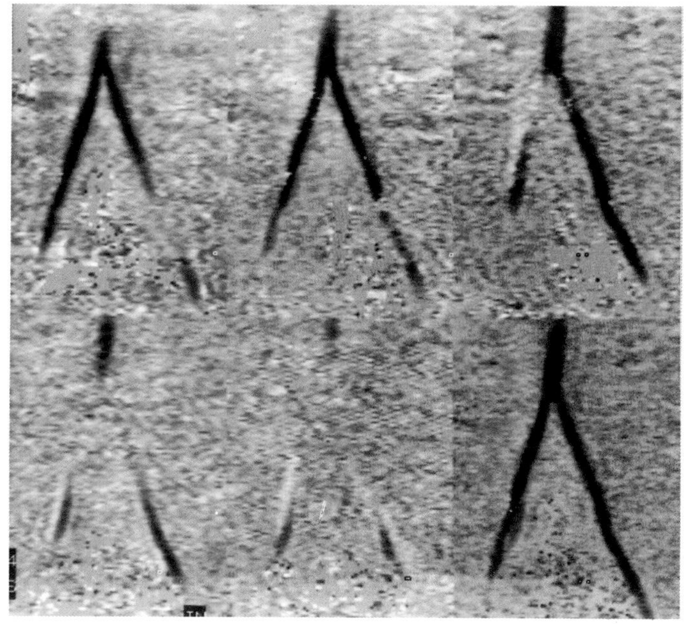

(a)

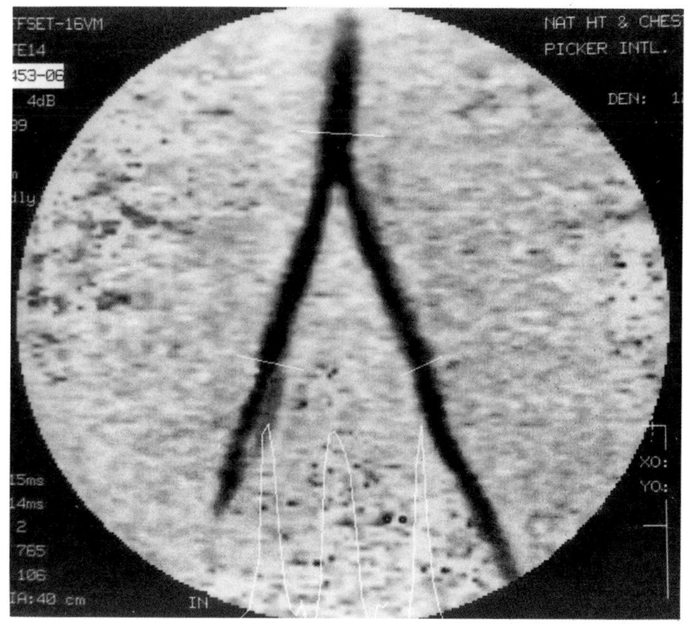

(b)

Figure 11.11. (a) Velocity mapping in contiguous 10 mm slices parallel to the abdominal aorta, and the right and left iliac arteries of a healthy volunteer. By taking the maximum velocity of each pixel, irrespective of which plane it is seen in, a projection image of the three vessels is constructed (bottom right). (b) The projection image is enlarged and the similar velocity profiles are seen indicating a normal vessel.

atherosis. Both components of the disease are closely linked, however, and both are adversely affected by hypercholesterolaemia, hypertension, and diabetes.

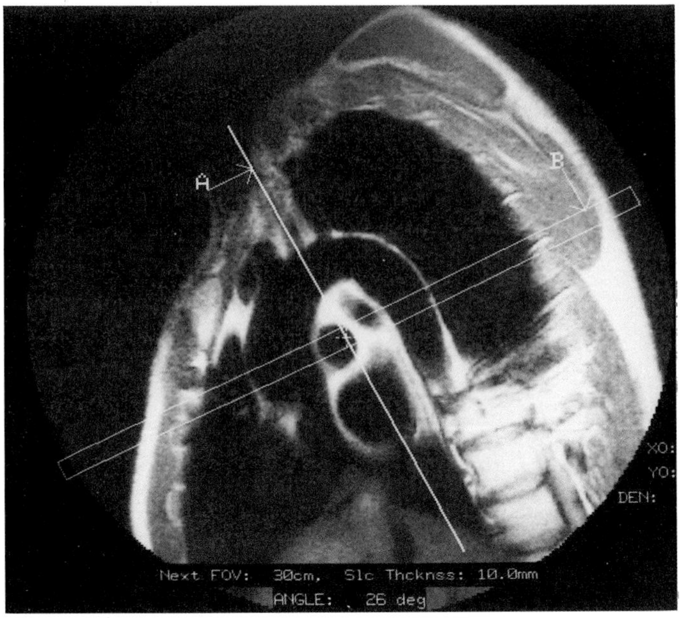

(a)

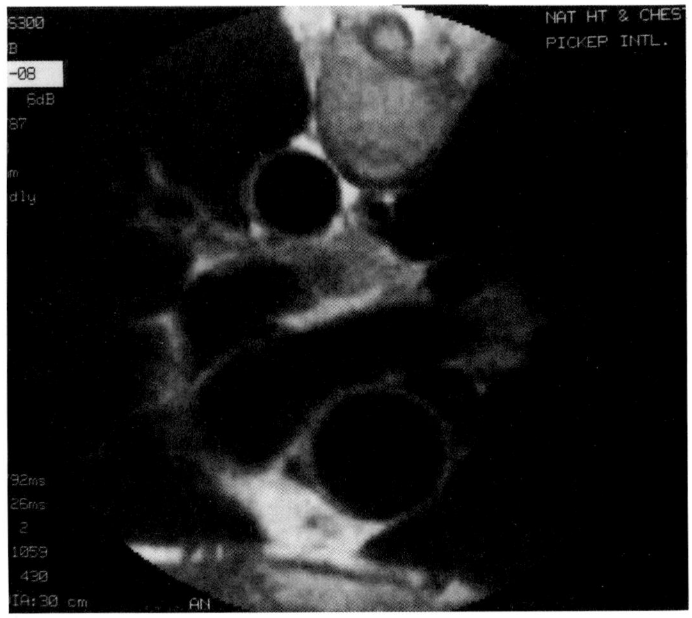

(b)

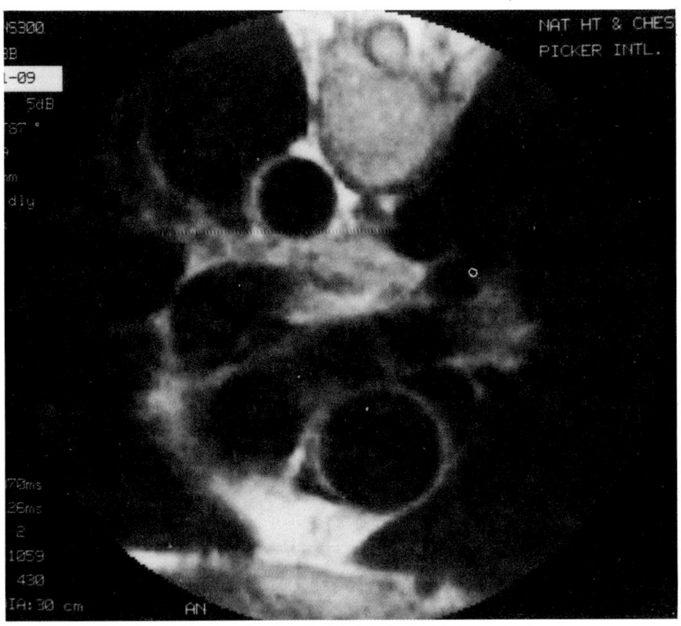

(c)

Figure 11.12. (a) Oblique image of the ascending aorta, aortic arch and descending thoracic aorta illustrating the sites where compliance is most easily measured. (b) Systolic and (c) diastolic images of the ascending and descending aorta showing good compliance in a 38-year-old normal volunteer. (Reproduced with permission from *Br Heart J* 1989; **62**: 90–96.)

That atherosis is reversible has been shown in several studies.[25] The reversal of coronary atherosis has been confirmed in animals[26,27] but reversal in humans is more difficult to demonstrate. Certainly, lesions in the peripheral circulation[28] and the coronary arteries[29] progress less rapidly following treatment of hyperlipidaemia, but regression has also been documented.[30] Regression is more readily achieved in early lesions,[31] hence the importance of early detection and treatment. Atherosis will however usually be well advanced before it has a significant effect upon arterial flow or flow reserve, and many patients present well before this stage with sudden death from thrombosis superimposed upon an active and fissured plaque that is not necessarily flow limiting.[32] For this reason, strategies that rely upon the detection of sclerosis may be better suited to detect patients at a stage of the disease when reversal of risk factors may be beneficial.

11.2.1 Aortic compliance

Compliance is the change in volume per unit change in pressure and it is a measure of stiffness and distensibility. The combination of elastic arteries and resistant arterioles constitutes a hydraulic filter enabling the intermittent cardiac output to be converted to a steady capillary flow. Part of the energy of left ventricular contraction produces forward flow during systole, but the remainder is stored as potential energy in the distended arteries. During diastole, elastic recoil converts this potential energy into forward flow. A fall in aortic compliance increases the impedance to ventricular ejection and decreases capillary blood flow.[33,34] Aortic compliance, therefore, is a determinant of left ventricular afterload and it is important in patients with ventricular disease.[35]

Magnetic resonance imaging provides a direct noninvasive way of studying regional aortic compliance.[10] Images can be acquired at end diastole and end systole through the thoracic aorta (figure 11.12) and the change in volume between diastole and systole can be measured. The pulse pressure is measured using a conventional sphygmomanometer. In normal subjects, the ascending aorta is the most compliant region and compliance falls more distally. In athletes, regional aortic compliance is higher than normal, and in patients with coronary artery disease under the age of 50 it is lower (figure 11.13). These changes are likely to be the result of structural changes in the aorta and they are a potential screening tool for the detection of vascular disease. Because there is overlap between normal compliance and compliance in patients with coronary artery disease, the test cannot have perfect sensitivity and specificity. Below the age of 50 however there is much less overlap and the test is more sensitive.

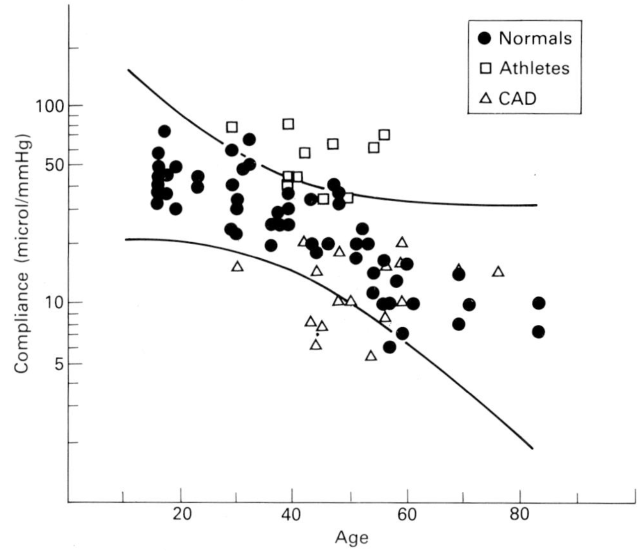

Figure 11.13. Ascending aortic compliance displayed using a logarithmic scale and plotted against age. The 95% confidence intervals in a group of normal volunteers are shown, and compliance can be seen to fall with age. In a group of athletes, compliance is abnormally high and in patients with coronary artery disease (CAD) it is low. (Reproduced with permission from *Br Heart J* 1989; **62**: 90–96.)

11.2.2 Aortic flow wave velocity

The repeated ejection of the ventricles generates pressure and flow waves in the aorta and pulmonary artery, and these pulsations are transmitted throughout the arterial tree.[36] The velocity of such waves depends principally on the distensibility and compliance of the vessel wall. If the vascular tree were rigid and blood incompressible, the motion of blood in the root of aorta would be transmitted peripherally instantaneously. Blood is indeed incompressible, but the vessels are distensible in varying degrees, and the flow wave velocity is therefore finite.

The flow wave velocity can be measured by Doppler ultrasound[37] or by magnetic resonance velocity mapping.[38] Although measurements cannot be made in the coronary arteries, the aorta is an ideal target because it is easy to image and because fatty streaks in the aorta and coronary arteries progress to raised lesions in parallel.[39] In the magnetic resonance technique, high temporal resolution (10 ms) velocity maps are acquired in a plane perpendicular to the ascending and descending aorta and the time taken for the flow wave to travel between the two points is measured (figure 11.14). Flow wave velocity increases with age and with blood pressure and there is an inverse relationship between flow wave velocity and regional compliance (figure 11.15). In the same way that aortic compliance may be used to detect vascular disease, flow wave velocity may also be a valuable parameter of the state of the arterial system.

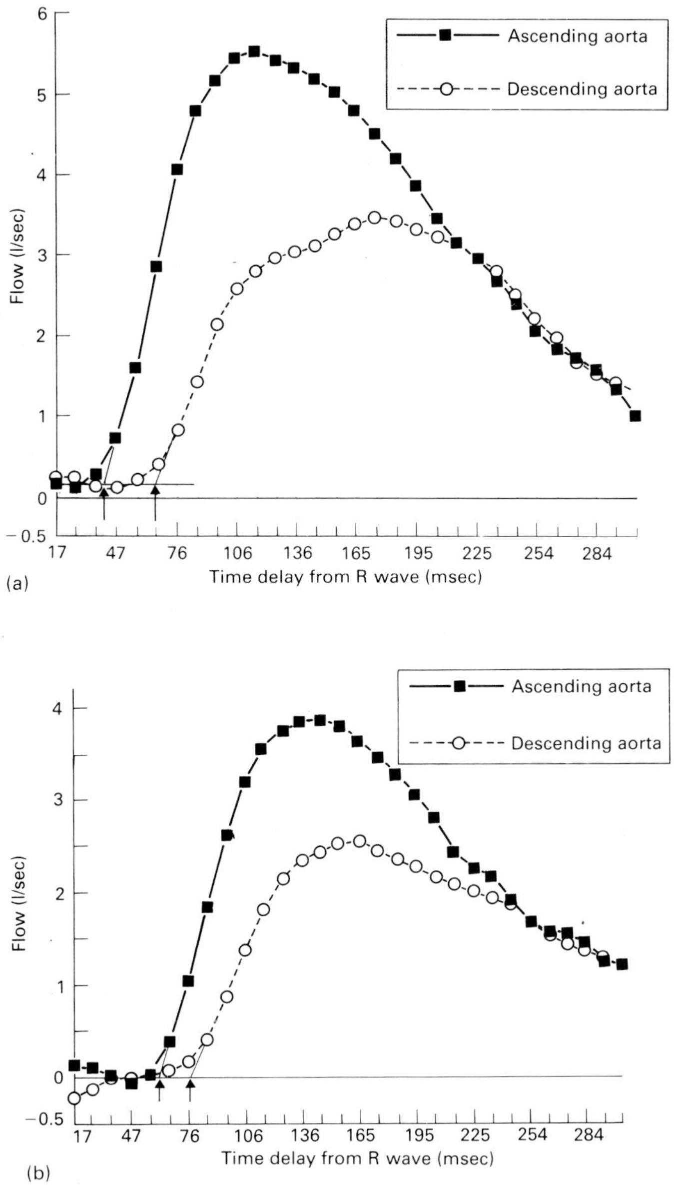

Figure 11.14. The foot of the flow wave is defined by extrapolation of the rapid upstroke of the flow wave to the base line. The transit time needed for the flow wave to propagate from a point on the mid-ascending aorta and a point on the mid-descending thoracic aorta can be then calculated. (a) Data obtained from a young normal subject with good aortic compliance. (b) Data obtained from an elderly normal subject with poor compliance and a reduced flow wave velocity. (Reproduced with permission from *Br Med Bull* 1989; **45**: 968–90.)

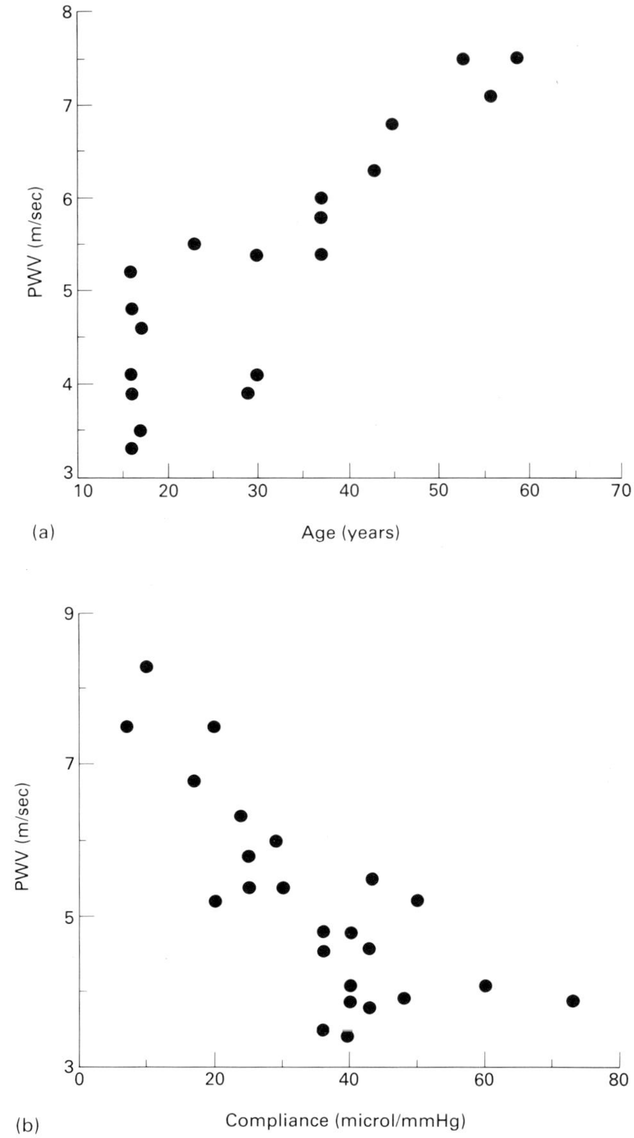

Figure 11.15. The pulse wave velocity (PWV) is directly related to age (a) and is inversely related to regional aortic compliance (b). (Reproduced with permission from *Br Med Bull* 1989; **45**: 968–90.)

11.2.3 The clinical importance of sclerosis

The clinical effects of sclerosis are subtle and it is not clear that it affects tissue perfusion in the same way as flow limiting atheroma.[40] Certainly, variations in compliance along an artery can lead to connective tissue overgrowth[41] and so local compliance changes could influence disease progression. In addition, aortic compliance is an important component of left ventricular afterload and reduced compliance will not only increase myocardial oxygen demand, but it may also reduce oxygen supply through its affect on the normal aortic diastolic backflow which aids coronary perfusion.[11,42,43] Similarly, reduced pulmonary arterial compliance may be a factor in the onset of right heart failure in patients with chronic lung disease.[44] Another area of clinical importance may be following surgical repair of aortic coarctation, where persistent systolic hypertension may be the result of more widespread structural changes in the aorta.[45]

References

1 *Report of the Working Group of Arteriosclerosis of the National Heart, Lung and Blood Institute*, volume 2. Washington: Government printing office, 1981 (DHEW publication No (NIH) 82–2035).

2 Clarkson TB, Weingnad KW, Kaplan JR, Adams MR. Mechanisms of atherogenesis. *Circulation* 1987; **76**: 1–20.

3 Virchow R. *Phlogose und thrombose im gefassystem, Gesammelte Abhandlungen zur wissenschaftlichen Medicin*. Frankfurt-am-Main: Meidinger Sohn 1856: 458.

4 Ross R. The pathogenesis of atherosclerosis—an update. *New Eng J Med* 1986; **314**: 488–500.

5 Band W, Goedhard WJ, Knoop AA. Comparison of effects of high cholesterol intake on viscoelastic properties of the thoracic aorta in rats and rabbits. *Atherosclerosis* 1973; **18**: 163–72.

6 Banga I, Balo J. Elasticity of the vascular wall. 1 The elastic tensibility of the human carotid as a function of age and arteriosclerosis. *Acta Physiol Acad Sci Hung* 1961; **20–21**: 237–47.

7 Farrar DJ, Green HD, Wanger WD, Bond MG. Reduction in pulse wave velocity and improvement of aortic distensibility accompanying regression of atherosclerosis in Rhesus monkey. *Circ Res* 1980; **47**: 425–32.

8 Mohiaddin RH, Firmin DN, Underwood SR, *et al.* Magnetic resonance chemical shift imaging of human atheroma. *Br Heart J* 1989; **62**: 81–90.

9 Mohiaddin RH, Longmore DB. MRI studies in atherosclerotic vascular disease: structural evaluation and physiological measurements. *Br Med Bull* 1989; **45**: 968–90.

10 Mohiaddin RH, Underwood SR, Bogren HG, *et al.* Regional aortic compliance studied by magnetic resonance imaging: the effect of age, training and coronary artery disease. *Br Heart J* 1989; **62**: 90–6.

11 Bogren HG, Mohiaddin RH, Klipstein RH, *et al.* The function of aorta in ischemic heart disease: a magnetic resonance and angiographic study of aortic compliance and blood flow patterns. *Am Heart J* 1989; **118**: 234–47.

12 Herfkens R, Higgins C, Hricak H, *et al.* Nuclear magnetic resonance imaging of atherosclerotic disease. *Radiology* 1983; **148**: 161–6.

13 Wesby GE, Higgins CB, Amparo EG, Hale JD, Kaufman L, Pogany AC. Peripheral vascular disease: correlation of MR imaging and angiography. *Radiology* 1985; **156**: 733–9.

14 Pykett I, Rosen L. Nuclear magnetic resonance: in vivo proton chemical shift imaging. *Radiology* 1983; **149**: 197–201.

15 Brateman L. Chemical shift imaging: a review. *Am J Roentgenol* 1986; **146**: 971–80.

16 Dixon T. Simple proton spectroscopic imaging. *Radiology* 1984; **153**: 189–94.

17 Hinks RS, Quencer RM. Multislice chemical shift imaging by slice-selection gradient reversal. *Magn Reson Imag* 1988; **6**: 22 (Abstract).

18 Wissler RW, Vesselinovitch D, Davis HR, Lambert PH, Bekermeier M. A new way to look at atherosclerotic involvement of artery wall and the functional effects. *Ann NY Acad Sci* 1985; **454**: 9–22.

19 Smith E. Development of atherosclerotic plaque. In: Shillingford J, Birdwood G (eds), *Impact of Research on the Practice of Cardiology*. London: British Heart Foundation, 1986; 1–5.

20 Potkin BN, Roberts WC. Effects of percutaneous transluminal coronary angioplasty on atherosclerotic plaques and relation of plaque composition and arterial size to outcome. *Am J Cardiol* 1988; **62**: 41–50.

21 Gotto AM. Regression of atherosclerosis. *Am J Med* 1983; **70**: 989–91.

22 Mohiaddin RH, Sampson C, Firmin DN, *et al.* MR anatomic and flow imaging in peripheral vascular disease. *Radiology* 1989; **173**: 321 (Abstract).

23 Aschoff L. In: Cowdry EV (ed). *Arteriosclerosis: a Survey of the Problem*. New York: MacMillan 1933: 1–8.

24 Roach MR, Burton AC. The reason for the shape of the distensibility curves of arteries. *Can J Biochem Physiol* 1957; **35**: 681–90.

25 Blankenhorn DH, Kramsch DM. Reversal of atherosis and sclerosis. *Circulation* 1989; **79**: 1–7.

26 Armstrong ML, Warner ED, Connor WE. Regression of coronary atheromatosis in rhesus monkeys. *Circ Res* 1970; **27**: 59–67.

27 Armstrong ML, Megan MB. Lipid depletion in atheromatous coronary arteries in rhesus monkeys after regression diets. *Circ Res* 1972; **30**: 675–80.

28 Duffield RG, Lewis B, Miller NE, Jamieson CW, Brunt JN, Colchester AC. Treatment of hyperlipidaemia retards progression of symptomatic femoral atherosclerosis: a randomised controlled trial. *Lancet* 1983; **ii**: 639–42.

29 Brensike JF, Levy RI, Kelsey SF, *et al.* Effects of therapy with cholestyramine on progression of coronary arteriosclerosis: results of the NHLBI Type II Coronary Intervention Study. *Circulation* 1984; **69**: 313–24.

30 Blankenhorn DH, Nessim SA, Johnson RL, Sanmarco ME, Azen SP, Cashin-Hemphill L. Beneficial effects of combined colestipol-niacin therapy on coronary atherosclerosis and coronary venous bypass grafts. *J Am Med Assoc* 1987; **257**: 3233–40.

31 Stary HC. Progression and regression of experimental atherosclerosis in rhesus monkeys. In Goldsmith EF, Morr-Hankowsky J (eds), *Medical Primatology*. Basel: S Karger, 1972: 356–67.

32 Hackett D, Davies G, Maseri A. Pre-existing coronary stenoses in patients with first myocardial infarction are not necessarily severe. *Eur Heart J* 1988; **9**: 1317–23.

33 Berne RM, Levy MN. *Cardiovascular Physiology*. London: CV Mosby Company, 1981: 94–7.

34 Wilcken DE, Charlier AA, Hoffman JI, Guz A. Effect of

alterations in aortic impedance on the performance of the ventricles. *Circ Res* 1964; **14**: 283–93.

35 Urschel CW, Covel JW, Sonnenblick EH, Ross J, Braunwald E. The effect of decreased aortic compliance on performance of the left ventricle. *Am J Physiol* 1968; **214**: 298–304.

36 Milner WR. *Hemodynamics*. Baltimore: Williams & Wilkins, 1982: 211–43.

37 Caro CG, Fish PJ, Goss DE. Effect of isosorbide dinitrate on arterial haemodynamics in man. *J Physiol* 1985; **365**: 93P.

38 Mohiaddin RH, Firmin DN, Underwood SR, *et al*. Magnetic resonance measurements of aortic flow wave velocity: the effect of age and disease. *Magn Reson Med* 1988; **7**: 180 (Abstract).

39 Atherosclerosis of the aorta and coronary arteries in five towns. *Bull WHO* 1976; **53**: 485–645.

40 Pickering G. Arteriosclerosis and atherosclerosis: the need for clear thinking. *Am J Med* 1963; **34**: 7–18.

41 Hasson JE, Megerman J, Abbott WM. Increased compliance near vascular anastomoses. *J Vasc Surg* 1985; **2**: 419–23.

42 Klipstein RH, Firmin DN, Underwood SR, Rees RSO, Longmore DB. Blood flow patterns in the human aorta studied by magnetic resonance. *Br Heart J* 1987; **58**: 316–23.

43 Bogren HG, Klipstein RH, Firmin DN, *et al*. Quantitation of antegrade and retrograde blood flow in the human aorta by magnetic resonance. *Am Heart J* 1989; **117**: 1214–22.

44 Bogren HG, Klipstein RH, Mohiaddin RH, *et al*. Pulmonary artery distensibility and blood flow patterns: a magnetic resonance study of normal subjects and of patients with pulmonary arterial hypertension. *Am Heart J* 1989; **118**: 990–9.

45 Rees RSO, Somerville J, Ward C, *et al*. Magnetic resonance imaging in the late postoperative assessment of coarctation of the aorta. *Radiology* 1989; **173**: 499–502.

Chapter 12
Magnetic Resonance Spectroscopy

BHEESHMA RAJAGOPOLAN AND GEORGE RADDA

Magnetic resonance imaging and spectroscopy provide complementary information about tissues *in vivo*, the first describing the anatomy of the heart and its mechanical function and the second describing the biochemistry of the cell. Although imaging is almost entirely confined to ^{1}H (proton) magnetic resonance, a number of different nuclei are of interest in spectroscopy, including ^{1}H, ^{31}P, ^{13}C, ^{23}Na and ^{19}F. The limitation of imaging to the proton stems from the fact that the concentration of water in biological tissues is 55 M (110 M protons), and so water and, to a lesser extent, fat provide all of the signal used to generate the images. There are many other hydrogen containing compounds present, including amino acids, lactate, creatine and phosphocreatine, but because they are only present in millimolar concentrations their signal is swamped by that from water.

In vivo magnetic resonance spectroscopy of the heart has also concentrated, until recently, on a single atom: ^{31}P. This is the naturally occurring isotope of phosphorus and it is part of high energy molecules such as adenosine triphosphate (ATP) and phosphocreatine (PCr), which are intimately involved with the viability of cells and their ability to perform mechanical and chemical work. In addition to ATP and PCr only inorganic phosphate (P_i), and a few mono (PME) and phosphodiesters (PDE) are detectable by ^{31}P spectroscopy. In contrast, ^{13}C or ^{1}H spectra of tissues *in vivo* have a multitude of spectral lines not only because there are many more chemical compounds contributing to the spectra but also because each chemical can contribute several lines because of magnetic interactions between nuclei (homonuclear or heteronuclear coupling) (figure 12.1). The problems of detecting millimolar concentrations of compounds in the presence of 55 M water in ^{1}H spectroscopy, or of identifying the many peaks caused by proton coupling in ^{13}C spectroscopy make their use *in vivo* much more difficult.

A large amount of information has been acquired in the last decade using phosphorus spectroscopy in isolated perfused rodent hearts and hearts of a variety of other animals *in vivo*, as well as of other tissues such as skeletal muscle, brain and liver.[1–4] The development of large bore magnets and of techniques for the spatial localisation of spectra has allowed phosphorus metabolism of the human heart to be studied *in vivo*.

12.1 The physics of magnetic resonance spectroscopy

The physics of magnetic resonance has been described in chapter 1 and general reviews are also available elsewhere.[5,6] It is appropriate however to consider some aspects that are relevant to spectroscopy. The frequency of precession or Larmor frequency (ν_0) of a sensitive nucleus in an applied magnetic field (B_0) is given by:

$$\nu_0 = \gamma . B_0 / 2\pi$$

where γ is the gyromagnetic ratio of the nucleus and $\gamma/2\pi$ for ^{1}H is 42.57 MHz/T. At 1.9 T which is a typical field strength for *in vivo* spectroscopy, the Larmor frequency of ^{1}H is 80 MHz, ^{31}P is 32 MHz, and ^{13}C is 20 MHz).

The same nucleus in different chemical environments experiences different fields because of shielding by surrounding electrons. At 2 T the Larmor frequencies of the phosphorus atoms of γ-ATP and PCr differ by about 100 Hz while at 4 T the difference is 200 Hz. Thus it can be seen that the separation between individual peaks increases with the applied field. It is convenient to express this chemical shift in units that are independent of field, and the ratio of parts per million (ppm) of the applied field is used with respect to a

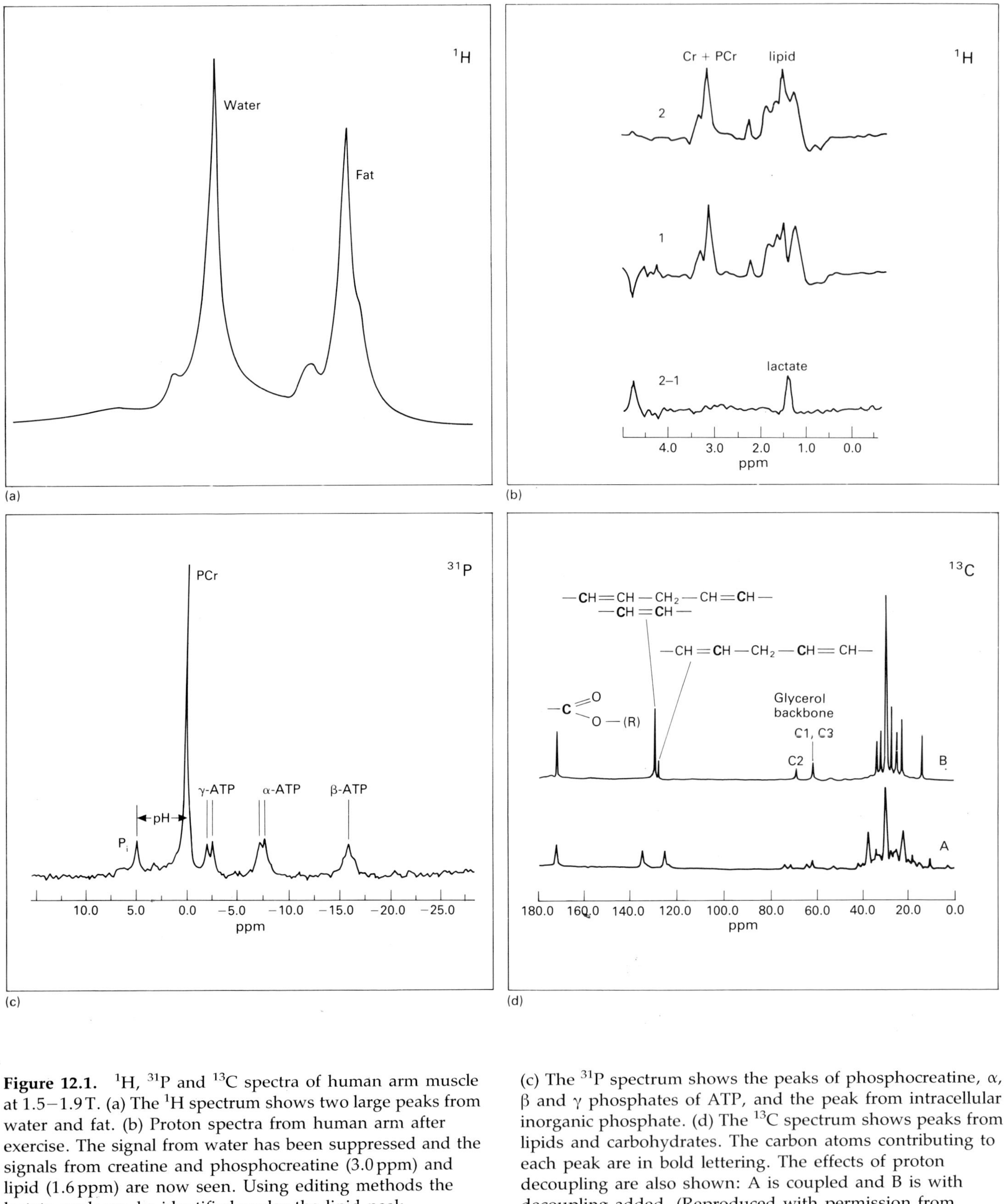

Figure 12.1. ^1H, ^{31}P and ^{13}C spectra of human arm muscle at 1.5–1.9 T. (a) The ^1H spectrum shows two large peaks from water and fat. (b) Proton spectra from human arm after exercise. The signal from water has been suppressed and the signals from creatine and phosphocreatine (3.0 ppm) and lipid (1.6 ppm) are now seen. Using editing methods the lactate peak can be identified under the lipid peak. (Reproduced with permission from Hetherington *et al.* 1989.) (c) The ^{31}P spectrum shows the peaks of phosphocreatine, α, β and γ phosphates of ATP, and the peak from intracellular inorganic phosphate. (d) The ^{13}C spectrum shows peaks from lipids and carbohydrates. The carbon atoms contributing to each peak are in bold lettering. The effects of proton decoupling are also shown: A is coupled and B is with decoupling added. (Reproduced with permission from Luyten *et al.*[43])

reference peak. Phosphocreatine is a convenient reference in cardiac spectroscopy.

$$\text{Chemical shift (ppm)} = (\nu - \nu_{ref})/\nu_{ref} \cdot 10^6$$

The Larmor frequency is also affected by interaction between nuclei in different chemical environments in the same molecule. Thus the α and γ phosphates each have two components separated by about 6 Hz at 2 T (homonuclear coupling) and the β phosphate is split into three components by interaction with the other two. Similar interaction can occur between different nuclei such as P–H or C–H (heteronuclear coupling) and this splitting of spectral lines causes individual peaks to be broadened making identification and quantification more difficult. In some cases (such as P–H or C–H) heteronuclear coupling can be removed by applying a second radio-frequency pulse of the appropriate frequency to the sample. For instance, to remove splitting of ^{13}C spectra caused by proton coupling, a radio-frequency pulse at the Larmor frequency of ^{1}H will collapse the broadened peaks into single lines.

The ability to resolve neighbouring peaks also depends upon T_2 relaxation times since T_2 determines peak width. Rapid transverse relaxation (short T_2) leads to broad spectral lines, the relationship being:

$$\Delta\nu_{1/2} = 1/\pi T_2$$

where $\Delta\nu_{1/2}$ is the width of the line in Hertz at half height. The effective T_2 (T_2*) is determined by the intrinsic T_2 and by field inhomogeneity, including the inhomogeneities caused by magnetic susceptibility variations within the tissue being examined, and all of these factors contribute to the broadness of spectral lines seen *in vivo*. Typical line widths for ^{1}H are 20 Hz in brain, and 30–40 Hz in liver and heart at 1.9 T, although widths down to 1–5 Hz can be achieved *in vitro*. Phosphorus line widths are roughly half that of the proton, being 10–15 Hz for ATP and PCr. Because the intrinsic T_2 of the tissue cannot be changed, the applied field must be as large as practical and as homogeneous as possible in order to maximise resolution between peaks. Thus, in contrast to magnetic resonance imaging where fields of 0.05 T and homogeneities of 100 ppm can be successfully used, a field of at least 1.5 T and homogeneity better than 0.1 ppm over the region of interest are necessary for spectroscopy. The United States Food and Drug Administration currently recommends an upper limit of 2 T for whole body magnets although at least four experimental 4 T whole body magnets are under development.

As well as increasing spectral resolution, a high field increases the signal to noise ratio of the spectra. This is particularly important for the spectroscopist because virtually all compounds of interest in biological tissues are present in millimolar concentrations or less, and the signal to noise ratio is inversely related to the square of the concentration. As an illustration, if one wanted to acquire a phosphorus image of the brain with the same resolution and signal to noise ratio as is commonly used in proton magnetic resonance imaging, the acquisition would take 10 000 years. The spectroscopist is forced to compromise and to accept larger volumes of interest and lower signal to noise than in imaging.

Although high magnetic fields are desirable for magnetic resonance spectroscopy, there are problems to be considered. High fields lead to high radio-frequency power deposition, and tissue heating may become significant. Artefacts caused by cardiac and vascular motion are greater at high field and susceptibility artefacts are also greater. Although preliminary studies at 4 T in man have not reported any major side effects, it is possible that the larger induced voltages may stimulate excitable tissues such as the retina or the brain (see chapter 14).

12.2 ^{31}P spectroscopy of the heart in animals

The effects of physiological and pathological perturbations on the ^{31}P spectra of isolated perfused rodent hearts have been studied in considerable detail.[7–9] Similar studies have been performed *in vivo* using surface coils placed on the exposed heart. Figure 12.2 shows a typical spectrum at 4.3 T of a rat heart perfused retrogradely using Langendorff's method. The peaks of the γ, α and β-phosphates of ATP, and of PCr and P_i can be identified, although the γ and α peaks contain a contribution from ADP and the α peak from NAD as well. Monoesters such as sugar phosphates, phosphocholine, phosphoethanolamine and phosphoserine partly overlap the P_i peak and the line widths in tissues are too large for them to be resolved from one another easily. The monoesters are present in micromolar concentrations and their contribution is small. When analysing ATP, the β-ATP peak is used in order to avoid contamination with ADP and NAD, but these compounds can be identified separately in high resolution spectra of myocardial extracts (figure 12.3).

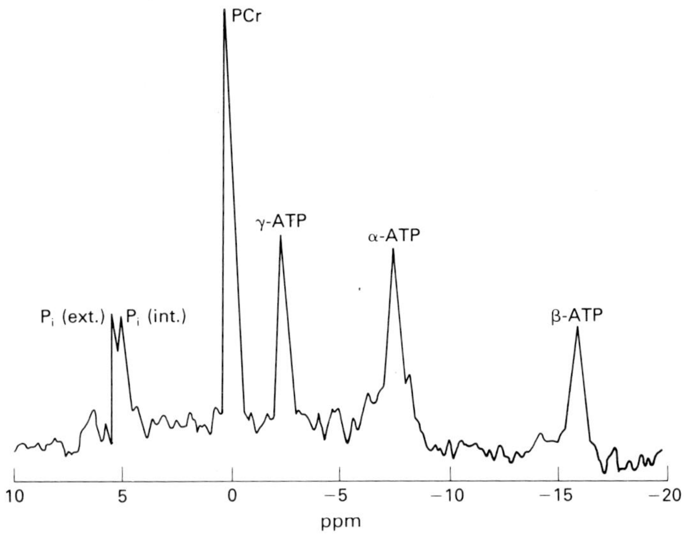

Figure 12.2. ^{31}P spectrum of a rat heart perfused with phosphate containing buffer. The single peak of PCr, the three peaks of ATP, and two P_i peaks (intracellular and extracellular) are seen. The separation of the P_i peaks is due to the pH difference between intracellular and buffer P_i.

Several important determinants of cardiac metabolism can be assessed: inorganic phosphate and ADP are important regulators of glycolytic and mitochondrial ATP synthesis and of muscle contraction, acidosis depresses myocardial function, and the ratio of ATP to ADP × P_i is a measure of the free energy available from the hydrolysis of ATP.

Intracellular pH is calculated from the chemical shift between P_i and PCr because the inorganic phosphate exists in equilibrium between HPO_4^{2-} and $H_2PO_4^-$ and the equilibrium is pH dependent. In solution there is a rapid exchange between the two forms and a net chemical shift is seen. From this, the proportion of the two species can be calculated and hence the pH.[10] Because the position of the PCr peak is pH independent at physiological pH, it is a convenient reference, and each laboratory has a reference curve to convert chemical shift between P_i and PCr to pH. Similar measurements using other species such as organic acids and deoxyglucose have shown that pH calculated from the chemical shift of P_i in perfused hearts represents cytoplasmic pH.

In order to calculate the absolute concentrations of other species, the spectra are acquired alongside a reference sample of an appropriate phosphate solution. Although the concentration of free ADP in most cells is too low to be detected, it can be calculated from the concentrations of other metabolites using the equation:

$$K_{eq} = \frac{[\Sigma ATP][creatine]}{[\Sigma ADP][H^+][PCr]}$$

where $K_{eq} = 1.66 \times 10^9\ \text{M}^{-1}$, Σ refers to sums of all free and metal complexed species, and the creatine is calculated from the total creatine measured in tissue samples. The concentrations of P_i and ADP obtained from freeze-clamped samples are often much higher than those obtained from magnetic resonance spectroscopy. This may be due to hydrolysis of phosphocreatine and ATP during the extraction procedure but in addition, magnetic resonance only detects mobile nuclei and does not detect nuclei that are restricted by attachment to large proteins. Because it is only the mobile species that are available for metabolism, spectroscopy is thought to be a much better measurement.

By modifying the isolated heart preparation so that the perfusate enters the left atrium and is ejected actively by the left ventricle, the heart can be studied under more realistic conditions. Alternatively, a balloon can be inserted into the left ventricle so that it contracts isometrically.[11] All of these models show similarities in their responses. If the heart is made globally ischaemic, PCr and pH fall in parallel with mechanical function (figure 12.4). With prolonged ischaemia, ATP may also fall and recovery depends upon the duration of ischaemia. Thus Bailey and colleagues have shown complete recovery after up to 12 minutes of ischaemia, but after longer periods, recovery is impaired, with mechanical recovery not necessarily following metabolic recovery (figure 12.5).[7] In hearts that recovered either totally or partially from an ischaemic insult, PCr rose dramatically often to levels greater than baseline, but ATP recovered more slowly (figure 12.6). This suggests an abnormal coupling between energy production and contraction because if necrosis was responsible for the observed changes, both PCr and ATP would have remained low.

The relationship between mechanical function and levels of PCr and ATP were more clearly demonstrated in Langendorff perfused guinea pig hearts by Brooks and colleagues.[12] They showed that when perfusion was decreased six-fold, the PCr to ATP ratio decreased three-fold and that the pressure developed by the left ventricle correlated closely with the ratio (figure 12.7). Metabolite concentrations can also be altered by factors unrelated to coronary perfusion. Thus, changing the substrate from glucose to pyruvate or acetate has been

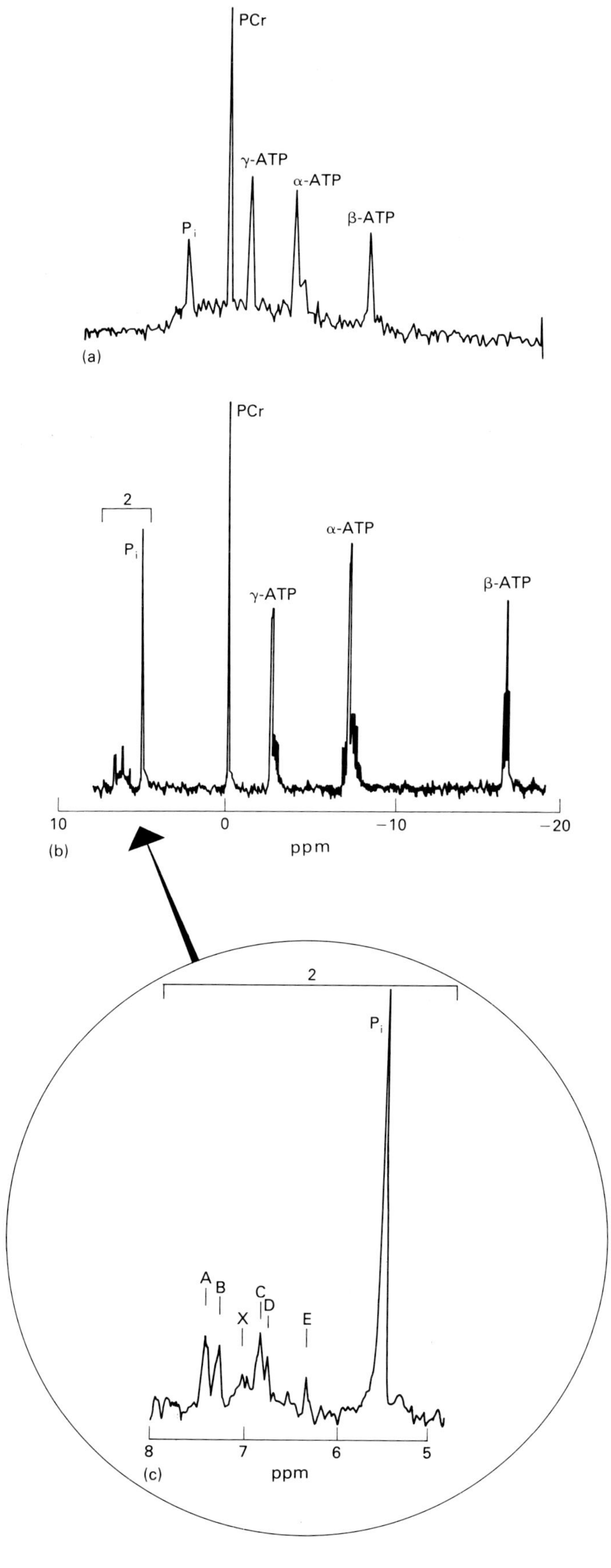

shown to increase PCr/ATP and PCr/P_i as PCr increases and P_i falls (figure 12.8).[13]

In addition to allowing measurements of metabolite concentrations, the steady state kinetics of some reactions, such as those catalysed by creatine kinase and ATP synthase, can be studied using the saturation transfer technique. In this technique, a selective radiofrequency pulse is applied to saturate the γ-ATP peak, which is thus labelled magnetically. The atom exchanges with the phosphate in creatine phosphate by a reaction catalysed by creatine kinase and with inorganic phosphate by a variety of reactions, and the rates of these reactions can be calculated from changes in peak intensities and relaxation times (figure 12.9).[14,15] The exchange of phosphorus between ATP and inorganic phosphate is particularly interesting because it reflects the conversion of ATP to chemical or mechanical work. If the oxygen consumption of the heart is measured, therefore, the efficiency of the conversion of oxygen and substrate to useful work can be assessed. Ugurbil and colleagues have used this technique to study mitochondrial ATP synthesis.[11] The number of phosphate ions converted to ATP for each molecule of oxygen consumed was 2.3–2.4, both in normal hearts and in hearts with significant postischaemic mechanical dysfunction, suggesting that mitochondrial uncoupling did not account for the dysfunction.

How far can the results from perfused hearts be extended to hearts *in vivo*? Spectra obtained using coils placed on the surface of exposed hearts[16–18] or catheter coils within the heart[19] are similar to those obtained *in vitro* (figure 12.10). ATP and PCr can be identified, but the P_i region is much more complex and an additional broad signal is seen between PCr and P_i. This is due to contributions from extracellular phosphate in blood and interstitial fluid and from 2,3-diphosphoglycerate (2,3-DPG) in red blood cells, and at fields less than 2T these peaks cannot be resolved easily. Editing techniques have been used to suppress the 2,3-DPG peak but in most *in vivo* studies P_i is too

Figure 12.3. ^{31}P spectrum of whole rat heart at 180 MHz (a) and of perchloric acid extracts (b,c). The splitting of the ATP peaks is seen in both spectra but the resolution is much better in the extract. Glucose-6-phosphate (A), glycerol phosphate and fructose-1-phosphate (B), phosphoethanolamine and fructose-6-phosphate (C), adenosine monophosphate (E), phosphocholine (E). Intracellular pH was 7.1. (Reproduced with thanks to Dr AM Seymour.)

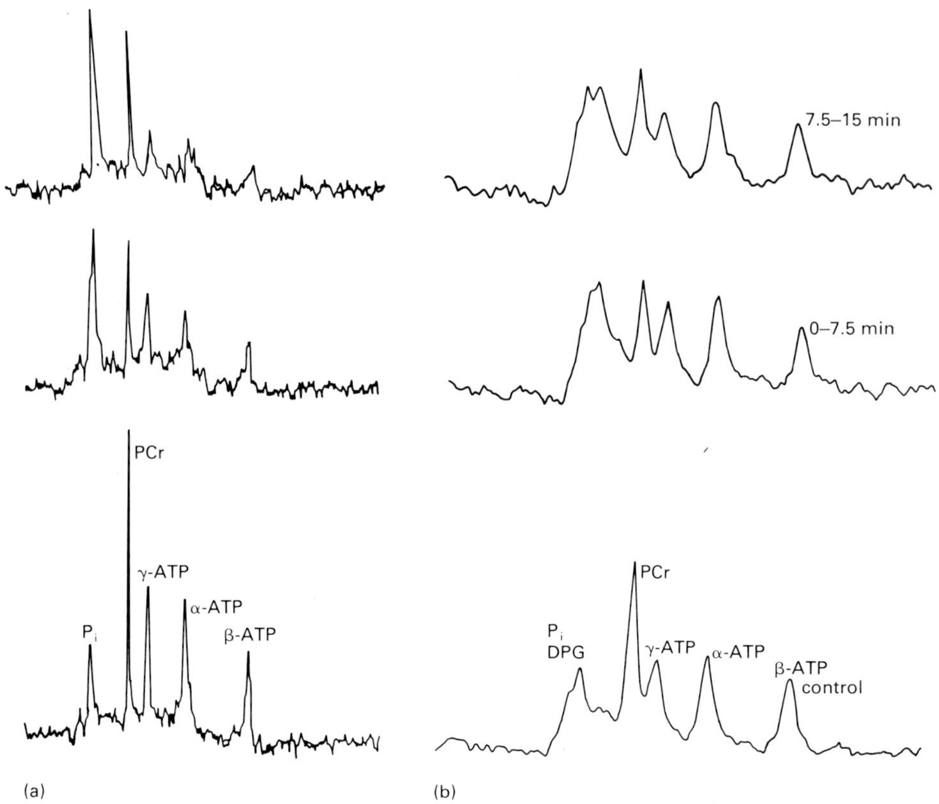

Figure 12.4. ^{31}P spectra of a globally ischaemic Langendorff perfused rat's heart (a) and a regionally ischaemic *in vivo* rabbit's heart (b). A solenoid coil was used in (a) and a surface coil in (b). There is rapid loss of PCr in both. Although there is loss of ATP in the rat, ATP changes little over 15 minutes in the rabbit. The P_i peak in the rat spectrum moves closer to PCr during ischaemia indicating intracellular acidosis. In the rabbit, intracellular P_i can only be identified in the third spectrum as the pH becomes sufficiently acid to move the P_i peak from the 2,3-DPG complex.

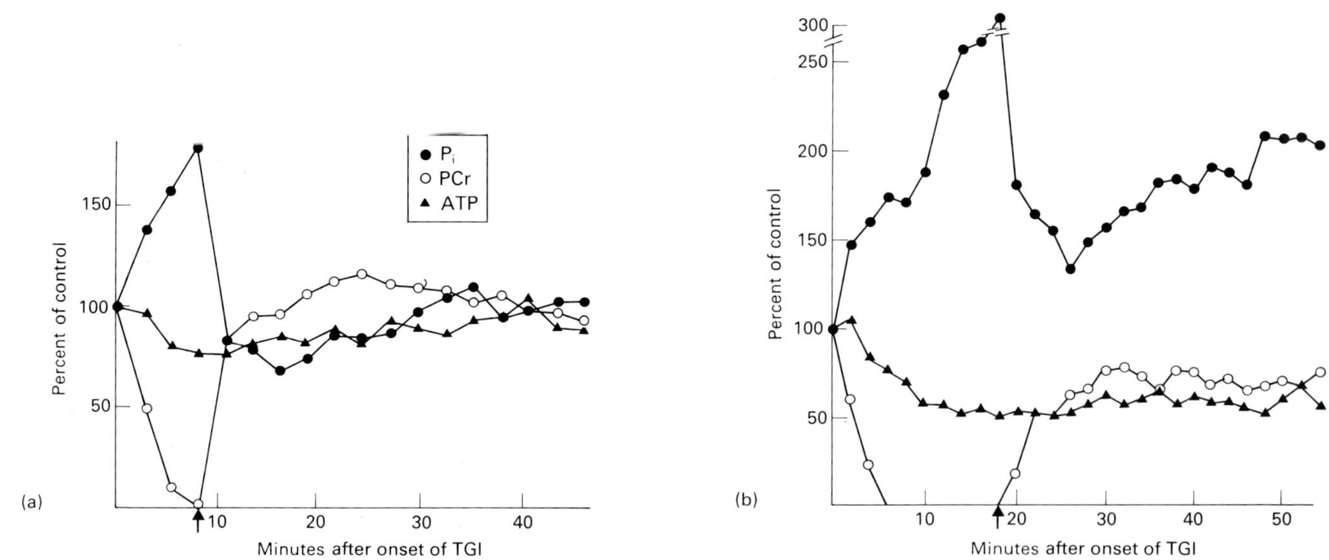

Figure 12.5. The effect of the duration of total global ischaemia (TGI) upon the metabolic recovery of Langendorff perfused rat hearts. The ischaemia is begun at time zero and abolished at the arrow (8 minutes in (a), 17 minutes in (b)). The full circles are P_i, open circles PCr, triangles ATP. Recovery of ATP is complete in (a) but it is impaired in (b). Other studies have found that there may be a correlation between loss of mechanical function and loss of ATP.

wide to allow differentiation of extracellular and intracellular phosphate without some other manoeuvre.[20] Saturation transfer is a possibility, with saturation of the γ-ATP peak which exchanges only with intracellular P_i, so that subtraction of control and saturated spectra allows the intracellular P_i to be measured. Using this

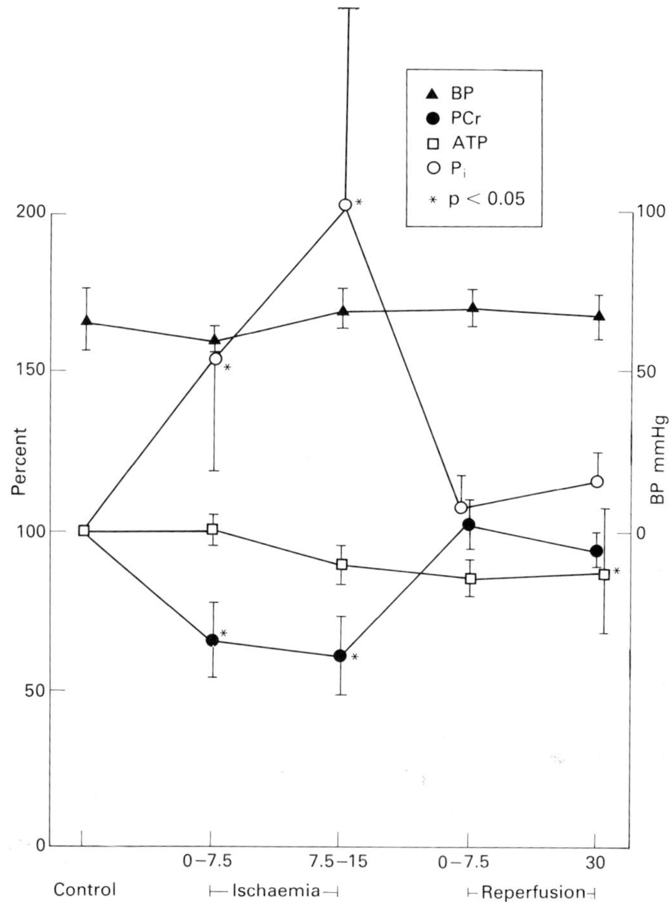

Figure 12.6. Changes in phosphorus metabolites following ischaemia in rabbit hearts *in vivo*. Spectra were obtained using a surface coil. PCr falls rapidly with the onset of ischaemia. ATP is only lost at the end of the ischaemic period. pH changes parallel PCr changes but with a little delay.

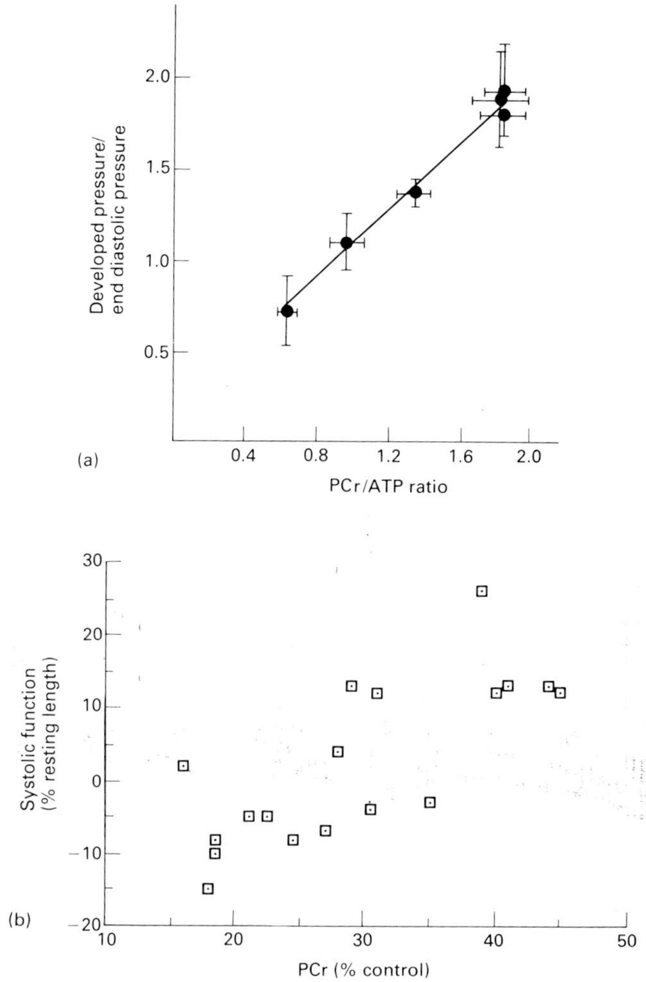

Figure 12.7. (a) The relationship between PCr/ATP and developed pressure in perfused guinea pig hearts. As flow is reduced, PCr falls. This is paralleled by a loss of mechanical function (b). Systolic function was measured *in vivo* in dog hearts using ultrasonic crystals. A similar relationship is found between PCr and mechanical function as in (a). ATP did not change significantly in the dog hearts. (Reproduced with permission from *J Mol Cell Cardiol* 1986; **18**: 149–55).

approach, Brindle and colleagues have shown the intracellular pH of hearts in open-chested dogs, cats and sheep to be between 7.0 and 7.2 (figure 12.11).[21] Unfortunately, the concentration of intracellular P_i cannot be estimated from the difference spectra, although at higher fields it may be possible to separate intracellular P_i from both extracellular P_i and 2,3-DPG (figure 12.12).

It is not possible to obtain absolute concentrations of metabolites because of the complex sensitivity profiles of surface coils,[22] but ratios of PCr to ATP or to P_i, if measurable, can be made.

12.3 ^{31}P spectroscopy of the human heart

Animal studies have indicated the potential of ^{31}P spectroscopy in humans but they have also highlighted some of the technical problems that need to be overcome. For spectroscopy to be of clinical value it is important to localise the spectra within the myocardium without contamination from skeletal muscle of the diaphragm or chest wall. Because of the relatively large volumes from which spectra must be acquired it is inevitable that they will be contaminated by a signal from intracavitary blood, and a method of examining intracellular P_i separately from extracellular P_i and 2,3-DPG is required. Finally, some form of stress will be essential in patients with coronary artery disease.

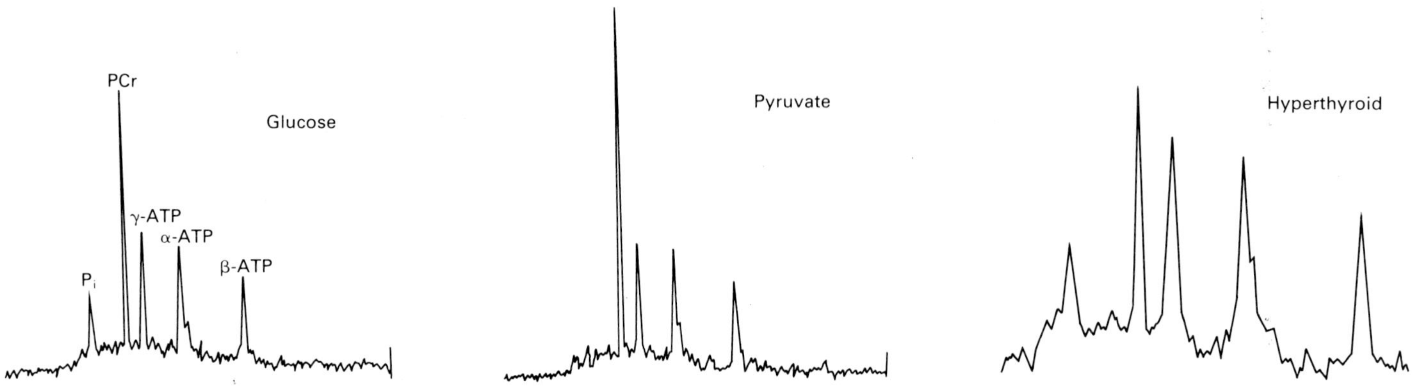

Figure 12.8. A comparison of ^{31}P spectra from rat hearts perfused with glucose and pyruvate as substrates, and from hearts from hyperthyroid animals. Note the differences in P_i between the glucose and pyruvate perfused hearts. As the preferred substrates are lipids and ketones, these studies imply that intracellular P_i is likely to be low.

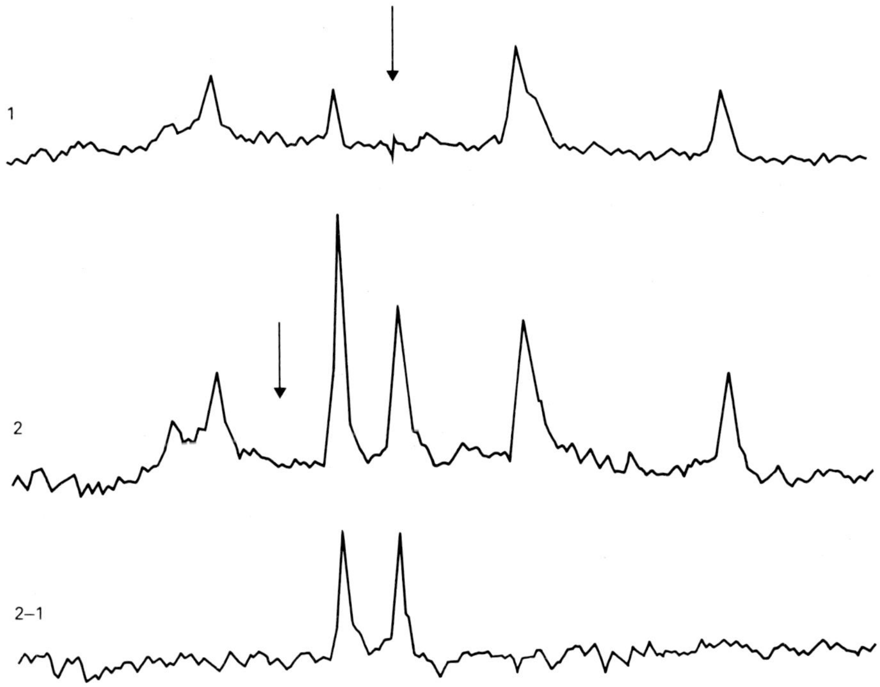

Figure 12.9. Saturation transfer experiment in a rat heart. Saturation of the γ-phosphate of ATP by a selective radio-frequency pulse at the frequency indicated by the arrow and allows the study of its transfer to both PCr (by creatine kinase) and to P_i (by ATP synthases and glycolytic exchange reactions). Spectrum 2 is the control spectrum which is irradiated at an equal and opposite distance from the PCr peak (arrowed). The subtraction (2–1) shows the exchange with PCr.

12.3.1 Localising strategies

Many different techniques have been described for localising the signal in magnetic resonance spectroscopy,[23] and they can be divided into three categories: those that use static field gradients (topical magnetic resonance),[24] those that use radio-frequency pulses and surface coils (rotating frame techniques, and depth pulses), and those that use pulsed gradients with or without frequency selective pulses. Topical magnetic resonance was used in early studies[25] but it has since been superseded. Of the others, only techniques known by the acronyms of PMRFI, DRESS, ISIS and also chemical shift imaging have been used successfully to obtain human heart spectra. PMRFI (phase modulated rotating frame imaging technique) uses a slice selective field gradient for localisation in one dimension and it relies upon the sensitivity profile of the surface coil to limit signal from the other two dimensions. DRESS (depth resolved surface coil spectroscopy) also uses the

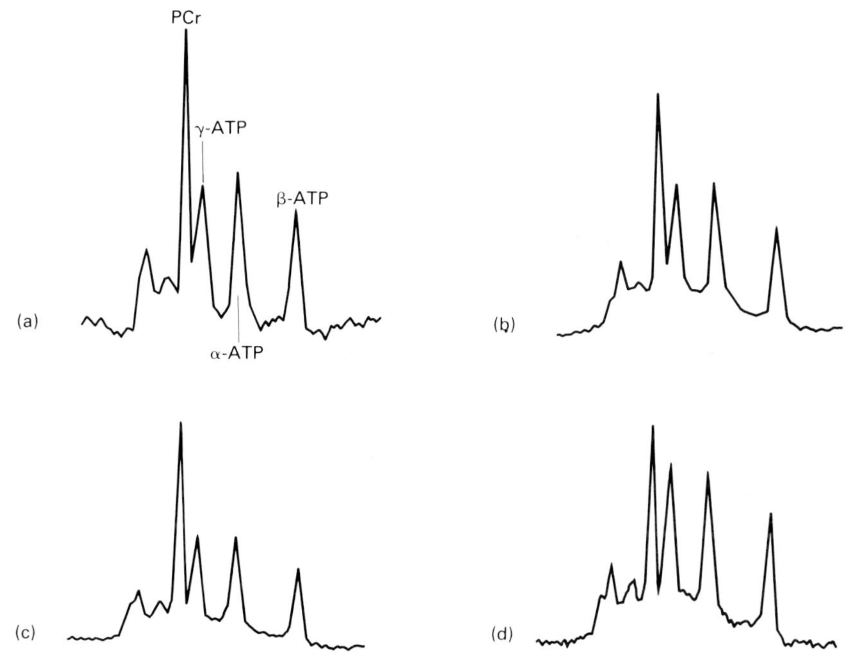

Figure 12.10. ^{31}P spectra acquired using surface coils placed over surgically exposed hearts. The spectra of dog hearts at 32 MHz (a) and of sheep (b), dogs (c) and cats (d) at 80 MHz are shown. There is a complex group of peaks in the P_i region because of erythrocyte 2,3-diphosphoglycerate (2,3-DPG). Note the variation in 2,3-DPG in the different species. In adult sheep, the signal is mainly red cell phosphate because the lamb loses the 2,3-DPG as it matures. The higher field spectra show partial resolution of this region. A broad peak is also seen between the P_i region and PCr, which has been attributed to diesters such as glycerophosphoryl-choline.

spatial selectivity of the surface coil but it depends on a pulsed field gradient for the third dimension. In ISIS (image selected *in vivo* spectroscopy) and chemical shift imaging, the signal can be obtained from anywhere within the sensitive volume but in the former this is limited to a preselected region, while in the latter, spatially resolved signal is obtained throughout the sensitive volume.

Magnetic field gradients are used to localise signal in the same way as in proton imaging but a complicating factor in spectroscopy is that chemical shift information must be preserved despite the frequency changes used to encode spatial information. At 1.5 T with gradients of 14 mT/m, the spatial shift corresponding to a chemical shift of 20 ppm is 2 mm, and since relatively large volumes are acquired, this can be ignored. In DRESS and ISIS, frequency selective pulses are used to select planes in space and the excitation band width (that is the range of frequencies excited) is inversely proportional to the pulse length. A compromise is therefore necessary because the pulse has to be long enough to be slice selective but short enough to excite all the chemical species of the nucleus of interest.

12.3.2 The phase modulated rotating frame imaging technique

For technical details the reader is referred to a number of recent publications,[26–30] but in summary the technique allows spectra to be acquired from slices of limited diameter at any required depth from the anterior chest wall. By examining slices at increasing depth it is possible to identify a slice in which the PCr/ATP ratio falls from the value of 4, typical of skeletal muscle, to 1.5 which is typical of myocardium. Phosphorus spectra of human heart obtained in this way are very similar to those obtained in animals but the inorganic phosphate region is poorly resolved because of contamination with signal from blood (figure 12.13).

The technique has been used in patients with hypertrophic cardiomyopathy and it has been shown that the abnormal muscle has a lower PCr/ATP ratio than normal muscle (figure 12.14).[31] These abnormalities may reflect an imbalance between blood supply and metabolic demand and it is possible that the hypertrophy is not accompanied by equivalent development of blood supply. Figure 12.15 shows another example in a teenager with hypertrophic cardiomyopathy affecting the septum. An abnormal diester peak is seen in the septum but not in the normal free wall. The diester region in liver and brain is known to have contributions from glycerophosphoryl-choline and glycerophosphoryl-ethanolamine, intermediates in the metabolism of membrane phospholipids, and this abnormal peak may therefore reflect an abnormality of membrane metabolism.

Conway and colleagues have studied the effects of exercise on cardiac metabolism in normal volunteers

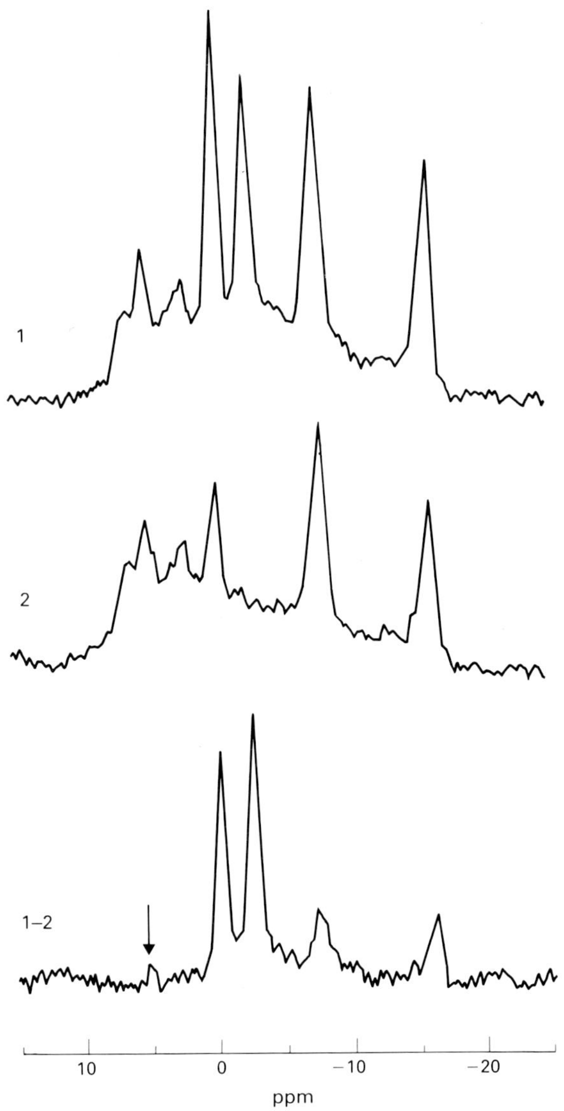

Figure 12.11. Determination of myocardial pH using the exchange of magnetisation between intracellular P_i and ATP. Spectrum 1 is the control spectrum and spectrum 2 shows the effect of irradiating the γ-ATP peak. In the subtraction spectrum (1−2) only the intracellular P_i should be visible (arrowed).

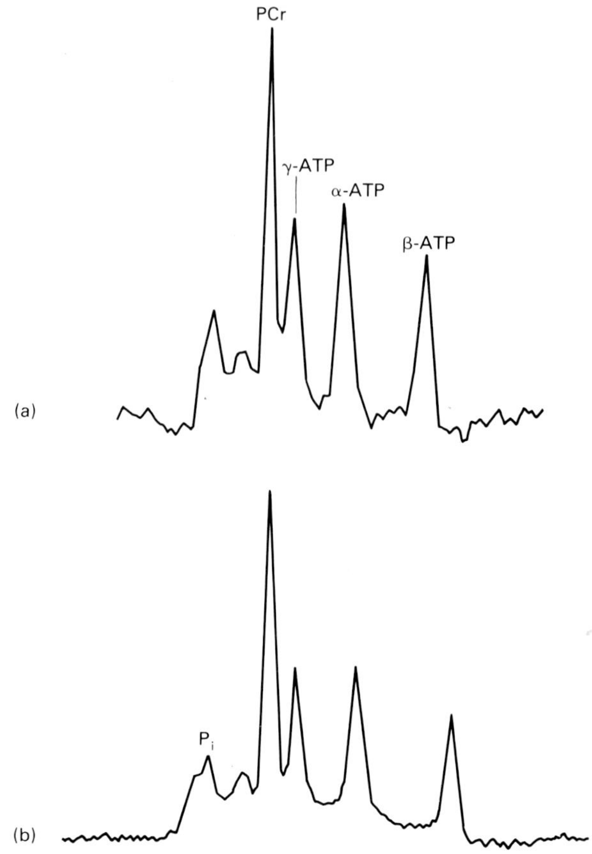

Figure 12.12. Comparison of dog heart spectra at 1.9 T (a) and at 4.7 T (b). The P_i region is a little better resolved at the higher field. Improvements in field homogeneity and proton decoupling may improve the resolution.

(figure 12.16).[32] The heart rate can be increased to levels equivalent to stage 1−2 of the Bruce protocol but it is necessary to maintain this level of exercise for 30 minutes during the acquisition. The myocardial PCr/ATP ratio is the same at rest and during exercise and intracellular pH is unchanged (figure 12.17). Thus there appears to be an increase in mitochondrial ATP production which matches the energy consumption of the heart during exercise, in contrast to skeletal muscle where significant changes in the levels of PCr, P_i and intracellular pH are seen.

12.3.3 Depth resolved surface coil spectroscopy

The DRESS technique has been developed and applied by Bottomley and colleagues and the reader is referred to other publications for details.[33–36] Like the PMRFI technique it allows spectra from slices at selected depths from a surface coil to be acquired.

In a study of 20 normal volunteers the PCr/ATP ratio was 1.6 and in 13 spectra the intracellular P_i could be identified with a mean PCr/P_i ratio of 8.8. In four patients with recent myocardial ischaemia, increases in P_i were observed and it appeared possible to differentiate epicardial from endocardial ratios (figure 12.18). If this increase in P_i is indeed due to intracellular P_i, then the findings would be of interest as elevated intracellular P_i has been blamed for the loss of mechanical function in ischaemic perfused animal hearts.

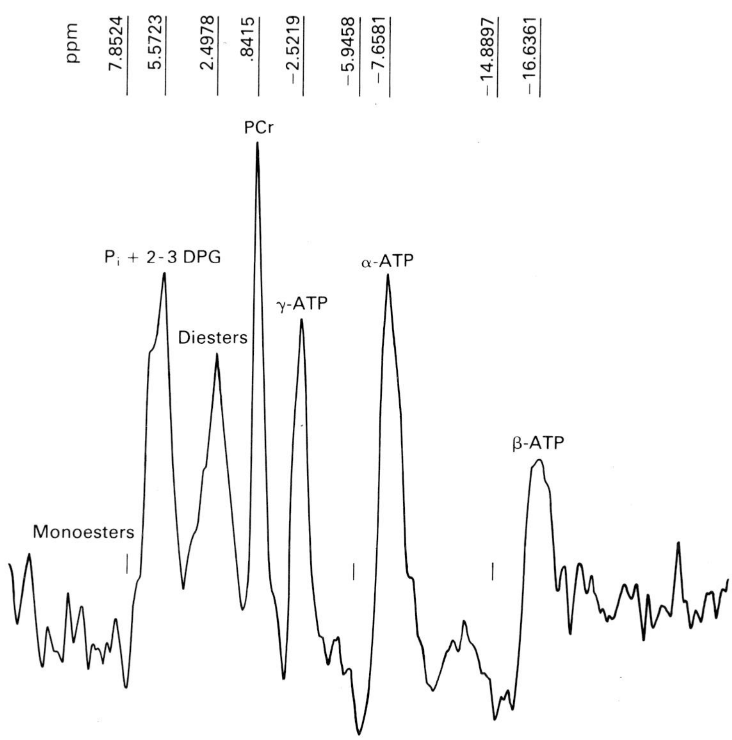

Figure 12.13. ^{31}P spectrum of a normal human heart obtained using the Fourier depth selection technique. The broad signal from intracellular and extracellular P_i and from 2,3-DPG is similar to the signal in animal hearts but the diester region is more prominent.

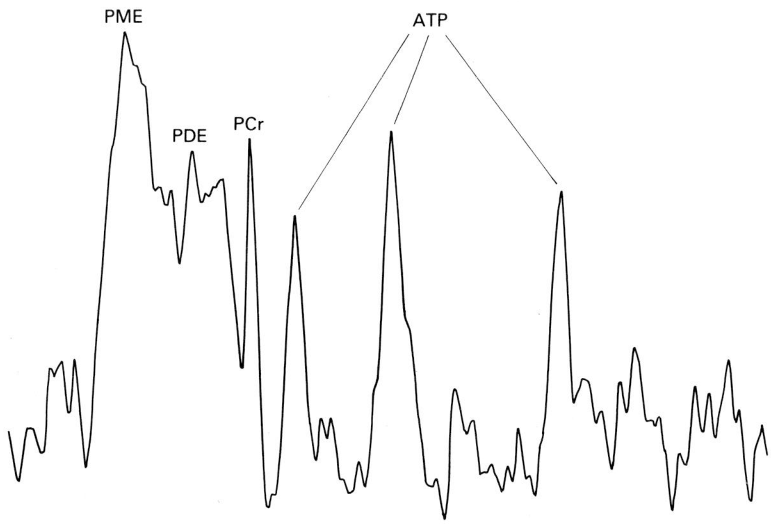

Figure 12.14. ^{31}P spectrum of the heart of a patient with hypertrophic cardiomyopathy involving the right ventricle. There is a low PCr/ATP ratio and abnormal diester and monoester peaks.

12.3.4 Image selected *in vivo* spectroscopy

ISIS uses three perpendicular magnetic field gradients to obtain spectra from eight overlapping planes and by appropriate additions and subtractions the spectrum from a selected volume is obtained.[37,38] Weiner and colleagues have used this technique to obtain ^{31}P spectra of human heart in normal volunteers, the selected volume being approximately 80 ml.[39] The mean PCr/ATP ratio was 1.33.

12.3.5 Chemical shift imaging

This technique provides a spectroscopic map of a selected slice and provides the most detailed metabolic map of the heart to date (figure 12.19).[40–42] It is diffi-

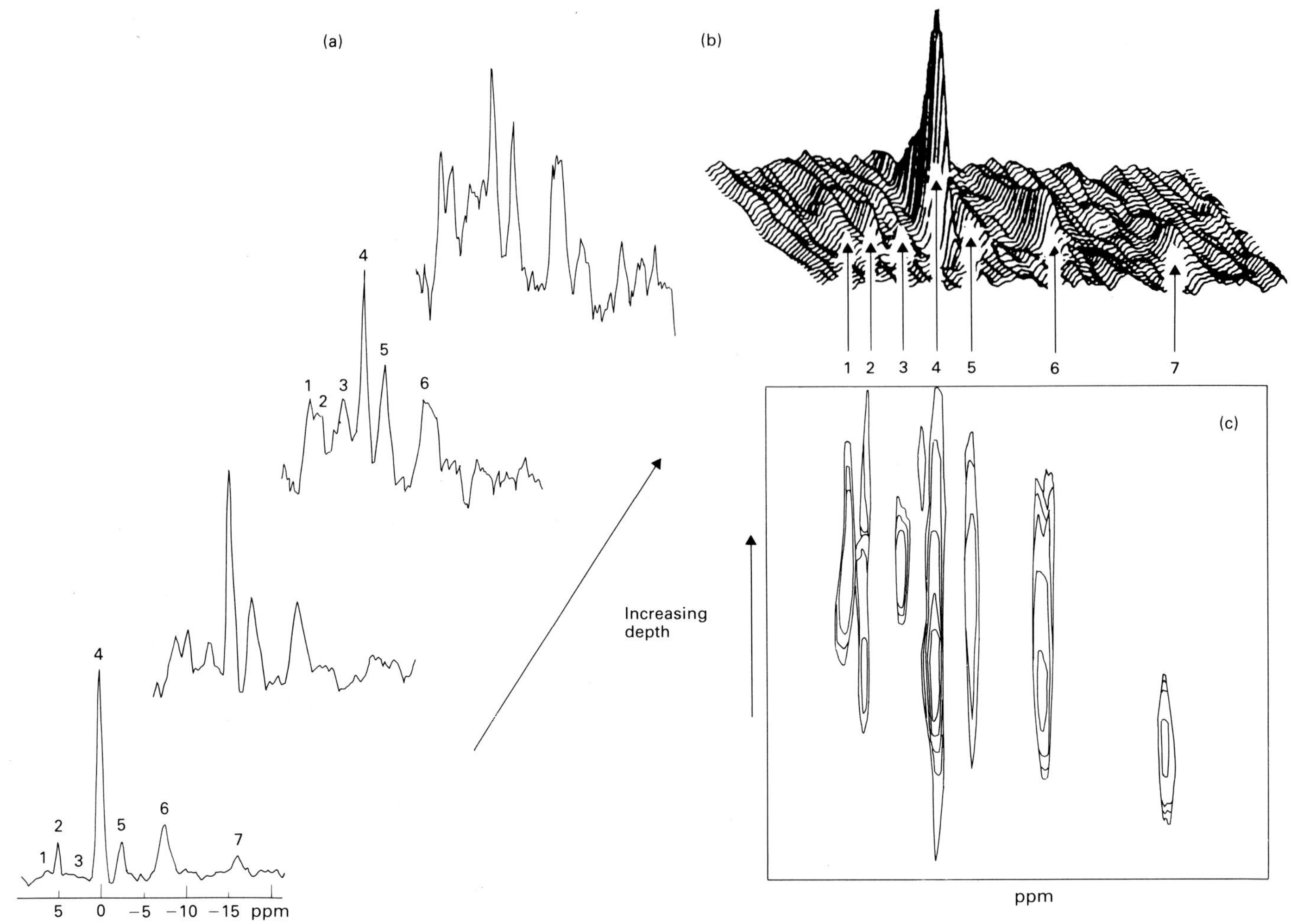

Figure 12.15. PMRFI of the heart of a teenager with hypertrophic cardiomyopathy. There is an abnormal diester peak in the septum. 1,2: 2,3-DPG and P_i, 3: diester, 4: PCr, 5: γ-ATP, 6: α-ATP, 7: β-ATP.

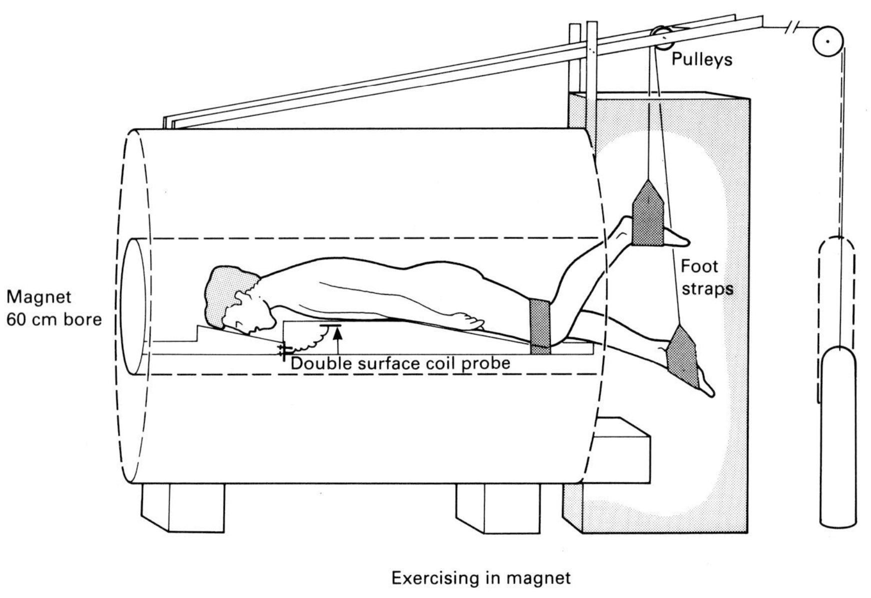

Figure 12.16. Device for exercising subjects in a whole body magnet while collecting spectra of the heart. (Reproduced with thanks to Dr. M. Conway.)

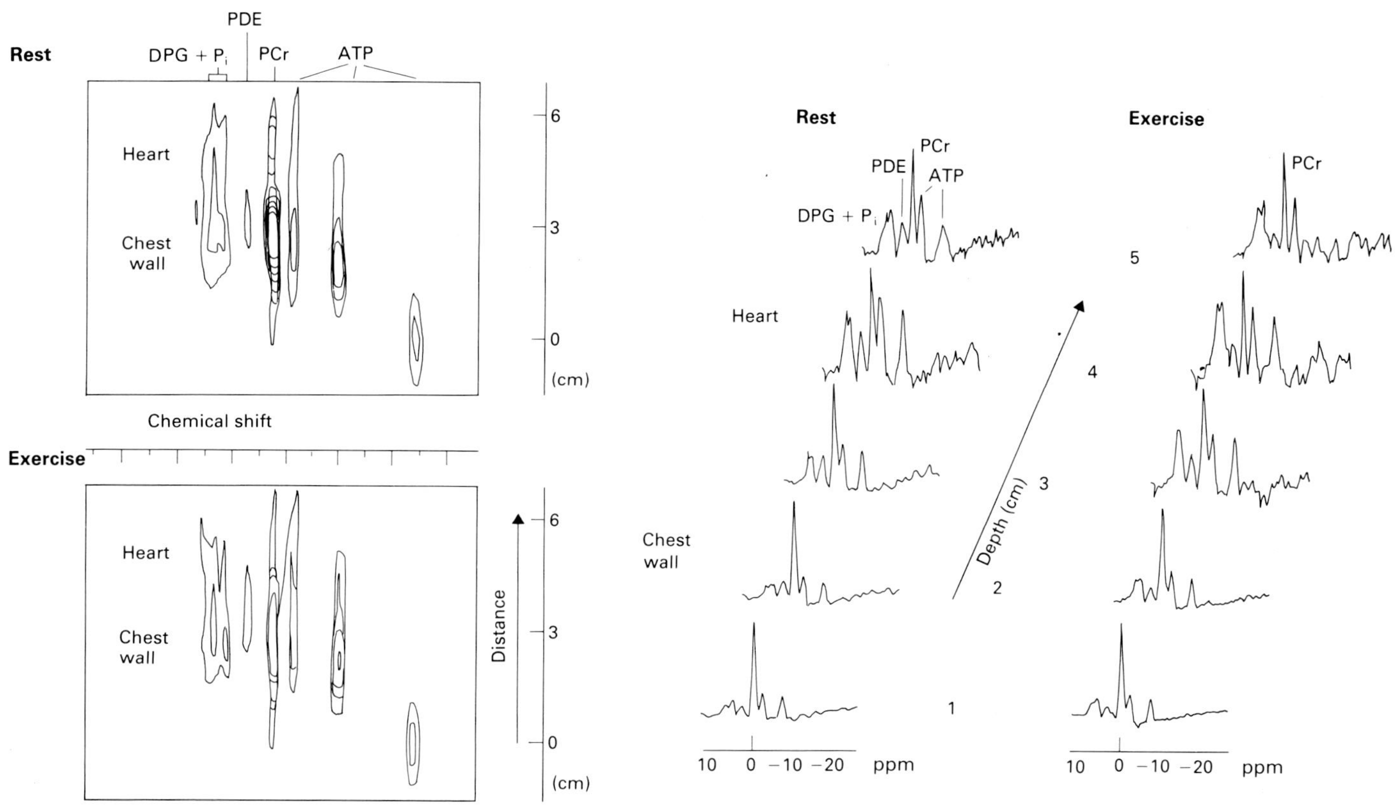

Figure 12.17. Images and selected spectra from a normal volunteer at rest and during exercise. There is no change with exercise. (Reproduced with thanks to Dr. M. Conway.)

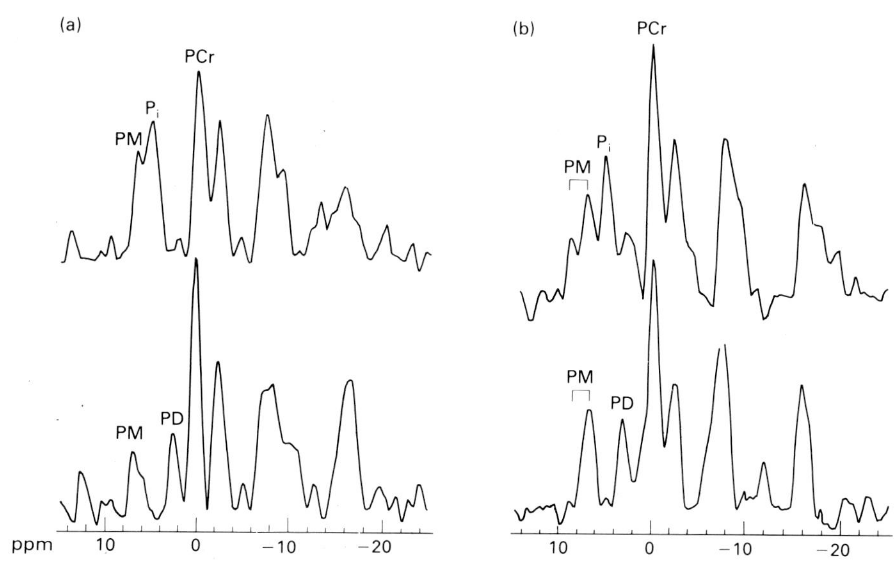

Figure 12.18. Human spectra of patients with myocardial infarction obtained using DRESS. Differences in the P$_i$ region in the endocardial slices (a) are apparent when compared with the epicardium (b). (Reproduced with permission from Bottomley *et al*.[36])

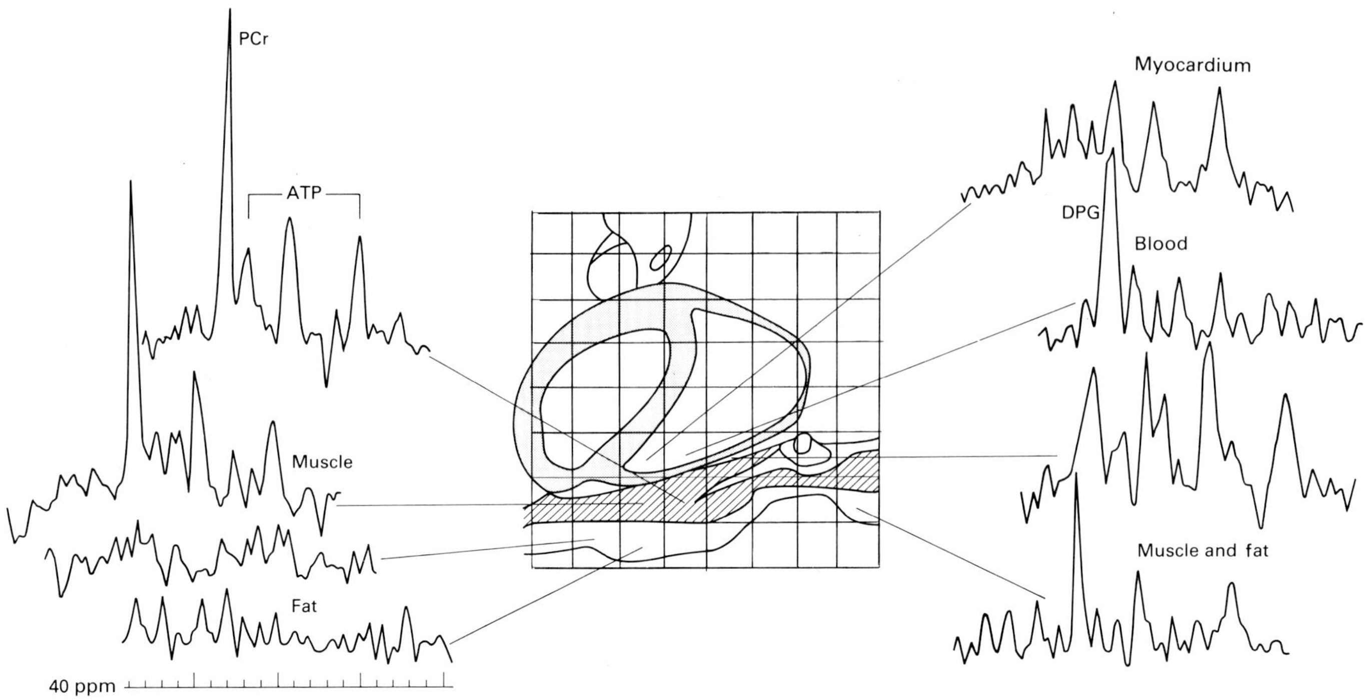

Figure 12.19. ^{31}P spectra of a normal human heart obtained using the chemical shift imaging method. (Reproduced with permission from Bottomley *et al.*[42])

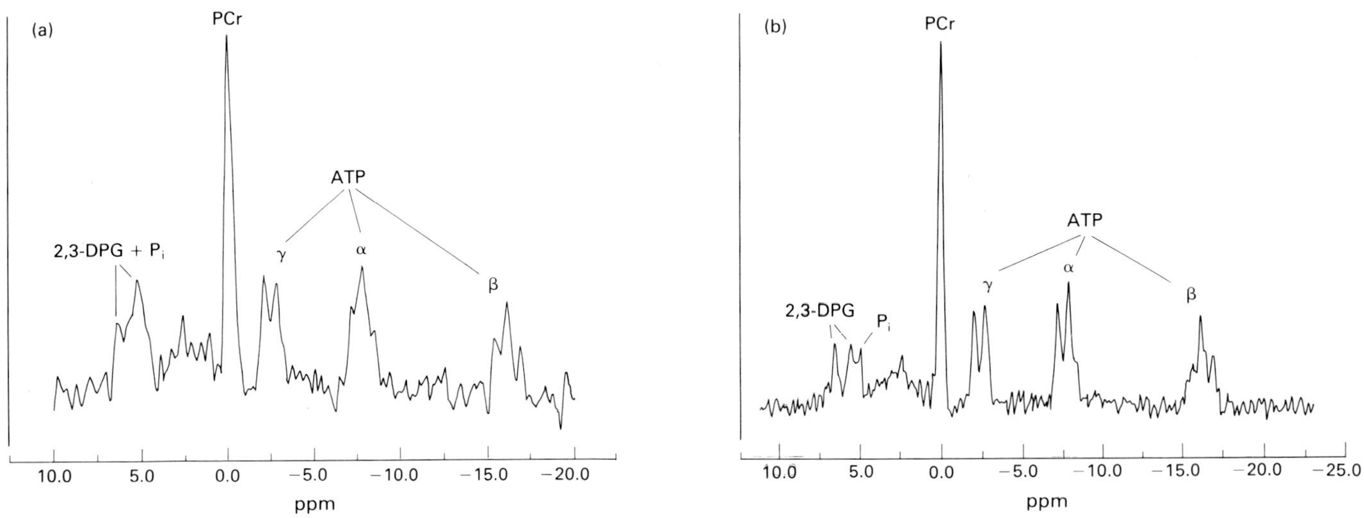

Figure 12.20. Coupled (a) and proton decoupled (b) spectra of a normal human heart. The P_i region is better defined even in the 1.5 T magnet. (Reproduced with permission from Luyten *et al.*[43].)

cult to apply at the moment without specially developed hardware.

12.4 Future directions

Den Hollander and colleagues have approached the problem of resolution and identification of myocardial P_i by using localised shimming procedures and proton decoupling.[43] They have succeeded in improving ^{31}P line widths to about 5 Hz and this degree of homogeneity allowed them to resolve the splitting of the ATP peaks caused by P—P coupling, and they have also resolved the P_i peak from 2,3-DPG (figure 12.20). Such techniques should be of particular value in the study of patients with ischaemic heart disease.

Absolute concentrations of metabolites are essential for the interpretation of the energy state of tissues. In order to achieve this, a clearly defined volume of interest is required, and the sensitivity of the transmitter and receiver coils must be accurately known. An alternative approach is to incorporate a calibration phantom into the coil, and using this approach in the ISIS technique, Roth and colleagues calculated ATP concentrations in the brain to be approximately 2.5 mM.[44] A similar approach has been used with the PMRFI technique in liver and brain and ATP concentrations were estimated to be 2.5 mM in normal brain and 1–1.5 mM in the centre of a meningioma.

12.5 Conclusions

Magnetic resonance spectroscopy is unique among non-invasive techniques applicable to clinical medicine in that it provides a description of the biochemistry of the living cell. Experiments on cellular extracts, whole cells and perfused organs have demonstrated that it is possible to obtain information about phosphorus, carbon, proton and sodium among the many nuclei that possess magnetic moments, and some of these studies have been extended to intact animals. It is also possible to obtain spectra of heart muscle in man in an acceptable time, and if only some of the *in vitro* experiments are extended to human hearts, valuable information for clinical management of a range of conditions will become available. The clinical problems wait to be solved, and it remains for magnetic resonance physicists and spectroscopists to rise to the challenge.

References

1 Radda GK. Potential and limitations of nuclear magnetic resonance for the cardiologist. *Br Heart J* 1983; **50**: 197–201.
2 Radda GK, Taylor DJ. Applications of nuclear magnetic resonance spectroscopy in pathology. In: Richter GW, Epstein MA (eds). *International Review of Experimental Pathology*. New York: Academic Press 1985: 1–58.
3 Radda GK. The use of NMR spectroscopy for the understanding of disease. *Science* 1986; **233**: 640–5.
4 Radda GK, Oberhaensli RD, Taylor DJ. The biochemistry of human diseases as studied by ^{31}P NMR in man and animal models. *Ann NY Acad Sci* 1987; **508**: 300–8.
5 Gadian DG. *Nuclear Magnetic Resonance and its Applications to Living Systems*. Oxford: Clarendon Press, 1982.
6 Morris PG. *Nuclear Magnetic Resonance Imaging in Medicine and Biology*. Oxford: Oxford University Press, 1986.
7 Bailey IA, Seymour AML, Radda GK. A ^{31}P-NMR study of the effects of reflow on the ischaemic rat heart. *Biochim Biophys Acta* 1981; **637**: 1–7.
8 Bailey IA, Radda GK, Seymour AML, Williams SR. The effects of insulin on myocardial metabolism and acidosis in normoxia and ischaemia: A 31P-NMR study. *Biochim Biophys Acta* 1982; **720**: 17–27.
9 Flaherty JT, Weisfeldt ML, Bulkley B, Gardner TJ, Gott VL, Jacobus WE. Mechanisms of ischaemic myocardial cell damage assessed by phosphorus ^{31}P nuclear magnetic resonance. *Circulation* 1982; **65**: 561–71.
10 Moon RB, Richards JH. Determination of intracellular pH by 31P magnetic resonance. *J Biol Chem* 1973; **248**: 7276–8.
11 Kingsley-Hickman PB, Sako EY, Mohanakrishnan P, *et al.* 31–P NMR studies of ATP synthesis and hydrolysis kinetics in the intact myocardium. *Biochemistry* 1987; **26**: 7501–10.
12 Brooks WM, Haseler LJ, Clarke K, Willis RJ. Relation between the phosphocreatine to ATP ratio determined by ^{31}P nuclear magnetic resonance spectroscopy and left ventricular function in underperfused guinea-pig heart. *J Mol Cell Cardiol* 1986; **18**: 149–55.
13 Matthews PM, Williams SR, Seymour AM, *et al.* A ^{31}P NMR study of some metabolic and functional effects of the inotropic agents epinephrine, ouabain and the ionophore R02–2985 (X537A) in the isolated perfused rat heart. *Biochim Biophys Acta* 1982; **720**: 163–71.
14 Matthews PM, Bland JL, Gadian DG, Radda GK. The steady state rate of ATP synthesis in the perfused rat heart measured by ^{31}P NMR saturation transfer. *Biochem Biophys Res Commun* 1981; **103**: 1052–9.
15 Shoubridge EA, Jeffry FMH, Keogh JM, Radda GK, Seymour AML. Creatine kinase kinetics, ATP turnover, and cardiac performance in hearts depleted of creatine with the substrate analogue β-guanidinopropionic acid. *Biochim Biophys Acta* 1985; **847**: 25–32.
16 Malloy CR, Matthews PM, Smith MB, Radda GK. In vivo ^{31}P NMR study of the regional metabolic response to cardiac ischaemia. *Adv Myocardiol* 1984; **6**: 461–4.
17 Malloy CR, Matthews PM, Smith MB, Radda GK. Influence of propranolol on acidosis and high energy phosphates in ischaemic myocardium of the rabbit. *Cardiovasc Res* 1986; **20**: 710–20.
18 Osbakken M, Ligeti L, Clark BJ, *et al.* Myocardial high energy phosphate metabolism in closed chest dog: creation of an animal model. *Magn Reson Med* 1986; **3**: 801–7.
19 Kantor HL, Briggs RW, Balaban RS. In vivo ^{31}P nuclear magnetic resonance measurements in canine heart using a catheter-coil. *Circ Res* 1984; **55**: 261–6.
20 Brindle KM, Rajagopalan B, Bolas NM, Radda GK. Editing of ^{31}P NMR spectra of heart in vivo. *J Magn Reson* 1987; **74**: 356–65.
21 Brindle KM, Rajagopalan B, Williams DS, *et al.* ^{31}P NMR measurements of myocardial pH in vivo. *Biochem Biophys Res Commun* 1988; **151**: 70–7.

22 Crowley M, Ackerman JJH. Enhanced surface coil spatial localisation with an inhomogeneous surface gradient. *J Magn Reson* 1985; **65**: 522.

23 Aue WP. Localisation methods for in vivo NMR spectroscopy. *Rev Magn Reson Med* 1986; **1**: 21–72.

24 Cresshull ID, Gordon RE, Hanley PE, *et al*. Localisation of metabolites in animal and human tissues using ^{31}P topical magnetic resonance. *Bull Magn Reson* 1981; **12**: 426.

25 Oberhaensli RD, Galloway GJ, Hilton-Jones D, *et al*. The study of human organs by phosphorus-31 topical magnetic resonance spectroscopy. *Br J Radiol* 1987; **60**: 367–73.

26 Blackledge MJ, Rajagopalan B, Oberhaensli RD, Bolas NM, Styles P, Radda GK. Quantitative studies of human cardiac metabolism by ^{31}P rotating-frame NMR. *Proc Natl Acad Sci USA* 1987; **84**: 4283–7.

27 Blackledge MJ, Styles P, Radda GK. Rotating frame depth selection and its application to the study of human organs. *J Magn Reson* 1987; **71**: 246–58.

28 Blackledge MJ, Styles P, Radda GK. The elimination of transmitter-receiver phase twist artifacts in the phase modulated rotating frame imaging experiment. *J Magn Reson* 1988; **79**: 176–83.

29 Blackledge MJ, Styles P. Effect of pulse angle imperfections and resonance offset in the phase modulated rotating frame spectroscopic imaging experiment. *J Magn Reson* 1988; **77**: 203–22.

30 Styles P. Passive isolation of double coil probes. *NMR in Biomedicine* 1988; **1**: 61–6.

31 Rajagopalan B, Blackledge MJ, Mckenna WJ, Bolas N, Radda GK. Measurement of phosphocreatine to ATP ratio in normal and diseased human heart by ^{31}P magnetic resonance spectroscopy using rotating frame depth selection technique. *Ann NY Acad Sci* 1987; **508**: 321–32.

32 Conway MC, Rajaopalan B, Massie B, *et al*. Evidence for a metabolic defect in skeletal muscle in heart failure from limb ischaemic studies. *Q J Med* 1987; **65**: 875–6.

33 Bottomley PA, Edelstein WA, Hart HR, Schenck JF, Scott-Smith L. Spatial localisation in ^{31}P and 13C NMR spectroscopy in vivo using surface coils. *Magn Reson Med* 1984; **1**: 410–3.

34 Bottomley PA. Non-invasive study of high energy phosphate metabolism in human heart by depth resolved ^{31}P NMR spectroscopy. *Science* 1985; **229**: 769–72.

35 Bottomley PA, Herfkens RJ, Smith LS, Brazzamano S, Blinder R, Hedlund LW. Non-invasive detection and monitoring of regional myocardial ischaemia in situ using depth resolved ^{31}P NMR spectroscopy. *Proc Natl Acad Sci USA* 1985; **82**: 8747.

36 Bottomley PA, Herfkens RJ, Smith LS, Bashore TM. Altered phosphate metabolism in myocardial infarction: P–31 MR spectroscopy. *Radiology* 1987; **165**: 703–7.

37 Ordidge RJ, Connelly A, Lohman JAB. Image selected in vivo spectroscopy (ISIS). A new technique for spatially selective NMR spectroscopy. *J Magn Reson* 1986; **66**: 283–94.

38 Connelly A, Counsell C, Lohman JAB. Outer volume suppressed image related in vivo spectroscopy (OSIRIS), a high-sensitivity localization technique. *J Magn Reson* 1988; **78**: 519–25.

39 Shaefer S, Gober J, Valenza M, *et al*. Nuclear magnetic resonance imaging-guided phosphorus–31 spectroscopy of the human heart. *J Am Coll Cardiol* 1988; **12**: 1449–55.

40 Brown TR, Kincaid BM, Ugurbil K. NMR chemical shift imaging in three dimensions. *Proc Natl Acad Sci USA* 1982; **79**: 3523–6.

41 Bottomley PA, Charles HC, Roemer PB, *et al*. Human in vivo phosphate metabolite imaging with ^{31}P NMR. *Magn Reson Med* 1988; **7**: 319–36.

42 Bottomley PA. Human in vivo NMR spectroscopy in diagnostic medicine: clinical tool or research probe? *Radiology* 1989; **170**: 1–15.

43 Luyten PR, Bruntink G, Sloff FM, *et al*. Broadband proton decoupling in human ^{31}P NMR spectroscopy. *NMR in Biomedicine* 1989; **1**: 177–83.

44 Roth K, Hubesch B, Meyerhoff DJ, *et al*. Noninvasive quantitation of phosphorus metabolites in human tissue by NMR spectroscopy. *J Magn Reson* 1989; **81**: 299–311.

Chapter 13
Magnetic Resonance Compared with other Imaging Techniques

GREGORY CRANNEY, CHAIM LOTAN AND GERALD POHOST

Previous chapters have demonstrated that magnetic resonance imaging is an extremely valuable technique in the cardiovascular system, but its dissemination in clinical practice has been slow compared with the rapid spread of imaging of static organs such as the brain, the spinal cord and the knee.[1] Several factors may account for this, including the need for cardiac triggering, the relatively long imaging times required, and the paucity of suitable software to display and analyse the dynamic data. The relative expense of the technique compared with, for instance, echocardiography has also hindered its spread. New developments have slowly altered the balance, however, including the development of oblique imaging planes, cine gradient echo imaging, and cine velocity mapping. There is now an increasing need to define the clinical role of cardiovascular magnetic resonance imaging, but few large studies have been undertaken because of the difficulties inherent in such analyses.[2]

In this chapter we compare magnetic resonance imaging with other imaging techniques, and in making this comparison it is important to remember the clinical value of the information provided by magnetic resonance, the ratio of risk to benefit for the patient, and the ratio of cost to effectiveness. Table 13.1 lists the technical advantages and disadvantages of magnetic resonance compared with other techniques for imaging the cardiovascular system.

13.1 The aorta

The strength of magnetic resonance imaging for the assessment of the thoracic and abdominal aorta is well established. It has the advantage of not requiring contrast agents or ionising radiation and it can be performed as an outpatient procedure. Serial examinations can easily be performed and the technique is ideal for long-term follow-up. Several studies have demonstrated the superiority of magnetic resonance over other techniques. In a combined retrospective and prospective study of 41 patients with a variety of aortic disease, Lois and colleagues[3] compared magnetic resonance imaging with computed X-ray tomography, ultrasound, X-ray angiography, and surgical findings, and they concluded that magnetic resonance provided sufficient information in all patients to obviate the need for further investigation.

13.1.1 Aortic dissection

Magnetic resonance imaging is a sensitive and specific method for the detection of aortic dissection (figure 13.1). Kersting-Sommerhoff and colleagues studied 54 patients with suspected aortic dissection and found the sensitivity of magnetic resonance imaging to be 96% for the detection of dissection.[4] In another study, Pernes and colleagues reviewed 30 patients with suspected or known chronic dissection and compared magnetic resonance with both computed X-ray tomography and X-ray aortography.[5] They found that magnetic resonance was more accurate in demonstrating an intimal flap than the other techniques but they did note difficulty in distinguishing between a thrombosed false lumen and an aneurysm with mural thrombus. Cranney and colleagues have suggested that gradient echo imaging improves the visualisation of the intimal flap,[6] and cine velocity mapping also helps in cases of doubt.[7]

13.1.2 Aortic aneurysm

The size and site of aneurysms can be accurately assessed using magnetic resonance imaging (figure 13.2).[8,9] Measurements of the aortic diameter, an important determinant of the need for surgery, correlate well with those obtained by other techniques.

Table 13.1. A technical comparison of different imaging techniques for the cardiovascular system

	MRI	X-ray angiography	Echo + Doppler	Radionuclide imaging	Ultrafast X-ray CT	PET
Invasive	N	Y	N	(Y)	(Y)	(Y)
Contrast medium	N	Y	N	N	Y	N
Ionising radiation	N	Y	N	Y	Y	Y
Real time imaging	(N)	Y	Y	N	Y	N
Stress imaging	(N)	(N)	(Y)	Y	Y	Y
Operator dependent	(N)	Y	Y	N	N	N
Unstable patients	(N)	Y	Y	Y	N	N
Spatial resolution	++	+++	++	+	++	+
Temporal resolution	++	+++	+++	++	++	+
Oblique imaging	+++	++	++	+++	+	+
Inpatient procedure	N	Y	N	N	N	N
Total imaging time	s	i	i	i	i	s
Cost	+++	+++	+	+	+++	++++

MRI = magnetic resonance imaging, CT = computed X-ray tomography, PET = position emission tomography. Y = yes, N = no, () = qualification, s = slow (> 30 min), i = intermediate (15–30 min).

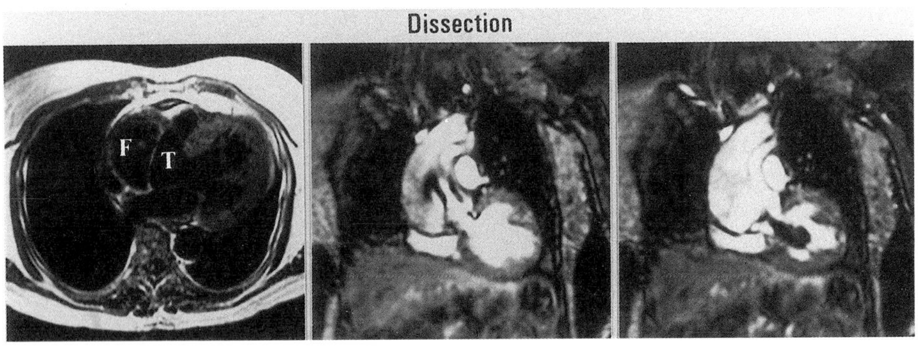

Figure 13.1. Aortic dissection. The transverse spin echo image at the level of the aortic valve (left) shows the true (T) and false lumens (F). In a systolic frame from the cine gradient echo acquisition (centre) a turbulent jet is seen entering the false lumen at the site of the intimal tear, and in the diastolic image (right) a jet of aortic regurgitation is seen.

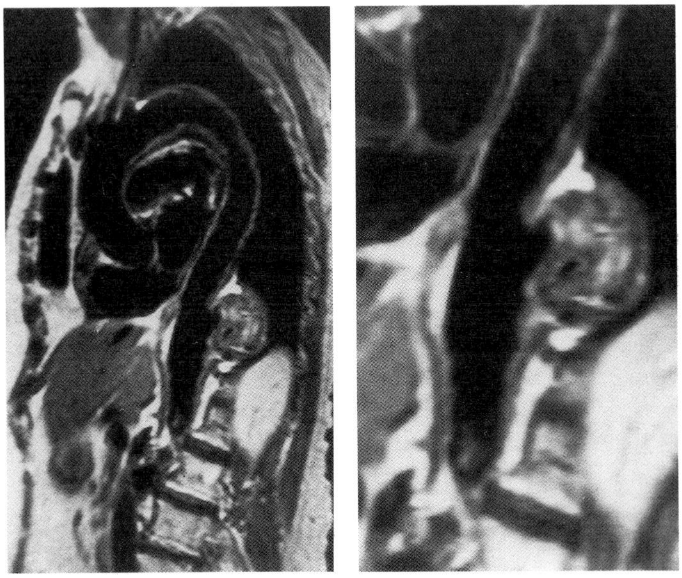

Figure 13.2. Oblique spin echo images showing a saccular aneurysm of the descending aorta filled with thrombus.

13.1.3 Conclusion

Magnetic resonance imaging appears superior to X-ray contrast aortography and computed tomography for thoracic aortic disease. It is likely to be most valuable in screening patients with a high risk of aortic disease, such as those with Marfan's syndrome, and in following patients with known disease. It has the potential to replace cardiac catheterisation and aortography when information about the coronary anatomy is not needed, but the ability to study patients with acute dissection will depend upon practical matters such as the siting of the magnet and expertise in the management of unstable patients. Early experience with transoesophageal echocardiography[10,11], suggests that this technique may also play an important role, particularly in sick patients who are unable to undergo magnetic resonance imaging.

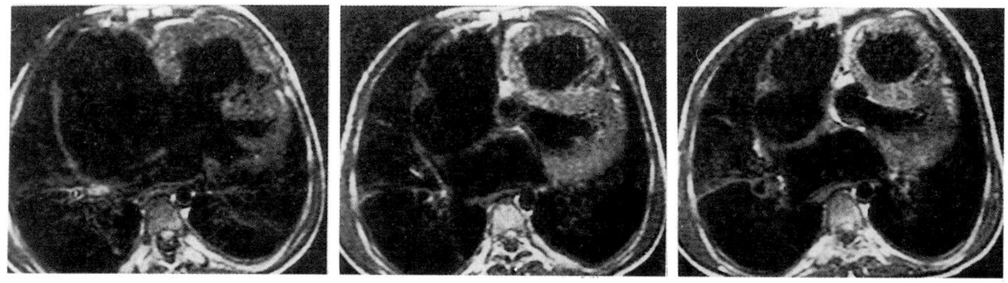

Figure 13.3. Atrioventricular canal defect. Contiguous transverse slices from inferior (left) to superior (right). There is a large defect at the crux of the heart and marked right ventricular hypertrophy.

13.2 Congenital heart disease

The high contrast and spatial resolution of magnetic resonance imaging and its ability to provide three-dimensional information make it an excellent technique for the investigation of congenital heart disease (figure 13.3). In an early review of 72 patients, Didier and colleagues were able to demonstrate the anatomy and relationship of the chambers and great vessels in all, and they correctly identify 44 of 47 abnormalities of the great vessels and 30 of 33 ventricular anomalies.[12] In a more recent study Chung and colleagues described their experience using spin echo and gradient echo imaging in 91 patients with a variety of defects.[13] The complete diagnosis was obtained in 81%, and partial information was obtained in a further 14%. Intracardiac shunts, incompetence of atrioventricular and semilunar valves, and surgical shunt patency were correctly diagnosed, and the visualisation of the right heart and the right ventricular outflow tract was comparable with X-ray angiography. They have also used cine imaging to follow children after surgical repair of cyanotic congenital defects and have shown that pulmonary artery obstruction, aneurysmal dilation of the right ventricular outflow tract, and superior venal caval obstruction are all well demonstrated.[14]

Congenital anomalies outside the heart are also well demonstrated, including the size and connections of the central pulmonary arteries in patients with pulmonary atresia,[15] and abnormalities of the ascending aorta and aortic arch (figure 13.4).[16,17] Simpson and colleagues showed that measurements of aortic diameter in 14 patients with aortic coarctation agreed closely with X-ray angiographic findings and they also observed an inverse correlation between the length of the turbulent jet observed on cine imaging and the angiographic severity of the coarctation.[18] Patients can be followed after balloon angioplasty of coarctation,[19] and magnetic resonance is superior to echocardiography for the detection of superior vena caval

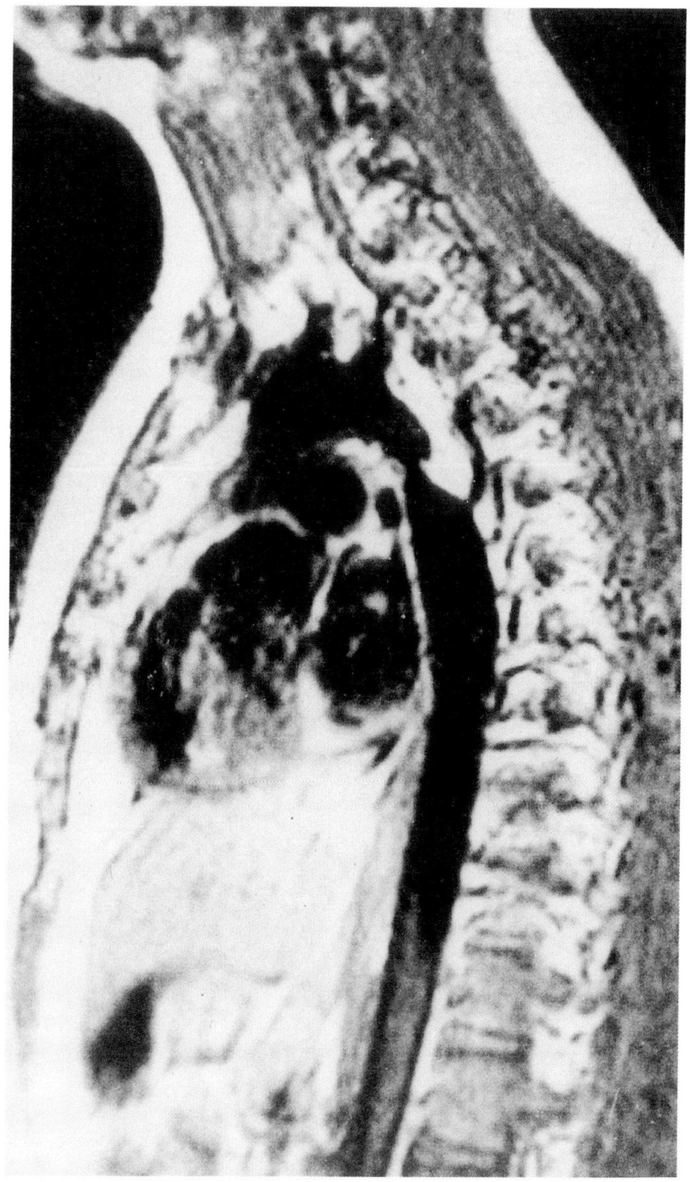

Figure 13.4. Sagittal image showing a discrete coarctation in the classical site just beyond the left subclavian artery. Collateral vessels are seen entering the descending aorta below the coarctation.

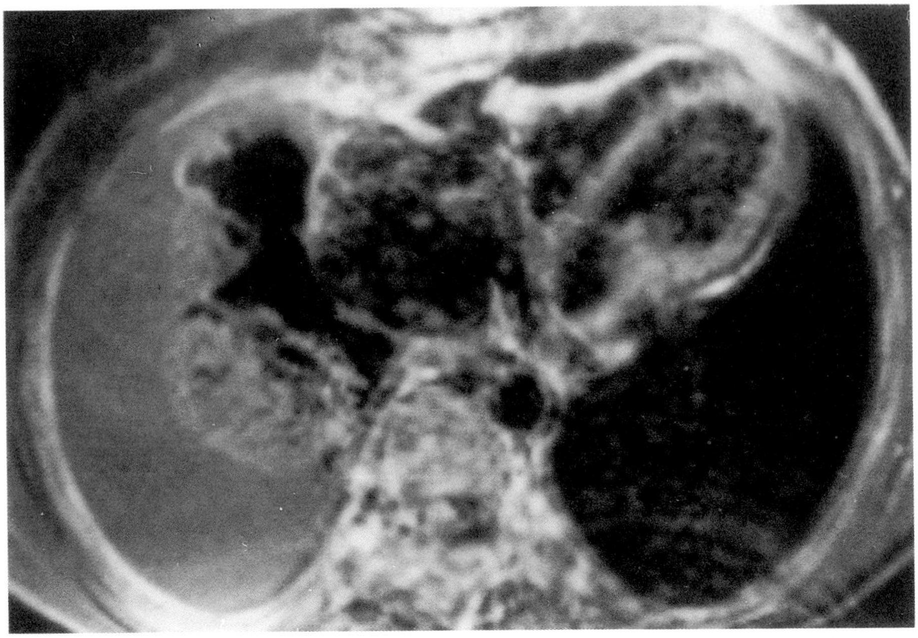

Figure 13.5. Constrictive pericarditis. The pericardium is thickened with loss of signal anteriorly because of calcification. The right atrium is dilated and the right ventricle is distorted. There is also a large right pleural effusion with collapse of the underlying lung.

obstruction after repair of transposition of the great arteries.[20]

The disadvantages of magnetic resonance compared with echocardiography include the difficulty of examining neonates without sedation and the thinness of the slices required to show small structures well. Whilst the former is not a significant problem, the latter is best achieved in high field machines.

In conclusion, magnetic resonance provides better anatomical information than any other technique, but echocardiography provides adequate information particularly in neonates and it is more widely available. The two are complimentary and there is no doubt that the combination can avoid the need for invasive investigation in selected cases. Magnetic resonance would be particularly helpful in those patients where assessment of the great vessels is important.

13.3 The pericardium

13.3.1 Constriction

The diagnosis of constrictive pericarditis is frequently a difficult clinical problem, but magnetic resonance imaging is helpful by virtue of its ability to show the pericardium and surrounding structures. The normal pericardium is usually seen in spin echo images as a 1–2 mm thick line of low signal intensity lying between the high intensity pericardial fat and the medium intensity myocardium or high intensity epicardial fat.[21] At high field strengths however the normal pericardium can be obscured by chemical shift artefact.

In a series of patients with pericardial constriction, pericardial thickening (exceeding 5 mm) was found in all five patients studied.[22] Associated findings included dilation of the right atrium and caval veins, a small tubular-shaped right ventricle and straightening of the ventricular septum (figure 13.5). In a subsequent series, a thickened pericardium was seen in six of eight patients with constrictive pericarditis and the authors suggested that magnetic resonance imaging was more reliable in differentiating constrictive pericarditis from restrictive cardiomyopathy than either echocardiography or X-ray computed tomography.[23]

13.3.2 Effusions and masses

Magnetic resonance imaging is helpful in assessing pericardial cysts, effusions, haematomas (figure 13.6), and tumours. Cysts are typically homogeneous with a low signal intensity on T_1 weighted images and higher signal intensity on T_2 weighted images. Calcification shows as reduced signal intensity but it cannot be identified confidently; this is in contrast to X-ray techniques.

13.3.3 Conclusion

Echocardiography remains the investigation of choice

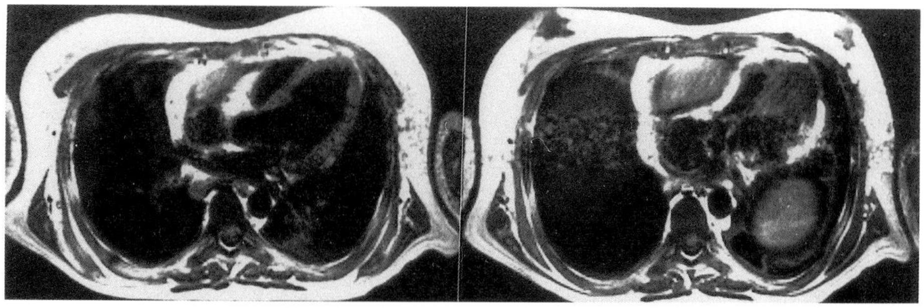

Figure 13.6. A traumatic loculated pericardial haematoma anterior to the right ventricle is distorting the right heart and there is also a haematoma below the left hemi-diaphragm.

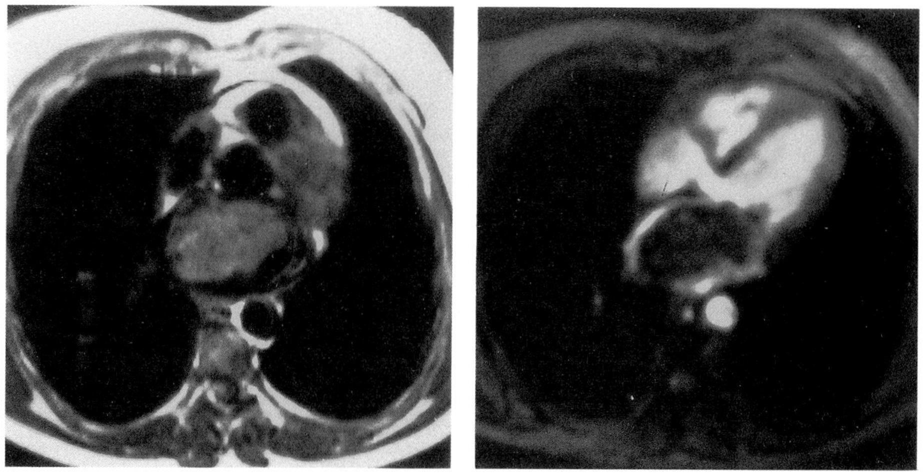

Figure 13.7. Large left atrial myxoma seen in both spin echo images (left) and gradient echo images (right). The tumour fills almost all of the left atrium and the posterior attachment is best seen in the gradient echo image.

in suspected pericardial effusion, but magnetic resonance imaging provides additional information in cases of doubt and occasionally effusions that are not seen by echocardiography may be detected. If pericardial constriction is suspected then magnetic resonance is clearly superior although echocardiography will still usually be performed as an initial investigation.

13.4 Cardiac and paracardiac masses

Intracavitary masses are best detected using a combination of spin echo and gradient echo images (figure 13.7). A number of studies have reported the effectiveness of magnetic resonance imaging.[24–26] Two studies have compared magnetic resonance with other imaging techniques. Freedberg and colleagues[27] looked at 14 patients with suspected tumours on echocardiography. In four patients with atrial myxomas and good quality echocardiograms, magnetic resonance did not contribute additional information but in the remaining ten patients, the tumour's relationship to other intracardiac structures or its extension to adjacent vascular and mediastinal structures was better seen. Winkler and colleagues[28] confirmed intracardiac masses in 15 of 34 patients believed to have masses on cross sectional echocardiography. The other 19 patients were found to have either normal morphology or an anatomical variant that had been misinterpreted by echocardiography.

The relative costs of magnetic resonance imaging and echocardiography suggest that echocardiography should be the initial investigation of suspected tumour in the majority of cases, but if the echocardiogram is equivocal or if more anatomical information is required (such as before surgery), then magnetic resonance imaging should be performed in addition.

13.5 Hypertrophic cardiomyopathy

Magnetic resonance imaging provides an assessment of myocardial thickness, a better appreciation of the distribution of hypertrophy than echocardiography,[29] and accurate measurements of left ventricular mass. Cine imaging demonstrates outflow tract obstruction by virtue of the signal loss generated by turbulence, but the measurement of intracavitary pressure gradients has not been achieved. The hope that magnetic resonance would provide a method of characterising the abnormal myocardium has not been fulfilled.

Echocardiography should still be considered the technique of choice for screening and for the assessment of patients with hypertrophic cardiomyopathy, while magnetic resonance imaging should be reserved for cases in which conclusive results can not be obtained.

13.6 Ventricular function

A knowledge of global left ventricular function is important in determining management and prognosis in patients with cardiac disease. Left ventricular ejection fraction is commonly determined by X-ray contrast ventriculography or by radionuclide ventriculography, and although the result is sensitive to both preload and afterload it is still a valuable parameter in a variety of cardiac disorders. End systolic volume is independent of preload and has been found to be an even better prognostic indicator after myocardial infarction[30] and in patients undergoing surgery for valvular regurgitation.[31] Routine measurement of left ventricular volumes has been hampered however by the lack of a reliable non-invasive technique, but magnetic resonance imaging now offers such measurements in both the left and the right heart.

The ability of magnetic resonance to measure left ventricular volume was recognised very early.[32] The accuracy of the technique has been discussed in chapter 5 and many studies have compared magnetic resonance with other techniques.[33–35] Several approaches have been used but they they can be summarised as multislice transaxial imaging,[36–40] multislice short axis imaging,[41–43] and single slice long axis.[44]

Regional ventricular function can also be studied. Underwood and colleagues examined 18 patients using coronal and sagittal planes and compared the findings with X-ray contrast ventriculography.[45] There was agreement in 68 segments analysed with 32 segments differing by only one grade out of four. Sechtem and colleagues examined 37 patients using transaxial spin echo images in multiple slices and there was a close correlation with echocardiography and X-ray ventriculography, although it was difficult to assess the inferior wall using this technique.[46] An alternative is to image in the short axis plane but this also has problems close to the base and the apex, where the myocardium moves through plane by a considerable amount.[47] In order to reduce imaging time and to avoid partial volume effects, Lotan and colleagues have used cine imaging in long axis planes[48] and found that all segments of the myocardium including the apex could be analysed adequately (figure 13.8).

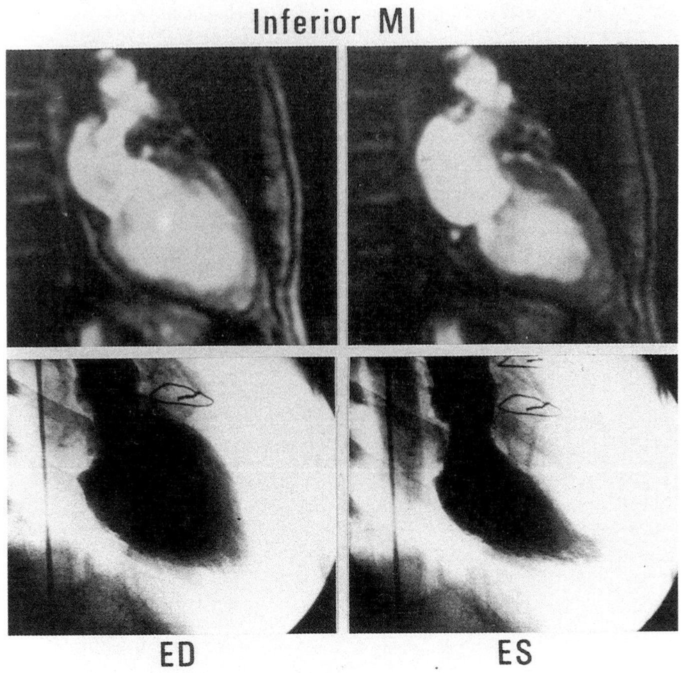

Figure 13.8. A comparison of cine gradient echo images (top) at end diastole (ED) and end systole (ES) with equivalent frames from the X-ray contrast ventriculogram in the right anterior oblique projection in a patient with previous inferior infarction. The magnetic resonance images show that in addition to inferior hypokinesis, the inferior myocardium fails to thicken. (Reproduced with permission from *J Am Coll Cardiol* 1989; **14**: 1721–9.)

Left ventricular hypertrophy is of prognostic significance in several cardiac disorders including hypertension and hypertrophic cardiomyopathy and magnetic resonance methods of measuring muscle mass have been discussed in chapter 5. The measurements have been validated in dog studies[49,50] but few studies have used the methods clinically. Echocardiography is less accurate and magnetic resonance is expected to be valuable in assessing left ventricular mass in patients with hypertrophy.

In conclusion, although echocardiography and radionuclide ventriculography provide important information about ventricular function, magnetic resonance imaging has the advantage of accuracy and of providing

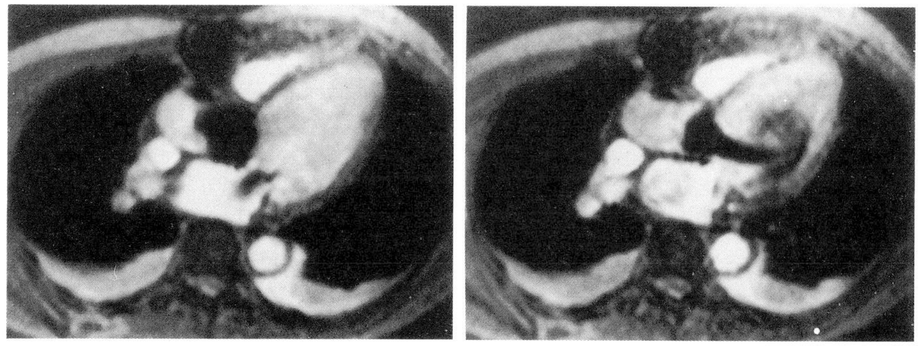

Figure 13.9. Systolic (left) and diastolic (right) gradient echo images in a patient with a prosthetic aortic valve and mitral and aortic regurgitation. The prosthetic valve produces a large area of signal loss but there is also a jet of mitral regurgitation in the left atrium in systole and a jet of aortic regurgitation in the left ventricle in diastole. There are also bilateral pleural effusions.

three-dimensional information. Its accuracy suggests that it should be used as the standard against which other techniques are judged, although its relative cost means that it will not always be used if only ejection fraction and wall motion are required.

13.7 Valvular regurgitation

An important clinical problem in the management of patients with valvular regurgitation is the best timing for surgery. The decision usually depends upon the symptoms, the degree of regurgitation, and upon left ventricular function. Magnetic resonance imaging has the potential to help in several ways.

Valve leaflets, while often seen on magnetic resonance images, are not usually seen well enough to provide pathological information. As a result, the diagnosis of conditions such as mitral valve prolapse and the visualisation of vegetations in infective endocarditis are better performed by echocardiography. In aortic regurgitation secondary to aortic root disease, however, magnetic resonance is particularly useful in defining the type and severity of the disease.

The ability of cine gradient echo imaging to detect turbulent jets has been discussed in chapter 7 (figure 13.9) and the severity of regurgitation can be estimated by measuring the area, depth, and persistence of the jet. The technique appears to be sensitive with no false negative results being found in two reported studies.[51,52] In addition, the area and direction of the jet have been shown to correlate well with Doppler echocardiography.[53] Pulmonary and tricuspid regurgitation can also be demonstrated but there have been no large comparative studies to date.

Like echocardiography, magnetic resonance imaging is a tomographic technique and two or more planes may be needed to appreciate fully the extent of the jet. For screening purposes, an angulated 'five chamber' plane intersecting the aortic and mitral valves and the left ventricular outflow tract detects the majority of left sided jets, and also allows a simultaneous assessment of left ventricular volumes and ejection fraction.[54] A more lengthy, but three-dimensional approach, is to acquire multiple contiguous cine images.

The comparative accuracies of magnetic resonance, Doppler echocardiography and X-ray contrast angiography have not been fully investigated. Doppler echocardiography is probably more sensitive, but it could be argued that it is too sensitive because physiological regurgitation can be detected in a large number of normal volunteers. The ability of magnetic resonance to determine regurgitant volume, left ventricular volume and muscle mass may give it an advantage over the other techniques.

Thus, although magnetic resonance provides similar diagnostic information to echocardiography, it is clear that the latter technique is less expensive, portable and it can be performed in sick patients more easily. If ejection fraction and a measure of regurgitant fraction are required then radionuclide ventriculography would be the simplest additional technique. Magnetic resonance gives reliable information, but it should be reserved for cases of doubt following the other investigations.

13.8 Valvular stenosis

Using cine magnetic resonance imaging, stenotic lesions manifest themselves by a region of signal loss distal to the valve. In aortic stenosis, this usually occupies the entire proximal ascending aorta to a varying distance from the valve (figure 13.10). With mitral

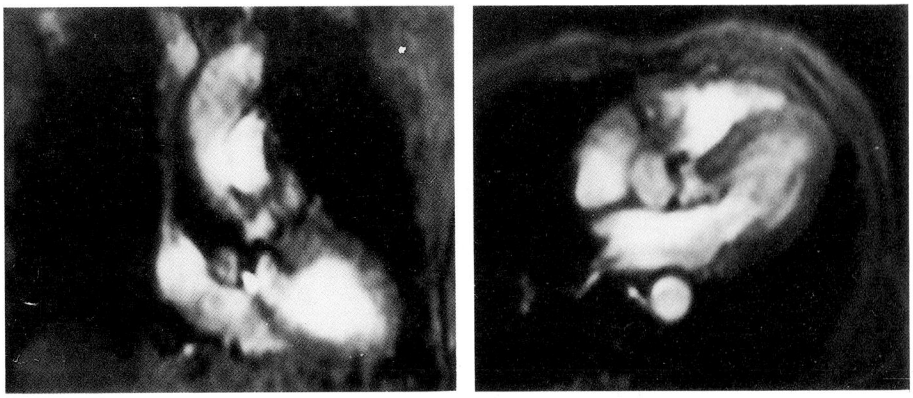

Figure 13.10. Coronal (left) and horizontal long axis (right) frames from a cine acquisition in aortic stenosis. There is a turbulent jet occupying the ascending aorta and a thickened valve with signal loss because of calcification.

Table 13.2. A comparison of imaging techniques in different diseases. The number of + signs indicates the clinical utility

	MRI	X-ray angiography	Echo + Doppler	Radionuclide imaging	Ultrafast X-ray CT	PET
Aorta	+++	+++	++	−	++	−
Pericardium	++	++	+	−	++	−
Intracardiac mass	+++	++	++	−	++	−
Extracardiac mass	+++	+	+	−	++	−
Ventricular function	+++	++	+	++	++	−
Myocardial ischaemia	+	+	−	+++	+	+++
Valvular stenosis	+	+++	+++	−	−	−
Valvular regurgitation	++	+	+++	+	+	−
Congenital heart disease	+++	++	+++	+	+	−
Peripheral angiography	++	+++	++	−	+	−
Coronary arteriography	−	+++	−	−	−	−

MRI = magnetic resonance imaging, CT = computed X-ray tomography, PET = position emission tomography.

stenosis, the signal loss may occupy the whole of the left ventricle during diastole. However, the area of signal loss does not appear to correlate well with the severity of stenosis because irregularity of the valve without stenosis can lead to turbulence and signal loss.[55]

An alternative approach is to use velocity mapping as described in chapter 10, and by using very short echo times (less than 5 ms), it is possible to maintain signal in these jets and to measure velocities in the valve orifice.[56] Comparative studies with Doppler ultrasound are awaited.

13.9 Summary

It is difficult to be dogmatic about the place of magnetic resonance for the solution of clinical problems, partly because of the lack of studies directly comparing it with other techniques and partly because of the evolving nature of the speciality. Table 13.2 summarises the strengths of different imaging techniques, and table 13.3 summarises the clinical role of magnetic resonance imaging in the most common cardiovascular conditions. Magnetic resonance is now the primary investigation for a number of conditions and in many others it either complements other investigations or it can be used as a secondary investigation if other techniques fail. Further developments in areas such as peripheral and coronary angiography, transplant re-

Table 13.3. A summary of the diagnostic role of magnetic resonance imaging in the most common cardiovascular conditions

Primary investigation	*Complementary investigation*
Thoracic aortic aneurysm	Complex congenital heart disease (adults)
Stable aortic dissection	Complex congenital heart disease (children)
Aortic coarctation	Intra-cardiac masses
Evaluation of central pulmonary arteries	Supra-valvular stenosis
Pericardial constriction	
Paracardiac masses	
Secondary investigation	*Research*
Abdominal aortic aneurysm	Peripheral angiography
Assessment of regional and global LV function	Coronary angiography
Assessment of right venticular function	Cardiac transplant rejection
Hypertrophic cardiomyopathy	Myocardial infarct sizing
Pericardial effusion	Assessment of myocardial perfusion
Valvular regurgitation	Myocardial tissue characterisation
Coronary artery bypass graft patency	Valvular stenosis

Primary: can be used as a first line diagnostic technique.
Complementary: will often provide additional information after other techniques.
Secondary: can be helpful when other techniques fail to provide diagnostic information.
Research: potential future applications but currently under investigation.

jection, and myocardial perfusion and viability can all be expected and will greatly increase the role of magnetic resonance.

References

1 Pohost GM, Canby RC. Nuclear magnetic resonance imaging: current applications and future prospects. *Circulation* 1987; **75**: 88–95.

2 Cooper LS, Chalmers TC, McCally M, Berrier J, Sacks HS. The poor quality of early evaluations of magnetic resonance imaging. *J Am Med Assoc* 1988; **259**: 3277–80.

3 Lois JF, Gomes AS, Brown K, Mulder DG, Laks H. Magnetic resonance imaging of the thoracic aorta. *Am J Cardiol* 1987; **60**: 358–62.

4 Kersting-Sommerhoff BA, Higgins CB, White RD, Sommerhoff CP, Lipton MJ. Aortic dissection: sensitivity and specificity of MR imaging. *Radiology* 1988; **166**: 651–5.

5 Pernes JM, Grenier P, Desbleds MT, de Brux JL. MR evaluation of chronic aortic dissection. *J Comput Assist Tomogr* 1987; **11**: 975–81.

6 Cranney GB, Lotan C, Helmcke F, Nanda NC, Pohost GM. Diagnosis of thoracic aortic dissection using nuclear magnetic resonance imaging — comparison with other imaging modalities (Abstract). *Aust NZ J Med* 1988; **18**: 362.

7 Bogren HG, Underwood SR, Firmin DN, *et al*. Magnetic resonance velocity mapping in aortic dissection. *Br J Radiol* 1988; **61**: 456–62.

8 Dinsmore RE, Liberthson RR, Wismer GL, *et al*. MRI of thoracic aortic aneurysms: comparison with other imaging methods. *Am J Roentgenol* 1986; **146**: 309–14.

9 Glazer HS, Gutierrez FR, Levitt RG, Lee JKT, Murphy WA. The thoracic aorta studied by MR imaging. *Radiology* 1985; **157**: 149–55.

10 Currie PJ. Transesophageal echocardiography—new window to the heart (editorial comment). *Circulation* 1989; **80**: 215–7.

11 Erbel R, Engberding R, Daniel W, *et al*. Echocardiography in the diagnosis of aortic dissection. *Lancet* 1989; **i**: 457–60.

12 Didier D, Higgins CB, Fisher MR, Osaki L, Silverman NH, Cheitlin MD. Congenital heart disease: Gated MR imaging in 72 patients. *Radiology* 1986; **158**: 227–35.

13 Chung KJ, Simpson IA, Newman R, *et al*. Cine magnetic resonance imaging for evaluation of congenital heart disease: role in pediatric cardiology compared with echocardiography and angiography. *J Pediatr* 1988; **113**: 1028–35.

14 Chung KJ, Simpson IA, Glass RF, Sahn DJ, Hessselink JR. Cine magnetic resonance imaging after surgical repair in patients with transposition of the great arteries. *Circulation* 1988; **77**: 104–9.

15 Rees RSO, Somerville J, Underwood SR, *et al*. Magnetic resonance imaging of the pulmonary arteries and their systemic connections in pulmonary atresia: comparison with angiographic and surgical findings. *Br Heart J* 1987; **58**: 621–6.

16 Kersting-Sommerhoff BA, Sechtem UP, Fisher MR, Higgins CB. MR of congential anomalies of the aortic arch. *Am J Roentgenol* 1987; **149**: 9–13.

17 Bisset GS, Strife JL, Kirks DR, Bailey WW. Vascular rings: MR imaging. *Am J Roentgenol* 1987; **149**: 251–6.

18 Simpson IA, Chung KJ, Glass RF, Sahn DJ, Sherman FS, Hesselink J. Cine magnetic resonance imaging for evaluation of anatomy and flow relations in infants and children with coarctation of the aorta. *Circulation* 1988; **78**: 142–8.

19 Soulen RL, Kan J, Mitchell S, White RI. Evaluation of balloon angioplasty of coarction restenosis by magnetic resonance imaging. *Am J Cardiol* 1987; **60**: 343–5.

20 Campbell RM, Moreau GA, Johns JA, *et al*. Detection of caval obstruction by magnetic resonance imaging after intra-atrial repair of transposition of the great arteries. *Am J Cardiol* 1987; **60**: 688–91.

21 Sechtem U, Tscholakoff D, Higgins CB. MRI of the normal pericardium. *Am J Roentgenol* 1986; **147**: 239–44.

22 Soulen RL, Stork DO, Higgins CB. MRI of constrictive pericardial disease. *Am J Cardiol* 1985; **55**: 480–4.

23 Sechtem U, Tscholakoff D, Higgins CB. MRI of the abnormal pericardium. *Am J Roentgenol* 1986; **147**: 245–52.

24 Amparo EG, Higgins CB, Farmer D, Gamsu E, McNamara M. Gated MRI of cardiac and paracardiac masses: initial experience. *Am J Roentgenol* 1984; **143**: 1151–6.

25 Boxer RA, LaCorte MA, Singh S, *et al*. Diagnosis of cardiac tumors in infants by MRI. *Am J Cardiol* 1985; **56**: 831–2.

26 Pizzarello RA, Goldberg SM, Goldman MA, *et al*. Tumor of the heart diagnosed by magnetic resonance imaging. *J Am Coll Cardiol* 1985; **5**: 989–91.

27 Freedberg RS, Kronzon I, Rumancik WM, Liebeskind D. The contribution of magnetic resonance imaging to the evaluation of intracardiac tumors diagnosed by echocardiography. *Circulation* 1988; **77**: 96–103.

28 Winkler M, Higgins CB. Suspected intracardiac masses: evaluation with MR imaging. *Radiology* 1987; **165**: 117–22.

29 Higgins CB, Byrd BF, Stark D, *et al*. Magnetic resonance imaging in hypertrophic cardiomyopathy. *Am J Cardiol* 1985; **55**: 1121–6.

30 White HD, Norris RM, Brown MA, Brandt PW, Whitlock RML, Wild CJ. Left ventricular end-systolic volume as the major determinant of survival after recovery from myocardial infarction. *Circulation* 1987; **76**: 44–51.

31 Borow KM, Green LH, Mann T, *et al*. End-systolic volume as a predictor of postoperative left ventricular performance in volume overload from valvular regurgitation. *Am J Med* 1980; **68**: 655–63.

32 Belenkov YN, Afonskaya NI, Pustovitova Demin NV, *et al*. Determination of the heart size in experimental animals with the help of tomography based on the principle of nuclear magnetic resonance. *Kardiologia* 1984; **24**: 16–18.

33 Longmore DB, Klipstein RH, Underwood SR, *et al*. Dimensional accuracy of magnetic resonance in studies of the heart. *Lancet* 1985; **i**: 1360–2.

34 Dilworth LR, Aisen AM, Mancini J, Lande I, Buda AJ. Determination of left ventricular volumes and ejection fraction by nuclear magnetic resonance imaging. *Am Heart J* 1987; **113**: 24–32.

35 Cranney GB, Lotan CS, Dean L, Baxley W, Bouchard A, Pohost GM. Left ventricular volume measurement using cardiac axis nuclear magnetic resonance imaging: validation by calibrated ventricular angiography. *Circulation* 1990; **82**: 154–63.

36 Osbakken M, Yuschok T. Evaluation of ventricular function with gated cardiac magnetic resonance imaging. *Cath Cardiovasc Diagn* 1986; **12**: 156–60.

37 Underwood SR, Klipstein RH, Firmin DN, *et al*. Magnetic resonance assessment of aortic and mitral regurgitation. *Br Heart J* 1986; **56**: 455–62.

38 Sechtem U, Pflugfelder PW, Gould RG, Cassidy MM, Higgins CB. Measurement of right and left ventricular volumes in healthy individuals with cine MR imaging. *Radiology* 1987; **163**: 697–702.

39 Sechtem U, Pflugfelder P, Higgins CB. Quantification of cardiac function by conventional and cine magnetic resonance imaging. *Cardiovasc Intervent Radiol* 1987; **10**: 365–73.

40 Utz JA, Herfkens RJ, Heinsimer JA, *et al*. Cine NMR determination of left ventricular ejection fraction. *Am J Roentgenol* 1987; **148**: 839–43.

41 Edelman RR, Thompson RT, Kantor H, Brady TJ, Leavitt M, Dinsmore R. Cardiac function: evaluation with fast-echo MR imaging. *Radiology* 1987; **162**: 611–5.

42 Pettigrew RI, Eisner RL, Ziffer JA, *et al*. Dynamic cardiac MRI using dual spin echoes. *Dynam Cardiovasc Imag* 1987; **1**: 214–9.

43 Pettigrew RI, Ziffer JA, Churchwell AL, Parks WJ, Baron M. Fast gradient echo imaging at 0.5 T: assessment of cardiac function and valvular dysfunction. *Dynam Cardiovasc Imag* 1987; **1**: 220–6.

44 Underwood SR, Gill CRW, Klipstein RH, Mohiaddin RH, Rees RSO, Longmore DB. Left ventricular volume measured rapidly by oblique magnetic resonance imaging. *Br Heart J* 1988; **60**: 188–95.

45 Underwood SR, Rees RSO, Savage PE, *et al*. Assessment of regional left ventricular function by magnetic resonance. *Br Heart J* 1986; **56**: 334–40.

46 Sechtem U, Sommerhoff BA, Markiewicz W, White RD, Cheitlen MD, Higgins CB. Regional left ventricular wall thickening by magnetic resonance imaging: evaluation in normal persons and patients with global and regional dysfunction. *Am J Cardiol* 1987; **59**: 145–51.

47 Zerhouni EA, Parish DM, Rogers WJ, Yang A, Shapiro EP. Human heart: tagging with MR imaging – a method for non-invasive assessment of myocardial motion. *Radiology* 1988; **169**: 59–63.

48 Lotan CS, Cranney GB, Bouchard A, Bittner V, Pohost GM. The value of cine nuclear magnetic resonance imaging for assessing regional ventricular function. *J Am Coll Cardiol* 1989; **14**: 1721–9.

49 Florentine MS, Grosskreutz CL, Chang W, *et al*. Measurement of left ventricular mass in vivo using gated nuclear magnetic resonance imaging. *J Am Coll Cardiol* 1986; **8**: 107–12.

50 Keller AM, Peshock RM, Malloy CR, *et al*. In vivo measurement of myocardial mass using nuclear magnetic resonance imaging. *J Am Coll Cardiol* 1986; **8**: 113–7.
51 Schiebler M, Axel L, Reichek N, *et al*. Correlation of cine MR imaging with two-dimensional pulsed doppler echocardiography in valvular insufficiency. *J Comput Assist Tomogr* 1987; **11**: 627–32.
52 Utz JA, Herfkens RJ, Heinsimer JA, Shimakawa A, Glover G, Pelc N. Valvular regurgitation: dynamic MR imaging. *Radiology* 1988; **168**: 91–4.
53 Plugfelder PW, Landzberg JS, Cassidy MM, *et al*. Comparison of cine MR imaging with Doppler echocardiography for the evaluation of aortic regurgitation. *Am J Roentgenol* 1989; **152**: 729–35.
54 Cranney GB, Benjellous H, Perry G, Lotan CS, Pohost GM. Simultaneous assessment of aortic regurgitation and left ventricular function using cine nuclear magnetic resonance imaging. (Abstract). *Aust NZ J Med* 1989; **19**: 567.
55 Underwood SR, Firmin DN, Mohiaddin, *et al*. Cine magnetic resonance imaging of valvular heart disease (Abstract). *Sixth Annual Meeting of the Society of Magnetic Resonance Imaging* 1987; 723.
56 Underwood SR. Cine magnetic resonance imaging and flow measurements in the cardiovascular system. *Br Med Bull* 1989; **45**: 948–67.

Chapter 14
The Safety of Magnetic Resonance in Cardiac Patients

BERTIL PERSSON AND FREDDY STÅHLBERG

14.1 Introduction

Magnetic resonance imaging is widely regarded as a safe and non-invasive procedure without any of the hazards associated with ionising radiation, and without the need for injection of iodine containing contrast media in order to distinguish the different structures of the heart. Until the appearance of magnetic resonance imaging, however, we had little practical experience of the safety implications of the magnetic fields and radio-frequency radiation to which the patient is exposed. There are good theoretical reasons for believing that the phenomenon of magnetic resonance itself would not interfere with the chemical properties of proteins and nucleic acids, since these are determined mainly by interactions between electrons and are unaffected by nuclear transitions between different spin orientations. There are, however, three other factors to be considered when evaluating the potential hazards of magnetic resonance: the effects of the static magnetic field, the rapidly changing magnetic field gradients, and the radio-frequency radiation used to induce nuclear transitions.

Common static magnetic fields used in imaging range from 0.02 to 2 T: on average, 10 000 times greater than the the Earth's magnetic field of approximately 0.00005 T. During imaging, rapidly changing gradients are imposed upon this magnetic field, the rate of change of field being of the order of 1 T/s. This induces currents in the body which could also have biological effects. The radio-frequency electromagnetic radiation is partly absorbed by the body and this might lead to local heating and other non-thermal effects.

This chapter summarises a more extensive review of the subject,[1] and pays special attention to factors of importance for the cardiac patient. Potential biological and health effects are discussed as well as guidelines for patient and occupational exposure. Consideration is also given to the safety of imaging patients with implanted electromagnetic and magnetic devices.

14.2 The static magnetic field

14.2.1 Mechanical effects

Many diamagnetic molecules will orient themselves with strong magnetic fields. They usually have a rod-like shape, and the effect is the result of anisotropic magnetic susceptibility. This leads to a torque on molecules such as DNA or retinal rods, which is proportional to the square of the applied field. The free energy of such molecules oriented at an angle to a magnetic field is small compared with thermal energy, and so the effect can be ignored. For small structures in fields up to 2 T at room temperature it is between 10^{-19} and 10^{-21} J, which is of the same order of magnitude as thermal energy (4×10^{-21} J).

Some biological species have permanent magnet moments which lead to much greater effects. An example is the magnetotactic bacterium in which approximately 2% of the dry mass is iron in the form of magnetite crystals (Fe_3O_4).[2,3] For iron the critical field gradient is 0.5 T/m and above this, the pull exerted by the magnetic field exceeds the pull of gravity.

Mechanical effects could also influence metallic prostheses, haemostatic clips and heart valves, all of which are relevant to the cardiac patient. Shellock has reviewed the literature concerning the magnetic properties of commonly used implants and, with the exception of four types of cerebral aneurysm clip, none is significantly affected by static magnetic fields below 2 T.[4] Previous clipping of cerebral aneurysms had been considered a contraindication to magnetic resonance imaging, but the point has been made that provided the clips used are known not to be ferromagnetic, then imaging can be performed safely.[5] With the possible

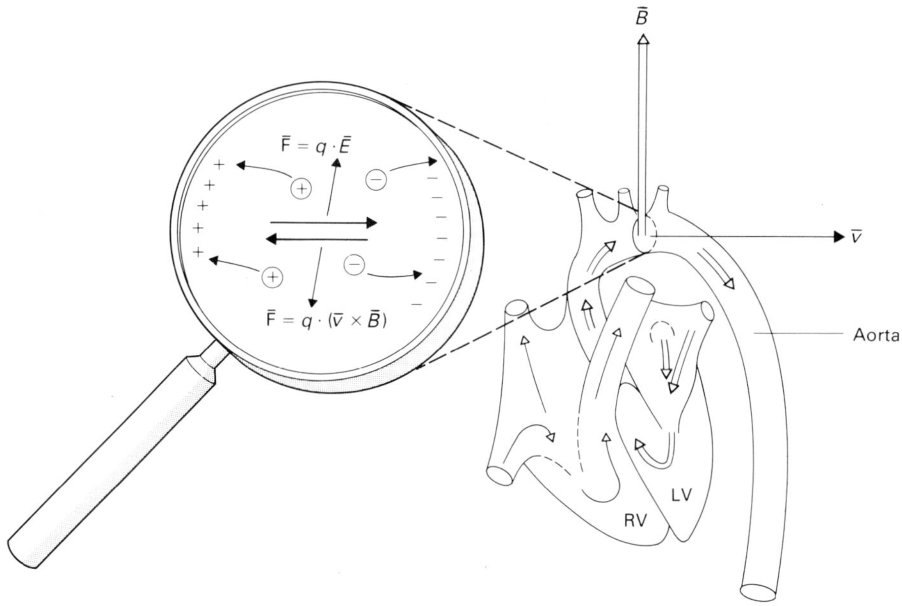

Figure 14.1. Flow through the aorta of velocity v in the presence of an applied field generates an electrical potential as illustrated in the magnified circle. The force separating ions of opposite charge, q, by virtue of their velocity, v, with respect the the magnetic field, B, is balanced by the restoring force of the electrical field, E, created by their separation.

exception of early Starr–Edwards valves (few of which are likely still to be implanted) all prosthetic valves are safe,[6–8] as are many other intravascular devices.[9,10]

14.2.2 Interactions with moving conductors

An electrical conductor moving with respect to a static magnetic field has a potential (and hence a current) induced in it and this effect is the basis of conventional electrical generators. When blood moves through a magnetic field, ions of opposite charge are acted upon by forces in opposite directions. These Lorentzian forces are balanced by attraction between charges, but the net effect is a potential across the vessel carrying the blood. This potential U can be calculated from the expression:

$$U = |\vec{v}| \cdot |\vec{B}| \cdot d \sin \theta$$

where $\vec{v}$ is the velocity of flow through a blood vessel of diameter d at an angle θ to a magnetic field $\vec{B}$. The situation is illustrated for the aorta in figure 14.1. By assuming a parabolic velocity profile in the radial direction, the average flow potential can be expressed as:

$$U = 16BQ \;/\; 3\pi d$$

From this it can be seen that the average flow potential varies linearly with the magnetic flux density B, and with the blood flow Q, and the potential will be largest in the major blood vessels around the heart and in the heart itself. Estimation of the potential for an adult in a magnetic field of 1.0 T with a cardiac output of 5.1 litres per minute and an aortic diameter of 3 cm, gives 4.8 mV. This would be applied across the whole diameter of the aorta and so the potential across individual excitable cells would be very much less than the normal depolarisation threshold of 40 mV. There is therefore no danger of such cells being depolarised, but the potential is superimposed upon the T wave of the electrocardiogram and this leads to an apparently large T wave in the magnet (figure 14.2).

The effects of static magnetic fields upon the electrocardiogram have been studied by several investigators.[11–16] Between 0.1 and 1.4 T, the T wave in the rat increases linearly and above 1.4 T the increase is more rapid, probably because of additional potentials in vessels smaller than the aorta.[12] Figure 14.3 shows the relationship between aortic flow potential and body weight in a series of studies of different animals.[11–13]

In addition to the potential induced by blood flow within the chest, another potential is induced by motion of the heart. Assuming a myocardial cross-sectional area of $20\,\text{cm}^2$ and a rate of contraction of 10 mm/s, this potential is between 6 and 13 mV/T with a current density of between 0.2 and 1.6 $\mu\text{A/cm}^2\text{/T}$. This is insufficient to depolarise myocardial cells or to fibrillate the heart.

The effect of very high static magnetic fields (between 7 and 10 T) on the electrocardiogram and the

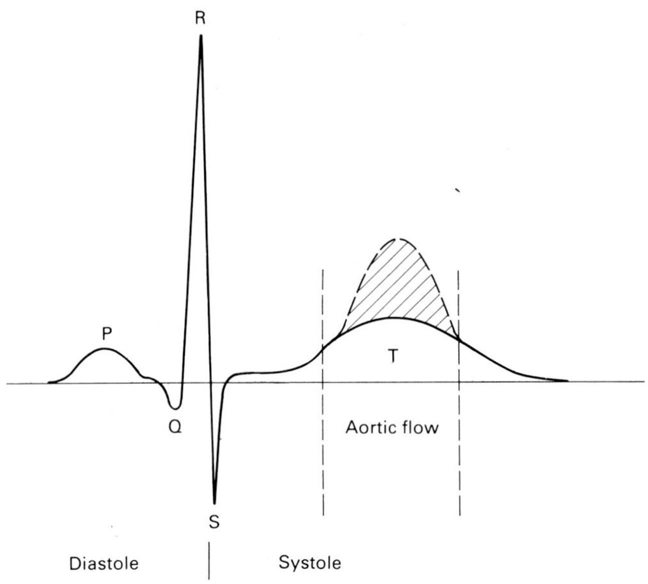

Figure 14.2. The potential generated by flow in the heart through an applied magnetic field is superimposed upon the T wave of the ECG, making it appear much larger than outside the field.

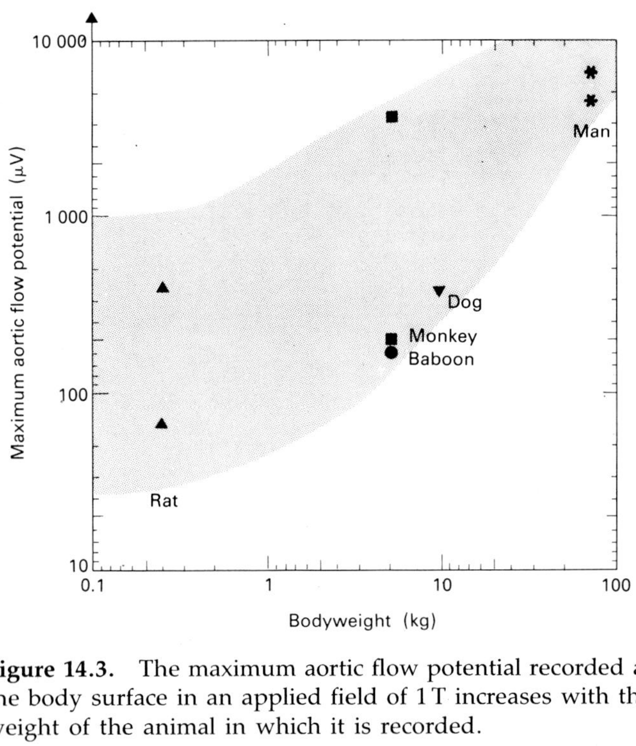

Figure 14.3. The maximum aortic flow potential recorded at the body surface in an applied field of 1T increases with the weight of the animal in which it is recorded.

heart rate of squirrel monkeys has been investigated by Beischer and colleagues.[17,18] The peak flow potential was estimated to be 50 mV across the aortic arch and the change recorded on the surface electrocardiogram was 0.7 mV. A 15 minute exposure to 10T had no discernible effect on heart rate, and exposure for several hours had no effect on respiratory rate or R wave amplitude, but there was a fall in heart rate and an increase in sinus arrhythmia.[19] There was no long-term effect. In a recent study of electrocardiographic changes at 1.5T, ST segment elevation was observed which was in some cases larger than the normal R wave, and this coincided with peak aortic flow.[20] Later negative deflections were also observed coinciding with peak flow through the mitral valve, but there were no clinical sequelae. In man, a 17% fall in heart rate has been observed in normal volunteers after 10 minutes at 2T, but no effect at 1T and no arrhythmias.[21,22]

14.2.3 Biological effects of static magnetic fields

There are examples of cellular structures with permanent magnetic moments in which significant magnetic orientation occurs. Some experimental observations are summarised in table 14.1; table 14.2 summarises the effects on whole cells. In several animal experiments biological effects of static magnetic fields have been reported, but detailed exposure measurements are lacking and it has not been possible to define a dose-response relationship. These effects are summarised in tables 14.3 and 14.4. The effects observed in humans are summarised in table 14.5. Although the delayed development of eggs and embryos from certain species is worrying, there have been no observations of similar effects in humans. Until more extensive studies have been performed, pregnant women should not be scanned without a strong medical indication, particularly in the first trimester of pregnancy during the period of active organogenesis.

14.2.4 Safety limits for static magnetic field exposure

Static magnetic fields are closely associated with particle accelerators as well as magnetic resonance scanners and early guidelines were drawn up for workers in this field. Details are given in table 14.6, but the limits are very conservative and the Stanford Linear Accelerator Group for instance has a limit of 0.02T for extended periods of exposure to whole body and the head. It is also stated that people with a history of mental problems, those with implanted electronic devices, pregnant women, and those with chronic medical problems such as sickle cell anaemia or heart disease should be excluded from exposure to magnetic fields above 0.2 T. The guidelines might also be applied to workers with clinical imagers although some of the latter exclusions may no longer be appropriate. For exposure of patients during clinical examinations the guidelines are more liberal and the West German, North American and Canadian authorities impose a limit of 2 T whereas the UK authority has a limit of 2.5 T.

Table 14.1. Orientation of diamagnetically anisotropic units

Structure	Magnetic field (T)	Effect observed	Reference
Chloroplasts	1–2	Orientation along the field	23
DNA	6	Orientation of 1% of molecules	24
Retinal rods	1	Orientation	25
Sickled erythrocytes	0.35	Orientation	26

14.2.5 Safety considerations for siting and shielding

In the area around a clinical magnetic resonance scanner there are magnetic fields which might interfere with cardiac pacemakers and which might be sufficiently powerful to turn ferromagnetic objects into projectiles. This area must therefore be supervised and restricted. A proposal for restriction limits is given below:

High magnetic field (>1.5 mT): inside this area, pacemakers might be disturbed, loose ferrous objects can move towards the magnet and small ferrous objects might become projectiles.

Caution–magnetic field (0.5–1.5 mT): area in which supervision of the entrance into a high magnetic field area should be maintained.

No supervision (<0.5 mT): outside the 0.5 mT area there is little or no risk for health and safety problems and this area thus does not need to be supervised.

Table 14.2. The cellular effects of static magnetic fields

Item	Magnetic field (T)	Exposure time	Effect observed	Reference
Bacteria, yeasts	0.3–1.5	2 days	No effects on growth rates	27–31
Human blood cells	1.0		No effects	32
Rabbit erythrocytes	0.5	15 min	Decrease in haemoglobin, haemoloysis, cell degeneration	33
Human blood (*in vitro*)	0.0023–1.8		Increased permeability and agglutination	34, 35

Table 14.3. Teratogenic effects of magnetic fields on eggs and embryos

Organism	Magnetic field (T)	Exposure time	Effect observed	Reference
Sea urchin	14	2 hr	Inhibited development of eggs from sea urchin	17
Frog embryo	1		Development retarded	36
Frog embryo	0.7		Development retarded	37
Fruit fly egg	0.3–0.4		Increased frequency of deformity such as withered wings	38
Chicken embryo	0.003		Development retarded	39
	0.0001		No effect	
Pigeon embryo	0.0005		Development retarded	39

Table 14.4. Biological effects of static magnetic fields on animals

Species	Magnetic field (T)	Exposure time	Effect observed	Reference
Rhesus monkey	4.6–9.7		Suppressed response rate to trained tasks	40
Rhesus monkey	2	65 hr	No haematological effect	41
Monkey	2	2 hr	Decrease in heart rate, increase in sinus arrhythmia, large T wave in ECG	17, 18
Mice	0.9	3 days	Increased urinary K^+ and Na^+, 25% increase in platelets	42
Mice	0.9	20 days	Increased urinary K^+ and Na^+, no increase in platelets	42
Mice	0.72	96 hr	Increased urinary K^+ and Na^+	43
Guinea pig	0.002–0.7	21 days	Transient morphological changes in testes, liver, kidneys, adrenals, and eye lens	37
Mice	0.59		Inhibited weight gain in young mice, weight loss in older mice	44
Rabbit	0.5	15 min	Reduced erythrocyte sedimentation rate	45
Mice	0.5	1 day	14% fall of liver K^+ 63% fall or renal Ca^+	46
Mice	0.5	3 days	3.5% rise of K^+, 12% fall of Ca^{2+}, 6% fall of Na^+ in blood	46
Mice	0.5	6 days	21% rise of liver K^+, normal renal Ca^{2+},	46
Mice	0.42–0.9	4–40 days	Fall in splenic megakaryocytes. Increase in liver mitoses. Adrenocortical lesions	47
Mice	0.42	14 days	Sensitisation to gamma radiation	48
Mice	0.42	4–5 weeks	Fall in white blood count	49
Mice	0.4		Delayed wound healing	50
Mice	0.3	12–46 days	Rejected tumour transplant	51
Mice	0.11	Continous	Increased appetite and activity	52
Rabbit	0.1	Unknown	Inhibits reaction to light or sound stimulus	53
Rats	0.04	13 days	Reduced fertility Increased stillborn	54
Cat	0.03	6 hr	Long-term effect on glia	53
Rabbit	0.03		Neuronal and glial damage	53
Rabbit	0.002–0.1	1–3 min	EEG alterations	53
Rats	0.02–0.12	1 month	No histological changes No change in leucocyte count	55

Table 14.4. (contd.)

Species	Magnetic field (T)	Exposure time	Effect observed	Reference
Rabbit	0.01		EEG unchanged	53
Worms	0.001		Mud snails and flat worms are sensitive to magnetic polarity	56
Pigeons	0.00005	Continous	Navigation hindered by attached magnet	57

The stray fields may deflect electron beams in cathode ray tubes, photo-multiplier tubes and image intensifiers. At low fields, this gives the appearance of a tilted image on a cathode ray tube, but as the field increases, curvature or wrapping of the image begins and ultimately the image may be deflected off the screen. The degree of distortion depends upon the relative orientation between the electron beam and the magnetic field. It is maximal when the field is perpendicular to the electron beam and zero if the two are parallel, and so the effect can be minimised by careful positioning of the screen or by magnetic shielding. Permanent damage to the screen does not usually occur although it may need degaussing before use outside the field. Stray fields can also alter magnetic memory devices such as computer disks, computer, audio and video tapes, and credit or bank cards. The effect is either inability to read the information or corrupted data. The degree of the problem depends upon local field strength and upon any motion of the magnetic medium through the field. The operation of mechanical devices such as cameras, analogue watches, electric motors and relays can be affected and they may slow or stop in the field because of magnetisation of the moving parts and induced eddy currents. The effect is not normally permanent although watches may need degaussing and the colour masks inside video cameras can be very sensitive and are best treated with respect. Devices with printed circuit boards are not affected by even quite high fields.

The safe distances for various devices in an axial direction from magnets of different strengths is illustrated in figure 14.4. The threshold values vary from relative tolerant (10–30 mT) for electric motors to

Table 14.5. Biological effects of magnetic fields on man

Magnetic field (T)	Exposure time	Effect observed	Reference
10	Short	Bitter coldness, aching bones, and feeling of ants moving on the hands	58
2	15 min	Slight sensation of pain in filled teeth	58
1.5		Taste sensation in mouth	59
0.5	3 days	No effect	59
0.25		No sensation, no change in pulse or respiration	60

Table 14.6. Recommended limits for occupational and clinical exposure to static field

Period of exposure	Field limit for head or whole body (T)	Field limit for arms and hands (T)	Reference
Unlimited	0.01–0.05		61
Less than 1 hr	0.5–1		61
Less than 15 min	1		61
Hr	0.02	0.2	62
Min	0.2	2	62
8 hr/day uniform	0.03	0.07	63
8 hr/day gradient	0.05–0.2/m	0.1–0.2/m	63
Clinical examination	2		64–66
Clinical examination	2.5		67, 68

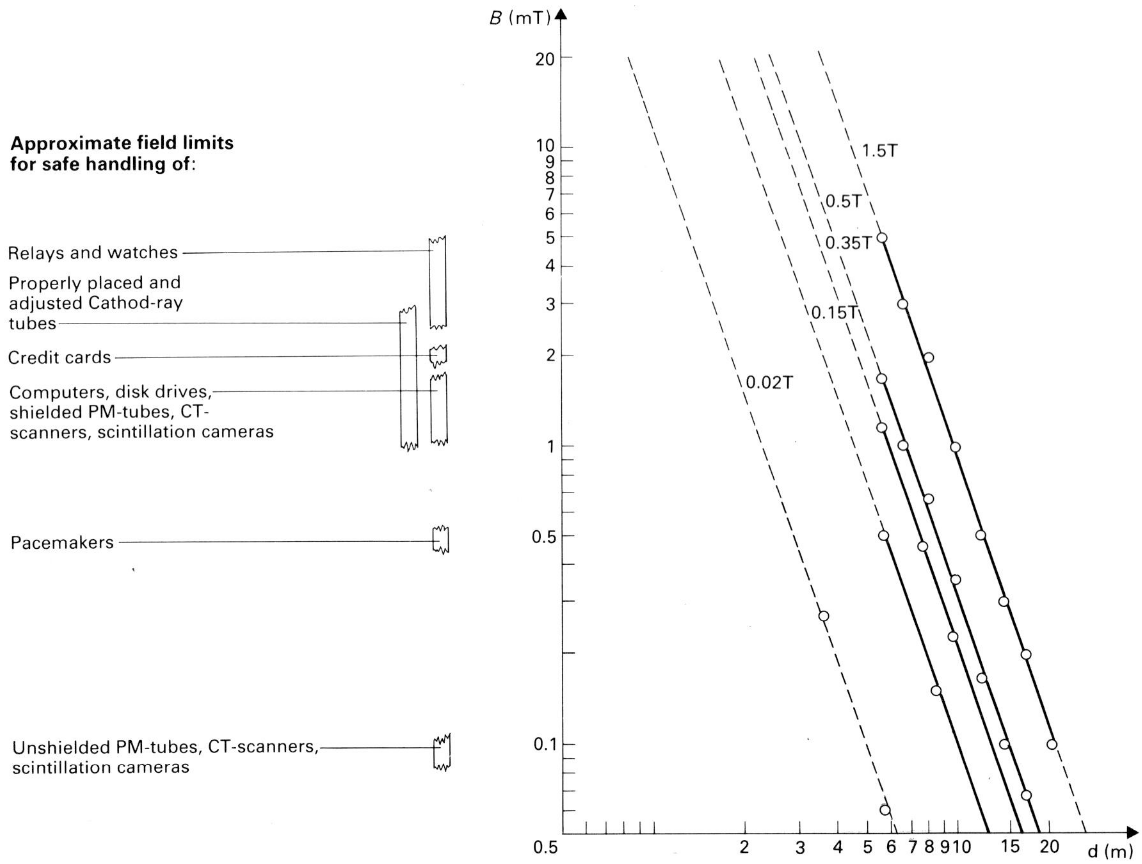

Figure 14.4. Plot of the magnetic field B (mT) with axial distance d (m) from magnets of different strengths. On the left is shown the safe distances for several sensitive devices.

extremely sensitive (below 10 mT) for photo-multipler tubes, CT-scanners and scintillation cameras. Such devices can be shielded by encasing them in μ metal or conetic which will provide protection from fields of 1 mT or less.

14.2.6 The effects of static magnetic fields on pacemakers

Protecting patients with implanted pacemakers from static and time varying magnetic fields is an important consideration when planning, installing and operating magnetic resonance scanners. Fortunately, outside the bore of the magnet, where only the static magnetic field has significant influence, the hazards are well understood and they are not severe.

Several generations of pacemakers are currently implanted. All modern pacemakers operate in the synchronous (or demand) mode; that is, an impulse is generated only when the native cardiac rate falls below a certain threshold. The simplest and oldest models have only analogue circuits, but the more advanced units have integrated circuits and are programmable. The pacemaker impulse usually has an initial magnitude of 5 V and a current of 0.75 mA. It is produced by discharging a capacitor, and its magnitude decays exponentially with a time constant of approximately 0.75 ms. The length of the lead to the endocardium of the right heart is about 0.6 m and its termination may be either unipolar or bipolar. A unipolar system uses the pacemaker casing as the electrical anode, and so the current returns through the body tissue, but a bipolar system provides a return path which is coaxial with the electrode lead. The coaxial lead has a platinum anode a few centimetres from the cathode at the tip of the lead.

Most pacemakers have a reed relay which can be closed by a 0.1 T magnet held externally. When the reed relay is closed, the pacemaker sensing system is bypassed and it is switched into asynchronous mode in which it pulses steadily at about 100/minute. As the battery discharges the rate slows to 85/minute and this is an indication for replacement of the pacemaker box. The reed relay will be closed by the field of a magnetic resonance scanner at between 1.7 and 4.7 mT depending on orientation. Although this conversion into fixed mode is unlikely to be hazardous, it may induce palpitation and a security zone should be established around magnets to alert patients. Limits of between 0.5 and 1.5 mT are recommended.

If a patient with a pacemaker is scanned the pacemaker will switch to asynchronous mode as soon as the patient is placed in the magnet, but there are more important considerations. Pacemakers have numerous ferromagnetic components and will experience a force or torque in a magnetic field. In particular, the lithium battery which constitutes the majority of the pacemaker volume will tend to align with the magnetic field. Apart from distorting the magnetic field and hence the image, this force is likely to be large enough to cause discomfort and possibly even displace the box. For this reason, patients with implanted pacemakers should not be examined, but there are additional implications from the magnetic field gradients used during imaging and these are discussed in the next section.

14.3 Magnetic field gradients

In order to obtain spatial resolution in magnetic resonance imaging, magnetic field gradients are applied in various directions and pulsed at various time intervals. The repetition rate of the gradient pulses is typically between 10 and 100 ms, and frequencies below 300 Hz are usually termed extremely low frequency (ELF). Magnetic fields in this range are present throughout the environment and they originate from both natural and manmade sources.

14.3.1 Physical interaction of varying magnetic fields with tissue

In biological objects exposed to time-varying, pulsed, or modulated magnetic fields, internal electric currents are generated according to Faraday's law of induction. These currents might in theory interfere with membrane potentials in nerves and other excitable tissues and might therefore induce biological effects.

In figure 14.5 we consider a loop of radius r in a human exposed to a time-varying field $\overline{B}$. According to

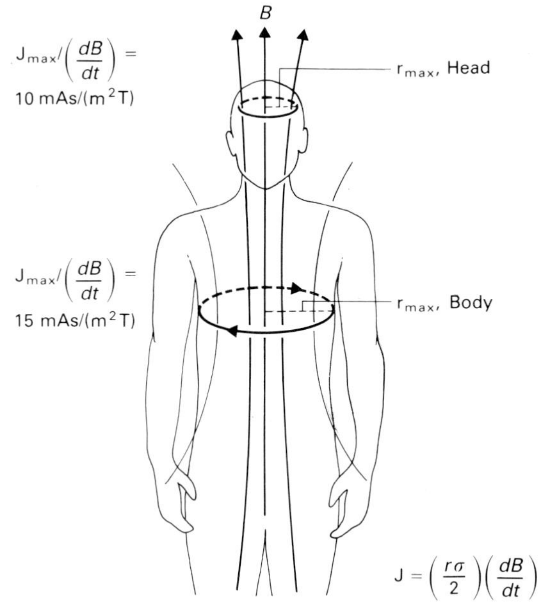

Figure 14.5. Circular eddy currents are induced in the body when placed in a magnetic field that varies with time.

Faraday, an electromotive force is induced around the loop:

$$emf = \oint \vec{E} \cdot dl = -\frac{d}{dt}\int \vec{B} = \frac{d\vec{B}}{dt} \cdot \pi r^2$$

The current density within the loop can be derived by Ohm's law and it is given by the equation:

$$J = \vec{E} \cdot \sigma = \frac{dB}{dt} \cdot \frac{r\sigma}{2} = \frac{dB}{dt} \cdot \text{constant}$$

If we assume the human head to have a radius of 0.1 m and the trunk of 0.15 m with an average conductivity of 0.2 S/m, then this constant for the head becomes 10 mA/s/m^2/T and for the trunk 15 mA/s/m /T.

In the same way that a changing magnetic field passing through a static object generates a potential within the object, motion of the object along a field gradient also generates a potential:

$$emf = -\frac{d\vec{B}}{dt} \cdot \pi r^2 = -\frac{d\vec{B}}{dx}\frac{dx}{dt} \cdot \pi r^2 = -G_x \cdot v_x \cdot S_x$$

where G_x is the magnetic field gradient, v_x the velocity, and S_x the cross-sectional area of the body in the x direction. For a body of cross sectional area 1 m^2 and velocity 1 m/s in a field gradient of 1 T/m, the induced potential will be 1 V and the current density 200 mA/m^2. This potential might be generated as a patient is pushed into the magnet, or in staff who are moving close to the magnet.

A change in cross sectional area of a body in a static field will similarly generate a potential:

$$emf = -\frac{d}{dt}\int_S \vec{B}\cdot\vec{dS} = -\vec{B}\cdot\frac{\Delta S}{\Delta t} = -B\cdot\nu\cdot\Delta S$$

where ΔS is the change in area and ν is the frequency of change. Such a potential might arise from respiration and it will be detected in the electrocardiogram, although it is typically only 25% of the potential induced by aortic flow.

14.3.2 The effects of varying magnetic fields

14.3.2.1 Physiological

It has been demonstrated that extremely low frequency magnetic fields can induce currents sufficiently large to excite normal neurones.[69,70] The best documented physiological effect arises from excitation of the retina which leads to the sensation of flashes of light known as magneto-phosphenes. The phenomenon was first described by D'Arsonval in 1893[71] and has subsequently been studied by many investigators.

Muscle fibres can be similarly affected and the most serious effect that could be anticipated is ventricular fibrillation, which could, in theory, be produced by fields with sufficently high rates of change. The threshold for ventricular fibrillation in dogs and humans is shown in figure 14.6.[72] Assuming that 1 T/s produces a current density of 1 μA/cm², the threshold in humans is likely to be approximately 500 T/s, but this threshold is a complex function of wave-form, amplitude, duration, and repetition rate. In practice, magnetic field changes during clinical imaging rarely exceed 10 T/s and so the threshold for ventricular fibrillation is never approached.

Table 14.7 summarises the literature of the physiological effects of changing magnetic fields.

14.3.2.2 Biological

A considerable amount of research has been performed on the effects of extremely low frequency electrical and magnetic fields on a variety of species over a wide range of field strengths. Much of the work has been carried out within the last decade and has been motivated by a concern for the possible biological effects of the fields experienced during magnetic resonance imaging. Almost every aspect of the health and function of a wide variety of plants and animals

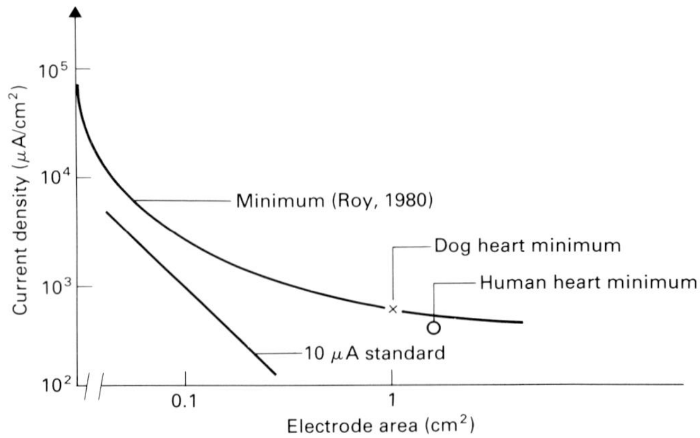

Figure 14.6. The relationship between current density and electrode area for induction of ventricular fibrillation in the dog and humans, according to Budinger and Roy *et al.*[72,76] If it is assumed that 1 T/s produces 1 μA/cm², then the threshold is probably over 500 T/s.

has been investigated, and some of the studies are summarised in table 14.8.

Claims of biological effects have been made many times, but few, if any, have been confirmed in independent laboratories. Although a few of the studies have been of very high quality, many of them suffer from poor experimental design and many of the observations are based upon a single experiment. The greatest burden that these studies have had to bear is that they have have the guidance of mechanistic models which characterise most of modern science.

14.3.3 Guidelines for human exposure to varying magnetic fields

Guidelines for exposure of patients to varying magnetic fields have been published in several countries.[64–68] Table 14.9 summarises these guidelines and in general the limits are very low. In the UK the guidelines are based on the induction of ventricular fibrillation and a limit of 20 T/s is recommended. Retinal stimulation can occur at values below this however and the North American and Canadian authorities recommend 3 T/s. In Germany, induced current density is chosen as the criterion and this must be below 30 mA/m² for pulse lengths of more than 10 ms and below 300 mA/m² for pulse lengths of less than 10 ms.

As described above, the varying magnetic fields applied during magnetic resonance imaging induce

Table 14.7. The physiological effects of changing magnetic fields

Species	Current density (A/m^2)	Exposure time and frequency	Effect observed	Ref.
Animals	10,000		Reversible nerve damage	72
Rats	100	180 μs	Stimulate thoracic muscle	73
Man	30	300 ms	Electroconvulsive therapy	74
Man	3		Ventricular fibrillation	75–77
Man	0.17	10–30 Hz	Direct current induces	78–80
Man	0.1	Weeks/ 30–60 Hz	Bone fracture repair	81
Man	0.02–0.05	20–30 Hz	Induction of magnetophosphenes	82,69
Man	0.000006	6 min	Increased latency of sensorimotor reactions	83
Man	0.000001	6 min	Increased reaction time	84

potentials in pacemaker leads. At a rate of change of 3 T/s the induced potential has been measured at 20 mV[104] and, since this may be sufficient to fibrillate the heart, this presents a further reason why such patients should not be scanned. Studies of the effects of scanning sequences on pacemakers have shown that in addition to switching the system to fixed mode as described above, some systems begin to pace at very rapid rates: up to 200/minute.[105–108] Clearly, this is yet another contraindication to scanning.

14.4 Electromagnetic radio-frequency fields

Radio-frequency and low-frequency electromagnetic fields are defined as being in the frequency range between 0 and 3×10^{12} Hz (figure 14.7).[112,113] In the radio-frequency range, interaction with the environment is described by Maxwell's equations, which describe the waves in terms of interrelated electric and magnetic fields. Although high power electromagnetic radiation (above 100 mW/cm^2) has considerable heating effect, controversy exists at powers below 10 mW/cm^2 where biological effects unrelated to the heating effect have been demonstrated. Even greater controversy exists over the existence and interpretation of resonance phenomena (the interference of reflected waves within the body leading to standing waves), which several investigators have demonstrated.

14.4.1 Interaction of radio-frequency fields with matter

There are three mechanisms involved in the interaction between electromagnetic fields and biological tissue:

- Displacement or drift of free charges (electrons, ions) caused by the electric field.
- Polarization of atoms and molecules.
- Orientation and polarisation of existing dipoles such as water and lipids.

The heating effect of electromagnetic radiation arises from the induced oscillations of free charges (conduction losses) and the relaxation of electric dipoles (dielectric losses) which leads to transfer of energy between the field and the tissue.[114] The rate at which power is absorbed is called the specific absorption rate (SAR), and it depends upon the electrical conductivity (σ) and density (ρ) of the tissue and the square of the electrical field strength ($\vec{E}$). For a sinusoidal wave the effective field strength is $E_0/\sqrt{2}$ where E_0 is the peak value. Thus:

$$\mathrm{SAR} = \sigma \cdot E_0^2 / 2\rho \qquad (\mathrm{W/kg})$$

Table 14.8. The biological effects of changing magnetic fields

Species	Magnetic induction (mT/s)	Exposure time	Effect observed	Ref.
Endocrine changes and altered hormonal responses				
Rabbit	8000	1 min	Effects on pancreatic calcium	85
Rat	1000	2 days	Effects on insulin secretion	86
Rat	1000	1 day		87
Mouse	600	33 min		88
Mouse	144–8000	3 days		89
Rat	0.14	100 days	Osteoblasts	90
Morphological tissue changes in adult animals				
Rat	2225	100 s		91
Rat	1000	5 hr		92
Guinea pig	1000	6.4 hr		37
Altered metabolism of carbohydrates, proteins and nucleic acids				
Rat	1000	24 hr		93
Rat	970	3 days		94
Drosophila	144–8000	1 hr		95
Chicken embryo	30	7 days		80
Human fibroblasts	9	2 days		96
Altered immune response to various antigens and lectins				
Mouse	1000	6 hr	Resistance to Listeria infection	97
Rat	6	3 hr		98
Human	5	28 days	Inhibition of lectin-induced lymphocyte mitogenesis	99
Alterations in the blood				
Human	250	4 hr	No effects	100
Monkey	40	1 day	No effects	101
Mouse	6.6	7 days	No effects	102
Human	4.5	1 day	Raised triglycerides	103

Figure 14.8 shows average specific absorption rates as a function of frequency for blood, skeletal muscle and myocardium as calculated by Grandolfo and colleagues.[115]

The situation is complicated by differing permittivities of different tissues which leads to reflections of electromagnetic radiation at interfaces. Extensive calculations of the distribution of specific absorption rate in various tissues have been made.[116,117] For such calculations it is important to know the electrical and geometrical characteristics of the irradiated body and the external exposure conditions, but the results have shown that the total amount and distribution of energy absorbed by the body depends strongly upon size, field frequency, and field orientation. Regions with small cross sectional area such as the neck and the extremities have a high specific absorption rate, and in the leg it is about five times the whole body average.

Absorption is increased at resonant frequencies, when the wave length of the radiation is twice that of the body dimension and standing waves are set up within the body. Whole body resonance occurs at about 47 MHz and partial body resonances occur at 150 MHz for the arms and 375 MHz for the head. Specific

Table 14.9. Guidelines for exposure to varying magnetic fields

Country	Pulse length (ms)	Current density limit (mA/m^2)	Induction limit (T/s)	Reference
UK	0.1	3000*	200	67, 68
	1	945*	63	
	>10	300*	20	
West Germany	1	300	30†	64
	10	30	3†	
USA		45*	3	65
Canada		45*	3	66, 109
USA	<30 MHz		0.060/v	110
Sweden	<10 MHz		0.025‡	111

* Derived from recommended induction levels using the relation for the human torso (1 T/s = 15 mA/m^2).
† Derived from recommended current density levels using the relation for the human head (1 T/s = 10 mA/m^2).
‡ At 0.5 m distance with $B \leq 50$ nT.

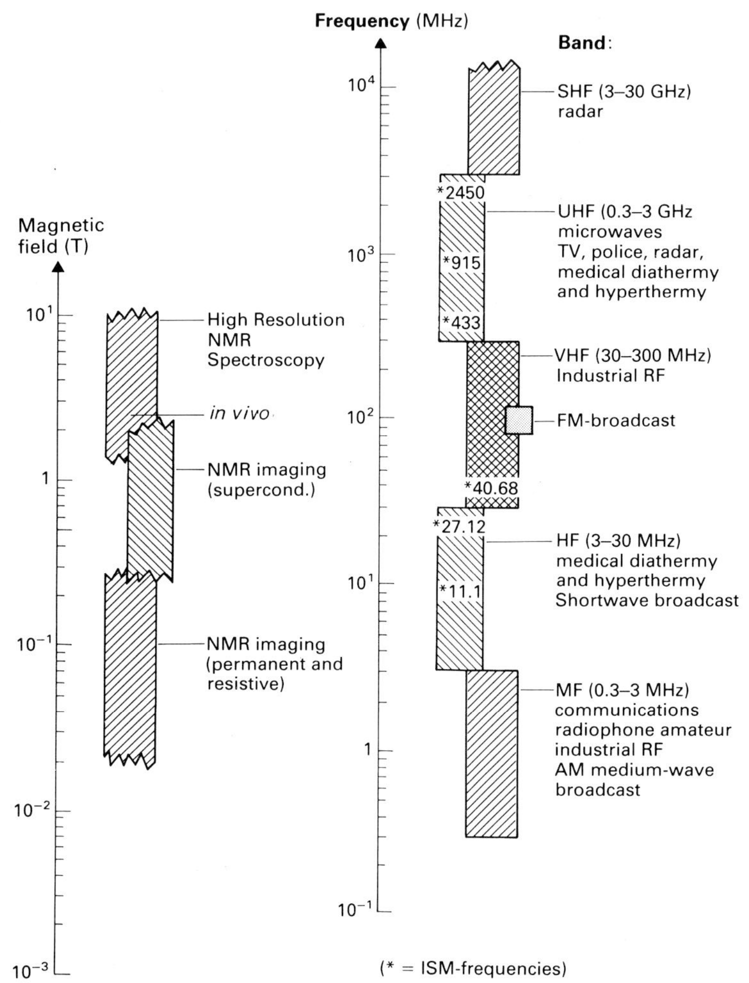

Figure 14.7. The spectrum of electromagnetic frequencies showing the frequencies used in clinical magnetic resonance imaging and spectroscopy in relation to other commonly used frequencies.

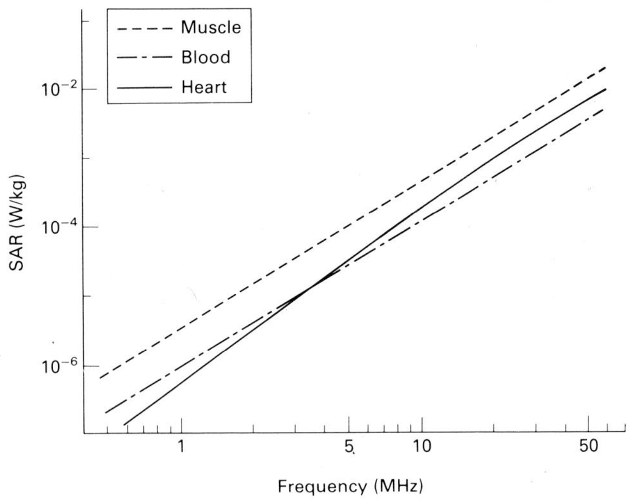

Figure 14.8. Average specific absorption rates for blood, skeletal muscle, and myocardium as a function of electromagnetic radiation frequency.[115]

absorption rates for the neck are relatively high throughout the frequency range of 100–400 MHz. The significance of resonance within the head has been emphasized by Hagmann and colleagues[118] who showed localised absorption at the front and back of the neck and in the basal region of the skull, with local specific absorption rates of two to four times the whole body average.

Table 14.10. Estimates of the biological effect of electromagnetic radio-frequency radiation at different specific absorption rates (SAR)

SAR (W/kg)	Biological effect
100	Increased embryonic and fetal resorptions, birth defects, postnatal weight loss, and reduced survival upon re-irradiation of the offspring of mice exposed during pregnancy
50	No mutation in bacteria, no enzyme effects, no change in lymphocyte transformation No effects on postnatal survival, adult body weight or longevity Increased potassium efflux and sodium influx from cells Increased response of the immune system
<6	Grey area: effects reported but unverified (90% involve behavioural, haematological or imunological effects, CNS structure or function, or hormone levels)
1.4	Core temperature increase <0.5°C
0.8–0.3	Normal thermoregulatory response
0.4	Unlikely to be associated with any effect
<0.4	No effect

14.4.2 Radio-frequency power absorption and tissue heating

In magnetic resonance examinations the body is subjected to a series of radio-frequency pulses, not necessarily evenly spaced, with pulse length τ and duty cycle $D = \tau/\mathrm{TR}$, where TR is the repetition time of the pulse train. The average power deposition P is given by the equation:

$$P = K \cdot \frac{\sigma v^2 R^2 D}{\rho \tau^2} \cdot \left(\frac{2\theta}{\pi}\right)^2 \quad (W/kg)$$

where $K = 6.8 \times 10^{-19}$ and θ is the inclination of the magnetisation vector.[119] The temperature rise caused by this power deposition is buffered by vasodilatation which increases heat loss from the body, but in some tissues, notably the lens of the eye, such homeostatic mechanisms are absent or limited.

A measurable rise in the temperature will occur if the rate of heat production or absorption exceeds the rate of heat loss. Changes in core temperature of up to 1°C can occur as a result of changing environmental or physiological conditions, and even greater changes occur pathologically. Sustained elevations of more than this might have an adverse effect however. The maximum expected temperature increase is obtained when no heat loss to the surroundings is considered and it can be calculated from the following equation:

$$\Delta T = \mathrm{SAR}.t \ / \ c_p$$

where c_p is the specific heat of tissue (3470 J/kg/°C), and t is the time of exposure (s). Thus, with an SAR of 2 W/kg applied for 10 minutes the maximum temperature rise would be 0.35°C. In practice of course this does not occur because of efficient thermo-regulatory mechanisms.

The heating of implanted metal objects in the body such as surgical clips, prosthesis, electronic or mechanical devices can also be estimated from the equations above. For instance, the radius of a metallic clip is 5 mm and of a joint prosthesis 25 mm, the electric conductivity of metals is of the order of 107 siemens (S), the density is 7700 kg/m^3,and the specific heat is about

Table 14.11. Non-thermal biological effects of electromagnetic fields at different frequencies in different biological levels of organisation

Man	Spark discharge perception	50 Hz
	Nerve excitation by induction	Mz
	Microwave heating	MHz–GHz
	Neuraesthenic syndrome	
Animal	Impaired peripheral nerve function and synaptic transmission in the rat	50 Hz
		MHz
	EEG changes in the rabbit	GHz
	Cloudy swelling and vacuole formation in brain	2450 MHz
	Teratogenic effects: impaired weight gain but few specific abnormalities	
Organ	Calcium efflux in chicken brain	50 Hz
	Calcium efflux in chicken and cat brain	MHz
	Bradycardia in the rat	GHz
	Endocrine function:	2450 MHz
	increased adrenocorticotrophic secretion	
	decreased thyrotrophic hormone secretion	
	decreased growth hormone secretion	
Cellular	On-off signals in frog retinal cells	50 Hz
	Nerve cell fatigue	MHz

Table 14.12. Guidelines for exposure to radio-frequency radiation during clinical magnetic resonance examinations

Country	Tissue mass	SAR limit (W/kg)	Reference
UK	Whole body (70 kg)	4	67, 68
	Local (≤ 1 g)	0.4	
	General public, 24 hr	0.03	
West Germany	Whole body (70 kg)	1	64
	Local (≤ 1 g)	5	
USA	Whole body (70 kg)	2	65
	Local (≤ 1 g)	0.4	
	General public, 24 hr	0.03	
Canada	25% body mass for ≤ 15 min	2	66, 109
	25% body mass for > 15 min	1	
USSR	Occupational exposure	0.012	145

450 J/kg/°C. Calculations using these values, and experimental data, show that the heating effect is negligible.

14.4.3 The biological effects of radio-frequency fields

The effect of radio-frequency fields upon biological tissues depends critically upon specific absorption rate. The most easily understood effect is of an increase in temperature which could occur in the absence of compensatory mechanisms at relatively low specific absorption rates. An increase of 0.5°C in core temperature is within the normal variation of the human body between sleep and maximal physical activity, and no adverse biological effects would be expected below this. Indeed, no effects have been reported on reproduction, fetal weight, growth, development, haematological and immunological values, hormone levels, and clinical chemistry.[120–129]

For the cardiac patient, the vasodilation which is part of the normal thermo-regulatory response should be considered, and the implications have been discussed by Rowell.[130] An increase in blood volume and cardiac output may occur with an increase in heart rate as well as changes in blood pressure and peripheral resistance. The vasodilatation that is part of the response is, on the whole, beneficial to the heart since it decreases afterload on the left ventricle. Only in patients who are volume depleted or hypotensive might it be expected to have an adverse effect. Tachyarrhythmias, and premature ventricle contractions have been reported in hyperthermia although there is no suggestion that clinical hyperthermia can occur during magnetic resonance imaging.[131,132]

Cataract induction is the most commonly reported irreversible effect of radio-frequency irradiation of humans. Over 50 cases have been attributed to microwave exposure, principally as a result of accidental occupational exposure, but there have been no reports associated with magnetic resonance imaging.

Non-thermal biological effects of microwave interaction with matter have been suggested by a number of investigators. Heller and Teixeira-Pinto,[133] for example, observed orientation of subcellular particles and micro-organisms along the lines of force in a radio-frequency electromagnetic field. However, this work has not been substantiated by other investigators at power densities below those associated with thermal effects.[134,135] Non-thermal effects would require particularly high field strengths of about 1 V/cm, unless cellular dimensions are well in excess of 100 μm.[136]

Table 14.10 summarises the relationship between measured or estimated specific absorption rates and reported effects, and table 14.11 summarises the effects of different frequencies of radiation. Experiments on rabbits have shown that the energy absorption in the eye sufficient to cause cataract is about 100 W/kg, resulting in a temperature rise of several degrees.[137] Similar values are associated in mammals with effects such as increased embryonic and fetal resorptions, birth defects, postnatal weight falls, and reduced survival on re-irradiation of the offspring of mice exposed during pregnancy.[138–140] Other studies at specific absorption rates between 10 and 45 W/kg report that human erythrocytes have increased electrophoretic mobility, potassium efflux, sodium influx, and hydrogen exchange.[141–143] Seaman and Wachtel[144] observed a threshold of 7 W/kg for the increased firing rate of aplysia pacemaker neurons. Almost all of the data showing no effect occur below 6 W/kg regardless of species or duration of exposure. Typical specific absorption rates for a multislice spin echo sequence are 0.16 W/kg at 0.5 T and 0.28 W/kg at 1.5 T, and so values during clinical imaging are significantly below the limit at which biological effects are known to occur. Commercial software normally bars the running of sequences that exceed 4 W/kg.

14.4.4 Exposure guidelines

Table 14.12 summarises the guidelines for exposure to radio-frequency radiation during clinical magnetic resonance examinations. Patients with cardiac pacemakers should not be scanned as explained in preceeding sections, although most pacemakers are shielded from radio-frequency interference by a titanium casing and a low-pass input filter with a 10 nF capacitor which protects against interference transmitted through the pacemaker lead in fields up to approximately 10 mW/cm^2. Patients with large metallic implants such as hip prostheses can be scanned although it is wise to discontinue the examination if discomfort is felt from the prosthesis.

References

1 Persson RBR, Ståhlberg F. *Health and Safety of Clinical NMR Measurements*. Florida: CRC Press, 1989.
2 Blakemore R. Magnetotactic bacteria. *Science* 1975; **190**: 377–9.
3 Frankel RB, Blakemore EP, Wolfe RS. Magnetite in freshwater magnetotactic bacteria. *Science* 1979; **203**: 1355–6.
4 Shellock FG. MR imaging of metallic implants and materials: a compilation of the literature. *Am J Roentgenol* 1988; **151**: 811–4.
5 Becker RL, Norfray JF, Teitelbaum GP, *et al*. MR imaging in patients with intracranial aneurysm clips. *Am J Neuroradiol* 1988; **9**: 885–9.
6 Soulen R, Higgins CB, Budinger TF. Magnetic resonance imaging of prosthetic heart valves. *Radiology* 1985; **154**: 705–7.
7 Shellock FG, Crues JV. High-field-strength MR imaging and metallic biomedical implants: an ex vivo evaluation of deflection forces. *Am J Roentgenol* 1988; **151**: 389–92.
8 Randall PA, Kohman LJ, Scalzetti EM, Szeverenyi NM, Panicek DM. Magnetic resonance imaging of prosthetic cardiac valves in vitro and in vivo. *Am J Cardiol* 1988; **62**: 973–6.
9 Teitelbaum GP, Bradley WG, Klein BD. MR imaging artifacts, ferromagnetism, and magnetic torque of intravascular filters, stents, and coils. *Radiology* 1988; **166**: 657–64.
10 Matsumoto AH, Teitelbaum GP, Barth KH, Carvlin MJ, Savin MA, Strecker EP. Tantalum vascular stents: in vivo evaluation with MR imaging. *Radiology* 1989; **170**: 753–5.
11 Gaffey CT, Tenforde TS. Changes in the electrocardiograms of rats and dogs exposed to DC magnetic fields.

In: *Lawrence Berkeley Laboratory Report, No 9085*, University of California, Berkeley 1979.
12 Gaffey CT, Tenforde TS. Alterations in the rat electrocardiogram induced by stationary magnetic fields. *Bioelectromagnetics* 1981; **2**: 357–70.
13 Gaffey CT, Tenforde TS, Dean EE. Alterations in the electrocardiograms of baboons exposed to DC magnetic fields. *Bioelectromagnetics* 1980; **2**: 209–18.
14 Tenforde TS, Gaffey CT, Moyer BR, Budinger TF. Cardiovascular alterations in macaca monkeys exposed to stationary magnetic fields: experimental observations and theoretical analysis. *Bioelectromagnetics* 1983; **4**: 1–9.
15 Togawa T, Okai O, Oshima M. Observation of blood flow EMF in externally applied strong magnetic fields by surface electrodes. *Med Biol Engn* 1967; **5**: 169–70.
16 Galle P, Cavellier JF. Effects and risks of using magnetic fields in magnetic resonance examination of man. *Radioprotection* 1985; **20**: 97–115.
17 Beischer DE, Knepton JC. Influence of strong magnetic fields on the electrocardiogram of squirrel monkeys (Saimiri sciureus). *Aerospace Medicine* 1964; **35**: 939–44.
18 Beischer DE. Vectorcardiogram and aortic blood flow of squirrel monkeys (Saimiri sciureus) in a strong superconductive electromagnet. In: Barnothy MF (ed). *Biological Effects of Magnetic Fields*, Vol 2. New York: Plenum Press, 1969: 241–59.
19 Beischer DE. Survival of animals in magnetic fields of 140,000Oe. In: Barnothy MF (ed). *Biological Effects of Magnetic Fields*, Vol 1. New York: Plenum Press, 1964: 201–10.
20 Mezrich R, Reichek N, Kressel HY. ECG effects in high-field MR imaging (Abstract). *Radiology* 1985; **157(P)**: 219.
21 Jehenson P, Duboc D, Lavergne T, *et al*. Change in human cardiac rhythm induced by a 2–T static magnetic field. *Radiology* 1988; **166**: 227–30.
22 Shellock FG, Crues JV. Temperature, heart rate and blood pressure changes associated with clinical MR imaging at 1.5T. *Radiology* 1987; **163**: 259–62.
23 Geacintov NE, Van Nostrand F, Becker JF, Tinkel JB. Magnetic field induced orientation of photosynthetic systems. *Biochim Biophys Acta* 1972; **267**: 65–79.
24 Maret G, Schickfus MV, Mayer A, Dransfeld K. Orientation of nucleic acids in high magnetic fields. *Phys Res Letters* 1975; **35**: 397–400.
25 Hong FT, Mauzerall D, Mauano A. Magnetic anisotropy and the orientation of retinal rods in a homogenous magnetic field. *Proc Natl Acad Sci USA* 1971; **68**: 1283–5.
26 Murayama M. Orientation of sickled erythrocytes in a magnetic field. *Nature* 1965; **206**: 420–2.
27 Gerencser VF, Barnothy MF, Barnothy JM. Inhibition of bacterial growth in fields of high paramagnetic strength. In: Barnothy MF (ed). *Biological Effects of Magnetic Fields*, Vol 1. New York: Plenum Press, 1964: 229–39.
28 Halpern MH, Green AE. Effects of magnetic fields on the growth of HeLa cells in tissue culture. *Nature* 1964; **202**: 717.
29 Jennison MW. The growth of bacteria, yeast, and moulds in a strong magnetic field. *J Bacteriol* 1937; **37**: 15–6.
30 Kimball GC. Growth of yeast in a magnetic field. *J Bacteriol* 1938; **35**: 103.
31 Leusden FP. Electric and magnetic effects on bacteria. *Zentr Bakeriol Parasitenk* 1929; **111**: 321–5.
32 Djordjevic Z, Lazarevic N, Djorkovic V. Studies on the hematologic effects of long-term, low-dose microwave exposure. *Aviat Space Environ Med* 1977; **48**: 516–8.
33 Gualtierotti T. Decrease of the sodium pump activity in the frog skin in a steady magnetic field. *Physiologist* 1964; **7**: 150.
34 Likhachev AI. Changes in the erythrocyte sedimentation rate of rabbits due to exposure of the central nervous system to a constant magnetic field. In: Barnothy MF (ed). *Biological Effects of Magnetic Fields*, Vol 2. New York: Plenum Press, 1969: 137–46.
35 Presman AS. *Electromagnetic Fields and Life*. New York: Plenum Press 1970.
36 Neurath PW. The effect of high gradient, high strength fields on the early embryonic development of frogs. In: Barnothy MF (ed). *Biological Effects of Magnetic Fields*, Vol 2. New York: Plenum Press, 1969: 177–87.
37 Toroptsev IV, Garganeyev GP, Gorshenina TI, Teplyakova NL. Pathologoanatomic characteristics of changes in experimental animals under the influence of magnetic fields. In: Kholodov YA (ed). *Influence of Magnetic Fields on Biological Objects*. NTIS report number JPRS 63038, Springfield, Virginia, 1974: 95.
38 Mulay IL, Mulay LN. Effects on Drosophila melongaster and S–37 tumor cells: postulates for magnetic fields interactions. In: Barnothy MF (ed). *Biological Effects of Magnetic Fields*, Vol 2. New York: Plenum Press, 1964: 146–69.
39 Veneziano PP. The effect of low intensity magnetostatic fields on the growth and orientation of the early embryo of gallus domesticus. *Dissertation Abstracts* 1965; **25**: 4319.
40 DeLorge J. Disruption of behaviour in mammals of three different sizes exposed to microwaves, extrapolation to larger animals. In: Stuchly SS (ed). *Proceedings of a Symposium on Electromagnetic Fields in Biological Systems* Edmonton, Canada: IMPI, 1979: 215–28.
41 Battocletti JH, Salles-Cunha S, Halbach RE, Nelson J, Sances A, Antonich FJ. Exposures of Rhesus monkeys to 20,000G steady magnetic field. Effect on blood parameters. *Med Phys* 1981; **8**: 115–8.
42 Barnothy MF, Barnothy JM. Magnetic fields and the number of blood platelets. *Nature* 1970; **225**: 1146–7.
43 Hanneman GD. Changes in sodium and potassium content of urine from mice subjected to intense magnetic fields. In: Barnothy FM (ed). *Biological Effects of Magnetic Fields*, Vol 2. New York: Plenum Press, 1969: 127–36.
44 Barnothy JM. Development of young mice. In: Barnothy MF (ed). *Biological Effects of Magnetic Fields*, Vol 1. New York: Plenum Press, 1964: 93–9.
45 Likhachev AI. Changes in the erythrocyte sedimentation rate of rabbits due to exposure of the central nervous system to a constant magnetic field. In: Barnothy MF (ed). *Biological Effects of Magnetic Fields*, Vol 1. New York: Plenum Press, 1969: 137–46.
46 Markuze II, Ambartsumyan RG, Chibrikin VM, Piruzyan

LA. Investigation of the PMP action on the alteration of electrolyte concentration in the blood and organs of animals. *Izv Akad Nauk SSSR, Ser Biol* 1973; **2**: 281.

47 Barnothy MF, Sumegi I. Effects of the magnetic fields on internal organs and endocrine system of mice. In: Barnothy MF (ed). *Biological Effects of Magnetic Fields*, Vol 2. New York: Plenum Press, 1969: 103–26.

48 Barnothy MF. Hematological changes in mice. In: Barnothy MF (ed). *Biological Effects of Magnetic Fields*, Vol 1. New York: Plenum Press, 1964: 109–26.

49 Barnothy JM, Barnothy MF, Boszormenyi-Nagy I. Influence of a magnetic field upon the leukocytes of the mouse. *Nature* 1956; **177**: 577–8.

50 Gross L, Smith LW. Effect of magnetic fields on wound healing in mice (Abstract). *Fed Proc* 1961; **20**: 164d.

51 Barnothy JM. Rejection of transplanted tumours in mice. In: Barnothy MF (ed). *Biological Effects of Magnetic Fields*, Vol 1. New York: Plenum Press, 1964: 100–8.

52 Russel DR, Hedrick HG. Preferences of mice to consume food and water in an environment of high magnetic field. In: Barnothy MF (ed). *Biological Effects of Magnetic Fields*, Vol 1. New York: Plenum Press, 1969: 233–40.

53 Kholodov JA, Alexandrovskaya MM, Lukjanova SN, Udarova NS. Investigation of the reactions of mammalian brain to static magnetic fields. In: *Biological Effects of Magnetic Fields*, Vol 2. New York: Plenum Press, 1969: 215–24.

54 Tarakhovsky ML, Samborskaya EP, Zadovozhnaya TD, Likhtenshtein EM. Effects of constant magnetic field on the course of pregnancy and progency development in albino rats. *Fizio Zh (Kiev)* 1969; **15**: 348.

55 Nahas GG, Boccalon H, Berryer P, Wagner B. Effects in rodents of a 1 month exposure to magnetic fields (200–1,200 gauss). *Aviat Space Environ Med* 1975; **46**: 1161–3.

56 Brown FA. Effects and after-effects on Planarians of reversals of the horizontal magnetic vector. *Nature* 1966; **209**: 533–5.

57 Keeton WT. The mystery of pigeon homing. *Sci Am* 1974; **231**: 96.

58 Beischer DE, Reno VR. Magnetic fields and man: where do we stand today? In: Pfisterer AM (ed). Special biophysical problems in aerospace medicine. *AGARD Conference Proceedings, part III*. 1971; **95**: 12.1–12.9

59 Beischer DE. Human tolerance to magnetic fields. *Astronautics* 1962; **7**: 24–48.

60 Peterson F, Kennelly AE. Some physiological experiments with magnets at the Edison Laboratory. *NY Med J* 1892; **56**: 729–32.

61 Interim standards for occupational exposure to magnetic fields. National Accelerator Laboratory, USA, 1979.

62 Limits on human exposure in static magnetic fields. Stanford Linear Accelerator Center, Stanford, USA, 1970.

63 Vyalov AM. Clinico-hygienic and experimental data on the effects of magnetic fields under industrial conditions. In: Kholodov YA (ed). *Influence of Magnetic Fields on Biological Objects*. Springfield, VA: National Technical Informational Service, report JPRS 63038, 1974: 163–74.

64 Bundesgesundheitsamt. Empfehlungen zur Vermeidung gesundheitlicher Risiken verursacht durch magnetisch und hoch frequente elektromagnetische Felder bei der NMR-tomographie und in-vivo NMR spectroskopie. Bonn: Carl Heymanns Verlag. *Bundesgesundheitsblatt* 1984; **27**: 92–6.

65 Bureau of Radiological Health, Food and Drug Administration. *Guidelines for Evaluating Electromagnetic Risk for Trials of Clinical NMR Systems*. FDA Publication HFX-460, Rockville, MD 20857, USA, 1982.

66 Environmental Health Directorate. *Recommendations to Ensure Protection of Patients and Operational Personel from Potential Hazard in Proton and NMR-imaging*. Environmental Health Directorate Publication No. 85–EHD–124, Ottawa, 1985.

67 National Radiological Protection Board. Exposure to nuclear magnetic resonance clinical imaging. *Radiography* 1981; **47**: 258–60.

68 National Radiological Protection Board. Revised guidance on acceptable limits of exposure during nuclear magnetic resonance clinical imaging. *Br J Radiol* 1983; **56**: 974–7.

69 Lövsund P, Nilsson SEG, Reuther T, Berg P. Magnetophosphenes. A quantitative analysis of thresholds. *Med Biol Eng Comput* 1980; **18**: 326–34.

70 Polson MJR, Barker AT, Freeston IL. Stimulation of nerve trunks with time-varying magnetic fields. *Med Biol Eng Comput* 1982; **20**: 243–4.

71 D'Arsonval MA. Action physiologique des courants alternatifs à grande fréquence. *Arch de Physiol* 1893; **5**: 401–8.

72 Budinger TF. Nuclear Magnetic Resonance (NMR) in vivo studies: known thresholds for health effects. *J Comput Assist Tomogr* 1981; **5**: 800–11.

73 Polson MJR, Barker AT, Freeston IL. Stimulation of nerve trunks with time-varying magnetic fields. *Med Biol Eng Comput* 1982; **20**: 243–4.

74 Fink M. *Convulsive Therapy: Theory and Practice*. New York: Raven Press 1979.

75 Roy OZ, Park GC, Stott JR. Intracardiac catheter fibrillation thresholds as a function of duration of 60 Hz current and electrode area. *IEEE Trans Biomed Eng* 1977; **BME–24**: 430–5.

76 Roy OZ. Technical note: summary of cardiac fibrillation thresholds for 60 Hz currents and voltage applied directly to the heart. *Med Biol Eng Comput* 1980; **18**: 657–9.

77 Watson AB, Wright JS, Loughman J. Electrical thresholds for ventricular fibrillation in man. *Med J Aust* 1973; **1**: 1179–82.

78 Barlow HB, Kohn HI, Walsh EG. The effect of dark adaption and of light upon the electric threshold of the human eye. *J Physiol* 1947; **148**: 376–81.

79 Budinger TF. *Indirect electrical stimulation of the visual apparatus*. Lawrence Radiation Laboratory Report, UCRL-18347. Berkeley, 1968.

80 Archer CW, Ratcliffe NA. The effects of pulsed magnetic fields on chick embryo cartilaginous skeletal rudiments in vitro. *J Exp Zool* 1983; **252**: 243–56.

81 Basset CAL, Pilla AA, Pawluk RJ. A non-operative salvage of surgically-resistant pseudarthroses and non-unions by pulsing electromagnetic fields. *Clinical Orthopaedics*

1977; **124**: 128–43.
82 Budinger TF, Cullander C, Bordow R. Switched magnetic fields thresholds for the induction of magneto-phosphenes (abstract). In: *Proceedings of the Third Annual Meeting*. Berkeley: Society of Magnetic Resonance in Medicine, 1984: 118–9.
83 Medvedev MA, Urazaev AM, Kulakov IUA. Effect of a constant and low frequency magnetic field on the behavioral and autonomic responses of the human operator. *Sov Neurol Psychiatry* 1978; **11**: 3–13.
84 Friedman H, Becker RO, Bachman CH. Effect of magnetic fields on reaction time performance. *Nature* 1967; **213**: 949–50.
85 Jolley WB, Hinshaw DB, Knierim K. Magnetic field effects on calcium efflux and insulin secretion in isolated rabbit islets of Langerhans. *Bioelectromagnetics* 1983; **4**: 103.
86 Sakharova SA. Ryzhov AI, Udintsev NA. Mechanism of the sympathoadrenal system's response to on time action of a variable magnetic field. *Kosm Biol Aviakosm Med* 1981; **15**: 52.
87 Udintsev NA, Moroz VV. Response of the pituitary-adrenal system to the action of a variable magnetic field. *Bull Eksp Biol Med* 1974; **77**: 51.
88 Riesen WH, Aranyi C, Kyle JL, Valentino AR, Miller DA. A pilot study of the interaction of extremely low frequency electromagnetic fields with brain organelles. In: *Compilation of Navy Sponsored ELF Biomedical and Ecological Research Reports, Vol 1*. Technical memorandum No 3 (IITRI project E6185). Bethesda: Naval Research and Development Command 1971.
89 Luben RA, Cain CD, Chen MCY, Rosen DM, Adey WR. Effects of electromagnetic stimuli on bone and bone cells in vitro: inhibition of responses to parathyroid hormone by low-energy low-frequency fields. *Proc Natl Acad Sci USA* 1982; **79**: 4180–4.
90 Ossenkopp KP, Koltek WT, Peringer MA. Prenatal exposure to an extremely low frequency, low intensity rotating magnetic field and increases in thyroid and testicle weight in rats. *Develop Psykobiol* 1972; **5**: 275–85.
91 Soldatova LP. Sequence of pathomorphological reactions to the effect of alternating magnetic fields. *Arkh Anat Gistol Embriol* 1982; **83**: 12–15.
92 Toroptsev IV, Soldatova LP. Pathomorphological reactions of cerebrocortical neural elements to alternating magnetic field. *Arh Patol (Moscow)* 1981; **43**: 33–6.
93 Udintsev NA, Kanskaia NV, Shchepetil'nifova AI, Ordina OM, Pichurina RA. Dynamics of cardiac and skeletal muscle lactate dehydrogenase activity following a single exposure to an alternating magnetic field. *Bull Eksp Biol Med* 1976; **81**: 670.
94 Kolodub FA, Chernysheva ON. Special features of carbohydrate-energy and nitrogen metabolism in the rat brain under the influence of magnetic fields of commercial frequency. *Ukr Biokhim Zh (Kiev)* 1980; **3**: 299.
95 Goodman EM, Greenebaum B, Marron MJ. Bioeffects of extremely low-frequency electromagnetic fields: variation with intensity, waveform and individual or combined electric and magnetic fields. *Radiat Res* 1979; **78**: 485–501.
96 Liboff AR, Williams T, Strong DM, Wistar R. Time-varying magnetic fields: effect on DNA synthesis. *Science* 1984; **223**: 818.
97 Odintsov YN. The effect of a magnetic field on the natural resistance of white mice to Listeria infection. *Tr Tomskogo Vaktsyn Syvorotok* 1965; **16**: 234–8.
98 Mizushima Y, Akaoka I, Nishida Y. Effects of magnetic field on inflammation. *Experientia* 1975; **21**: 1411–2.
99 Conti P, Gigante GE, Cifone MG, *et al.* Reduced mitogenic stimulation of human lymphocytes by extremely low frequency electromagnetic fields. *FEBS Lett* 1983; **162**: 156–60.
100 Sander R, Brinkman, J, Kuhne B. Laboratory studies on animals and human beings exposed to 50 Hz electric and magnetic fields. In: *Proceedings of an International Congress on Large High Voltage Systems*. Paris, 1982: paper 36–01.
101 DeLorge JO. *Operant Behaviour of Rhesus Monkeys in the Presence of Extremely Low Frequency, Low Intensity Magnetic and Electric Fields: Experiment 2*. Pensacola: Naval Aerospace Medical Research Laboratory, publication NAMRL–1179, 1973.
102 Fam WZ. Biological effects of 60 Hz magnetic field on mice. *IEEE Trans Magn* 1981; **MAG–17**: 1510–3.
103 Beischer DE, Grissett JD, Mitchell RR. Exposure of man to magnetic fields alternating at extremly low frequency. In: *Naval Aerospace Medical Research Laboratory, report number NAMRL–1180*, Pensacola, 1973: 1–31.
104 Pavlicek W, Geisinger M, Castle L, *et al.* The effects of nuclear magnetic resonance on patients with cardiac pacemakers. *Radiology* 1983; **147**: 149–53.
105 Pavlicek W, Geisinger M, Castle L, *et al.* The effects of nuclear magnetic resonance on patients with cardiac pacemakers. *Radiology* 1983; **147**: 149–53.
106 Fetter J, Aram G, Holmes DR, Gray JE, Hayes DL. The effects of nuclear magnetic resonance imagers on external implantable pulse generators. *PACE* 1984; **7**: 720–7.
107 Zimmerman BH, Faul DD. Artifacts and hazards in NMR imaging due to metal implants and cardiac pacemakers. *Diagn Imag Clin Med* 1984; **53**: 53–6.
108 Hayes DL, Holmes DR,Gray JE. Effect of 1.5 tesla nuclear magnetic resonance imaging scanner on implanted permanent pacemakers. *J Am Coll Cardiol* 1987; **10**: 782–6.
109 Environmental Health Directorate. *Guidelines on Exposure to Electromagnetic Fields from Magnetic Resonance Clinical Systems*. Environmental Health Directorate Publication No 85–EHD–124, Ottawa, 1986.
110 American Conference of Governmental Hygienists. Comments on proposed new threshold limit values for low frequency (ELF) magnetic fields. *Bioelectromagnetic Society Newsletter*, 1988.
111 National Institute of Radiation Protection, POB 60204, S–104 01, Stockholm, 1986.
112 Sams HW. *Reference Data for Radio Engineers, 5th edition*. New York: International Telephone and Telegraph Corporation, 1968.
113 International Telecommunication Union. *Radio Regulations, 1981 Revision*. Geneva: International Telecommunication Union, 1981.

114 Johnson CC, Gay AW. Nonionizing electromagnetic wave effects in biological materials and systems. *Proc IEEE* 1972; **60**: 692–718.

115 Grandolfo M, Vecchia P, Ghandi O. Calculation of RF power deposition in MRI of the human torso. *Magn Reson Med* (In press).

116 Schwan HP, Piersol GM. The absorption of electromagnetic energy in body tissues. Part I: Biological aspects. *Am J Phys Med* 1954; **33**: 370–404.

117 Schwan HP. Electrical properties of bound water. *Ann NY Acad Sci* 1965; **125**: 344–54.

118 Hagmann MJ, Gandhi OP, D'Andrea JA, Chatterjee I. Head resonance: numerical solutions and experimental results. *IEEE Transactions* 1979; **27**: 809–13.

119 Bottomley PA, Edelstein WA. Power deposition in whole-body NMR imaging. *Med Phys* 1981; **8**: 510–2.

120 Berman E, Kinn JB, Carter HB. Observations of mouse fetuses after irradiation with 2.45GHz microwaves. *Health Phys* 1978; **35**: 791–801.

121 Berman E, Carter HB, House D. Tests of mutagenesis and reproduction in male rats exposed to 2450 MHz (CW) microwaves. *Bioelectromagnetics* 1980; **1**: 65–76.

122 Djordjevic Z, Lazarevic N, Djorkovic V. Studies on the hematologic effects of long-term, low-dose microwave exposure. *Aviat Space Environm Med* 1977; **48**: 516–8.

123 Guillet R, Michaelson SM. The effects of repeated microwave exposure on neonatal rats. *Radio Sci* 1977; **12**: 125–9.

124 Johnson RB, Mizumori S, Lovely RH. Adult behavioral deficit in rats exposed prenatally to 918MHz microwaves. In: Mahlum DD, Sikov MR, Hacket PL, Andrew FD (eds). *Developmental Toxicology of Energy Related Pollutants*. Washington: DOE Symposium Series 47, 1978: 281–99.

125 Lovely RH, Myers DE, Irradiation of rats by 918MHz microwaves at 2.5 mW/cm^2: Delineation the dose-response relationship. *Radio Sci* 1977; **12**: 139–46.

126 Michaelson SM, Guillet R, Heggeness FW. Influence of microwave exposure on functional maturation of the rat. In: Mahlum DD, Sikov MR, Hacket PL, Andrew FD (eds). *Developmental Toxicology of Energy Related Pollutants*. Washington: DOE Symposium Series 47, 1978: 300–16.

127 Milroy WC, Michelson SM. Thyroid pathophysiology of microwave radiation. *Aerospace Med* 1972; **43**: 1126–31.

128 Smialowicz RJ, Kinn JB, Elder JA. Perinatal exposure of rats to 2450 MHz (CW) microwave radiation: effects on lymphocytes. *Radio Sci* 1979; **14**: 147–53.

129 Wangemann RT, Cleary SF. The in vivo effects of 2.45GHz microwave radiation on rabbit serum components and sleeping times. *Radiat Environ Biophys* 1976; **13**: 89–103.

130 Rowell LB. Cardiovascular aspects of human thermoregulation. *Circ Res* 1983; **52**: 367.

131 Houdas Y, Ring EFJ. *Human Body Temperature: its Measurement and Regulation*. New York: Plenum Press, 1982.

132 Hugander A, Gillis WK, Robbins IH. Whole body hyperthermia in the treatment of neoplastic disease. In: *Hyperthermia Monograph*, Bhaba Atomic Reseach Centre, Bhaba, India, 1985.

133 Heller KH, Teixeira-Pinto AA. A new physical method of creating chromosomal aberrations. *Nature* 1959; **183**: 905–6.

134 Schwan HP. Interaction of microwave and radiofrequency radiation with biological systems. In: Cleary SF (ed). *Biological Effects and Health Implications of Microwave Radiation*. US Public Health Service Publication, No BRH/DBE 70–2. Washington: Government Printing Office, 1970: 13–20.

135 Michaelson SM. Microwave biological effects. An overview. *Proc IEEE* 1980; **68**: 40–9.

136 Schwan HP. Classical theory of microwave interactions with biological systems. In: Taylor LD, Cheung AY (eds). *The Physical Basis of Electromagnetic Interactions with Biological Systems*. University of Maryland, 1957: 91–112.

137 Kramar PO, Harris C, Gay AW, Emery AF. Mechanism of microwave cataractogenesis in rabbits. In: Johnson CC, Shore ML (eds). *Biological Effects of Electromagnetic Waves*, Vol 1. HEW Publication (FDA) 77–8010, 1976: 49–60.

138 Rugh R, Ginns EI, Ho MS, Leach WM. Responses of the mouse to microwave radiation during gestrous cycle and pregnancy. *Radiat Res* 1975; **62**: 225–41.

139 Rugh R. Are mouse fetuses which survive microwave radiation permanently affected thereby? *Health Phys* 1976; **31**: 33–9.

140 O'Connor ME. Mammalian teratogenesis and radiofrequency fields. *Proc IEEE* 1980; **68**: 56–60.

141 Ismailov ES. Mechanism of effects of microwaves on erythrocyte permeability for potassium and sodium ions. *Biol Nauki* 1970; **21**: 58–60.

142 Ismailov ES. Infrared spectra of erythrocyte ghosts in the region of the amide I and amide II bands on microwave irradiation. *Biofizika* 1976; **21**: 940–2 (English translation, *Biophysics* 1977; **21**; 961–3).

143 Ismailov ES. Effect of ultrahigh frequency electromagnetic radiation on the electrophoretic mobility of erythrocytes. *Biofizika* 1977; **22**: 493–8 (English translation, *Biophysics* 1978; **22**: 510–6).

144 Seaman RL, Wachtel H. Slow and rapid responses to CW and pulsed microwave radiation by individual Aplysia pacemakers. *J Microwave Power* 1978; **13**: 77–86.

145 *Temporary Sanitary Rules for Working with Centimetre Waves*. Ministry of Health Protection of the USSR, 1958.

Chapter 15
The Future of Magnetic Resonance in Cardiology

DONALD LONGMORE

Exactness is difficult to achieve and small errors are bound to occur. I warmly commend the physician who makes small mistakes; infallibility is rarely to be seen. Most doctors seem to me to be in the position of poor navigators. In calm weather they can conceal their mistakes, but when overtaken by a mighty storm or a violent gale, it is evident to all that it is their ignorance and error which is the ruin of the ship. So it is with the sorry doctors who are in the great majority. They cure men but slightly ill, in whose treatment even the biggest mistakes would have no serious consequences. Such diseases are many and much more common than the more serious ones. When doctors make mistakes over such cases, their errors are unperceived by the layman, but when they have to treat a serious and dangerous case, a mistake or lack of skill is obvious to all and vengeance for either error is not long delayed.

These words, 2410 years old, are fresh and pertinent today. The thinking of Hippocrates sired ethical, diagnostic and curative medicine practised for two millennia. Now there is the opportunity to use the new information from magnetic resonance to move into the new era of preventing cardiovascular disease.

15.1 Calm weather

During the last hundred years, the medical profession has weathered waters ruffled by many advances, none of which have come from within the profession but all of which have changed medical practice. These include anaesthetics from chemists, organ transplantation from biologists, X-rays from physicists, antibiotics from chemists, steroids from biochemists, the contraceptive pill from pharmacologists, extracorporeal circulation from engineers, pacemakers from electronics engineers, and implants from metallurgists and plastics technologists. In this book are described the advances made in magnetic resonance, which was initially developed by physicists and chemists.

15.2 The storm to come

The quantum leap in technology in the Western world during and following World War II brought the computer and developments in communication such that information could no longer be withheld from the masses. Better education and higher standards of living have raised public expectation from medicine. Survival is no longer the prime consideration, it has been supplemented by the desire for a better quality of life.

The ever more enlightened general public are beginning to ask for better medical care and they have a track record of stimulating progress. Two stories of lay concern leading to medical discoveries illustrate the point.

In Old Lyme Connecticut in 1975,[1] a worried mother drew the attention of state health department officials to the fact that at least 12 children in the village were suffering from an illness which had been diagnosed as juvenile rheumatoid arthritis. Another mother complained to the Yale rheumatology clinic about an epidemic of arthritis in her family. To the community's health surveillance machinery this seemed ridiculous. Who had ever heard of an epidemic of arthritis? The parents demanded that the mystery be investigated. By 1977, it had been established that there was an epidemic of 'Lyme summer arthritis' appearing several weeks after a papule on the skin following a tick bite. A spirochaete was found in the tick and there were antibodies and similar spirochaetes in the patients, fortunately sensitive to antibiotics.

In 1934 a farmer in Wisconsin decided that he could no longer tolerate the fact that cows frequently bled uncontrollably, even from the smallest cuts. The farmer took a dead cow and a pail of still liquid blood to the university, where Dr Paul Link became interested and traced the trouble to bishydroxy-coumarin (or dicoumarol), a substance in spoiled clover closely related to coumarin which gives new-mown grass its attractive smell. Dicoumarol works by upsetting the liver's synthesis of prothrombin. (One wonders incidentally, how far a similarly affected farmer would have got if his nearest university had been Harvard or Yale or Oxford or Cambridge. How many college porters could have directed him where to take a pail of abnormal blood and a dead cow? This farmer succeeded because he turned up after normal working hours and found Link still at work—a good way to select a dedicated worker.)

The lesson from these episodes, is that public disquiet can sometimes be considerably more effective than medical 'knowing better' in bringing problems to light. The enlightened public are now asking why they pay more and more for medical care, and the management of vascular catastrophes such as stroke has not advanced significantly in two millennia, certainly not since the time of Galen. More significant may be the fundamental questions asked by governments of less affluent countries about the efficacy of 20th century medicine aimed at curing established disease. Should they invest a large proportion of their small GDP copying western high technology medicine? Is it cost effective? Or, should they skip this phase and concentrate on using modern technology like magnetic resonance prevention?

The answer to these first order questions so relevant to the future of cardiovascular magnetic resonance must lie in detailed analysis of the efficacy of the management of occlusive vascular disease, the most common cause of death in the Western world. In the UK and the USA, approximately half of all deaths are due to acquired occlusive vascular disease causing myocardial infarction and stroke. Has modern cardiology made any impact on the incidence of acquired cardiovascular disease? Has the coronary vein graft operation actually reduced the mortality from coronary disease or does the combination of operative mortality and cerebral damage following open heart surgery outweigh the benefits?

There is certainly no discernable relationship between survival rates and the proportion of the national wealth spent on curative medicine. The USA spends 9.2%, Holland 8.6%, Norway 7.6%, Australia 7.6% Denmark 7.4%, France 7.2%, Switzerland 6.9% Italy 6.3%, West Germany 5.7% the UK 5.4% and Japan 4.4%; yet the life span is similar, with the exception of Japan where it is 5 years longer and increasing. The US spending the largest proportion of its GDP and the UK nearly the lowest, are at the top of the list of premature deaths from occlusive vascular disease whereas France, a high spender, and Japan, the lowest spender, are at the bottom. Life expectancy in Japan has increased rapidly. Between 1965 and 1986 it rose by 7.5 years for men and 8 years for women.[2]

Hospital based medical training is set on the premise that curative medicine (which can be life saving in the individual) has an overall impact on disease. Is this assumption valid? The conquest of tuberculosis by mass X-ray diagnosis and treatment with antibiotics is often quoted as a classic example. The reality is different, the incidence of TB fell steadily in the UK from the time when records began in 1831 (figure 15.1). There were small increases during both world wars but otherwise there are no demonstrable changes, certainly none due to medical intervention. Attempts to control the disease included the Public Health Acts, the sanatorium movement, sending the sufferers to the Alps, artificial pneumothorax, phrenic crush, thoracoplasty, mass X-ray, streptomycin and the later more effective antibiotics.

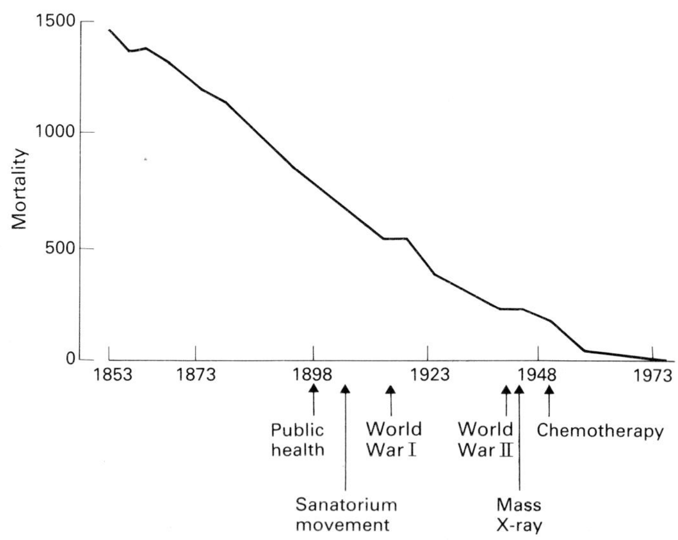

Figure 15.1. The decline of tuberculosis in the UK from 1853 to the present time. There is no detectable effect of medical intervention although there was a rise associated with both world wars. The initial slope of the graph suggests that tuberculosis should have been eliminated by 1948. The final elimination of a disease or its reduction to insignificant levels in a country is always difficult and there is a tail off when the numbers become small. The influence of magnetic resonance cardiovascular diagnosis should reduce the incidence of occlusive vascular disease in a similar pattern.

It is clear that unless medicine takes every opportunity to mitigate the effects of the major killing diseases, it is at risk of being overtaken by the storm of protest forecast by Hippocrates not about mistakes, lack of skill or the will to try harder, but about the way it conducts its affairs now that there is a viable alternative.

The factors which influence the adoption of beneficial new ideas in medicine will be examined in detail in this chapter. It discusses the way ahead based on what has already been achieved and reviews, without inhibition from established prejudices, the constraints on logical progress due to both the inevitable pitfalls and the avoidable hurdles.

15.3 A new instrument for accurate navigation

The problem which has faced medicine has been the lack of information about disease. It has been impossible to steer a course towards the kind of care wanted by the public because it has been impossible to learn about the natural history of the major killing cardiovascular diseases. Magnetic resonance properly used will enable the transition from the medicine practised by Hippocrates, the sometimes ineffectual management of end state disease, first to better management of established disease, and then to prevention. That these changes will take place is beyond question, however when they will happen and how many lives will be wasted before it does remain an enigma.

15.4 Predicting the future

There are accepted ways of predicting how new technology can be applied to medicine including the well known Delphi forecasting method. This depends on panels of experts whose opinions are combined and re-edited by the contributors. This method has a shortcoming; the experts have to be informed about the new ideas and technologies to take them into account. Forecasting however can be uncannily accurate. In 1969 the Office of Health Economics published a Delphic forecast[3] in which 40 experts (including the author) forecast amongst the many predictions routine lung transplants, widespread use of the female contraceptive pill, addiction as an increasing social problem, treatment of mental disease in the community, methods of determining the sex of a baby before birth, little fundamental improvement in the management of established neurological disease and 'studies of acceleration of blood in the aorta making it possible to carry out automated predictive studies bringing benefits by reorienting the medical profession to a predictive approach to heart disease'. It also forecast new, more powerful diagnostic machines.

Worse than using flawed methods of forecasting, major manufacturers of magnetic resonance machines (who strongly influence their application) do not appear to use any information wisely. One major manufacturer seeks advice from a panel of customers using existing equipment thereby depending on neuroradiologists and orthopaedic surgeons for advice about development of cardiovascular machines; another relies on feedback from their sales force. No wonder that their machines are just the wrong side of the fine dividing line between just not working satisfactorily and optimised for cardiovascular work.

The most reliable forecasts depend on a combination of knowledge of what has gone before, influencing the arrival at the present position, with informed conjecture about the future.

'The further you look back in history the further ahead you can see.' Winston S Churchill.

Wise industrialists have learnt to begin by asking not 'where do we want to be two decades from now?' but 'where would it be possible for us to be?' From a thorough survey of the possible futures they pick those that currently suit their purposes best and they start making the necessary changes—in organisation, staffing, training, investment, reserves, mergers, research, and so on. From time to time they review their original decisions, modify them if necessary, and check their current progress toward these rationally chosen and rationally modified goals. Medicine could be very like that too, and there has already been a study of the future of medicine, bioengineering and fundamental biology. We need not lack for basic, serious, and well-informed prediction. Unfortunately, those who control the destiny of medicine are all too apt to ask 'where do we want to be' questions and, of course, to get 'pie in the sky' answers. We should begin by asking 'what would it be possible for us to achieve, say, between now and the end of the century?' Much more analysis is required if cardiovascular magnetic resonance is to turn promise into performance.

It is vital also to have a clear understanding of where we should be. For example, the answer to where we could be in cardiac magnetic resonance, with minimal effort and maximum certainty, might be a method of detecting cardiac sarcoidosis at an early stage: an interesting (and important to the few sufferers) outcome. Alternatively, the answer could be a method of assessing stunned myocardium following reperfusion. Answers to these questions would make little difference to the future of *homo sapiens*. With a little more effort the answer could and should change to a strategy promising the early detection of occlusive vascular disease, an understanding of its natural history, monitoring the efficacy of preventive and therapeutic measures leading to a significant reduction in mortality and morbidity from the disease process.

This book details the present status of cardiovascular magnetic resonance, and fortunately, it is not necessary to gaze very far back into the mists of time to forecast the future. Indeed such remarkable progress has been made since the beginning of the decade when magnetic resonance imaging was first applied to the heart that it is difficult to order all the advances which have followed each other so rapidly. The lead times to publication in specialist and general journals vary so widely and there has been so much parallel development of the more obvious ideas that attributing the less important developments correctly to the many workers is impossible. The sources of the seminal ideas can however be attributed to a few real pioneers. The basic physics was often described in theory and later applied practically by others. An example is the description of the principle of phase mapping by Moran and the overcoming of the technical difficulties by Firmin, Bailes and others.

A detailed review of the developments of the past 6 years and a step by step deduction of what could be achieved by the end of the century carries the risk of narrowing the imagination, and any forecast must take into account where we are likely to be by the end of the century, which differs from where we should be. Furthermore it is a foolish doctor who tries to prognosticate. One is reminded of the unfortunate surgeon who told Sir Francis Chichester that he had 6 months to live with a lung cancer and had to watch this great adventurer set record upon record of feats of endurance for over 30 years. Forecasts of optimism are at risk too. 'Doctor, doctor, the man you just told was completely fit has dropped dead on the steps.' 'Quick, turn him round so that it looks as though he is coming in'.

Instead of embarking on a detailed tour through the circulation using an arbitrary classification, because atheromatous arterial disease is numerically the most important, only the arteries will be considered in detail.

15.5 Vascular magnetic resonance imaging

The contributions of the different forms of magnetic resonance to the investigation of the arterial tree are considered separately.

15.5.1 Static imaging

The aorta and the major arteries are well seen on gated images and these will continue to be used to diagnose many congenital and acquired conditions such as Marfan's disease and dissecting aneurysm. The diagnosis of vascular disease from tomographic images suffers the disadvantage of imaging a tortuous structure with a straight plane. Three-dimensional representation is essential (see below).

Although the arterial tree is well seen on triggered images, it is important to appreciate the limitations of the technology. Triggered acquisition does not solve all the problems of cardiac motion, although it is adequate in the peripheral circulation. The cardiac cycle is rarely regular, varying with respiration which itself is irregular. The effect of these irregularities combined with the cybernetic control of cardiac output which causes it to overpump for a period of time and then to switch to a period of underpumping, is to degrade conventional images which average data from many cardiac cycles. For this reason, real-time imaging will eventually replace static imaging, although the limitations of the signal to noise ratio may force a compromise in spatial resolution.

15.5.2 Cine imaging

The value of cine imaging lies in the qualitative impression of flow patterns and turbulence that is given by variations in signal strength. This coupled with velocity mapping and three-dimensional display is likely to provide the first important contribution of magnetic resonance to the non-invasive detection of disease. The coronary arteries are unlikely to be imaged in this way (see real-time imaging, below).

15.5.3 Magnetic resonance angiography

There is no difficulty in producing angiograms of static vessels down to branches approximately 1 mm in diameter. This approach however relies upon images of the arterial lumen to detect a disease which affects the wall, and it is not ideal. It also shares all the problems of interpretation and inter-observer variability familiar to radiologists. Unless combined with cine imaging and velocity mapping, it is unlikely to provide reliable information. An anatomical assessment of a vessel is also seriously flawed when it is more important to have a functional assessment. Blood is a non-Newtonian fluid, altering its viscosity in response to shear stresses. Vessels which appear angiographically to have an adequate lumen may have an internal configuration which under critical changes in flow will cause turbulence, dissipating energy into sideways forces instead of forward flow.

If there were a relationship between the number of manufacturers' exhibits of three-dimensional carotid and cerebral angiograms and their clinical value, the observer could be forgiven the impression that magnetic resonance angiography is the way ahead. The manufacturers' path is not necessarily the one of greatest clinical value, however, and the success of angiography will depend on who controls the direction of research. The 'turf' battle is discussed later in this chapter. If radiologists are responsible there will be a brief fashion for angiography lasting until its limited clinical value is appreciated. If physicists deeply involved in developing the technique are in charge, they risk becoming so engrossed that they may fail to distinguish between an absorbing technical exercise and the way ahead. If cardiologists run cardiovascular magnetic resonance, the far more informative quantitative measurement and visualisation of the vessel wall will prevail from the beginning.

15.5.4 Velocity mapping

Velocity mapping overcomes many of the limitations of angiography. Studies of back flow in the aortic root indicate that the functional ostia of the coronary arteries may arise several centimetres above the anatomical ostia and in normal subjects the back flow divides into two streams destined for the ostia.[4,5] Abnormal back flow may be used to study coronary disease but this indirect method will be displaced by direct measurement of coronary flow in the vessels as soon as they are reliable.

An important physiological fact that can be used to detect and quantify disease is that the velocity in paired vessels such as the carotids, the renal or iliac arteries, and the coronary arteries is the same in each. If circumstances change, the size of the vessel adjusts to maintain a constant velocity. The artery supplying an arterio-venous shunt enlarges for instance rather than the velocity of blood increasing. See figure 15.2. The patient had a partially resolved left iliac vein thrombosis caused by thromboangiitis obliterans migrans (Burger's disease). He had previously had a right below-knee amputation. The smaller size of the iliac artery on the right can be seen but the arterial velocities on both sides are identical. In contrast the high velocity in the acutely stenosed left iliac vein is seen.

15.5.5 Atheroma and chemical shift

Chemical shift analysis of atheromatous plaques in the larger vessels is already practical and these will be used as the test-bed for improved chemical shift analysis techniques which will then be applicable to smaller vessels and moving vessels like the coronary arteries.

15.5.6 Real-time imaging

Although conventional imaging techniques all give satisfactory results in the peripheral arteries, a thorough examination is time consuming and rapidly moving arteries such as the coronaries are less reliably seen. When real-time imaging can be used with similar resolution, it will displace conventional magnetic resonance sequences. An example will be examination of the renal arteries for stenosis in patients with hypertension. This is not done at present partly because the patients are not referred but mostly because of the time taken with conventional imaging to locate the renal vessels and to measure velocity in a number of slices along them at the same phase of the cardiac cycle.

15.5.7 Three-dimensional imaging, image enhancement and automation

Three-dimensional acquisition and display are essential for the examination of a tortuous arterial tree and will enable intravascular and intracardiac intervention. The clinical application of three-dimensional imaging depends upon the successful development of rapid imaging techniques and the development of automated edge tracking, area growth and image enhancement.

The combination of rapid imaging and fast three-dimensional image reconstruction will make 'catheter tip' surgery under magnetic resonance vision feasible. Initially this will be done in peripheral arteries, later it

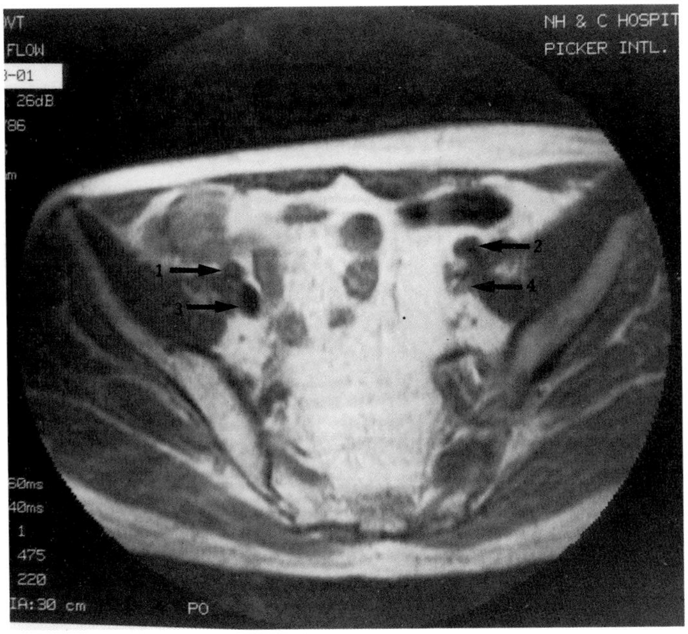

(a)

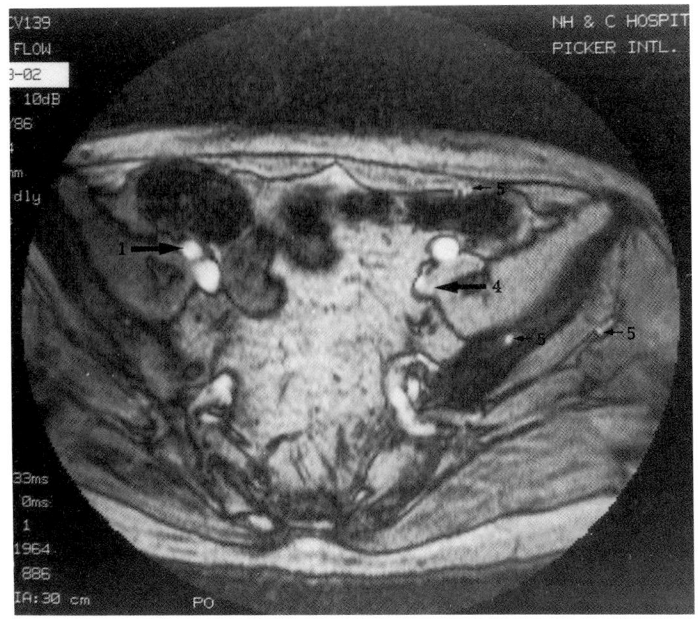

(b)

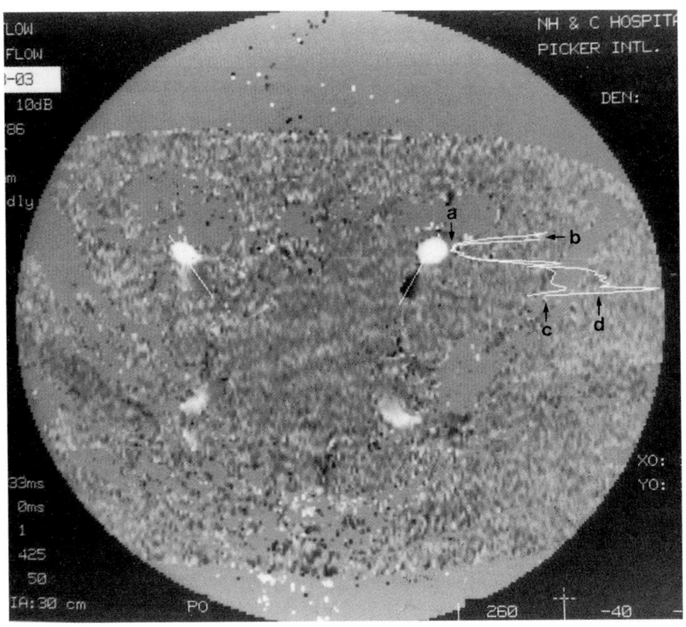

(c)

Figure 15.2. (a) A spin echo image across the pelvis of a patient with a swollen, painful left leg due to thrombo-angiitis obliterans migrans (Burger's disease). The right external iliac artery (1) is small, the left iliac artery (2) is normal in size, the right common iliac vein (3) is normal and the left common iliac vein (4) is partially occluded.

(b) The corresponding gradient echo image. The smaller size of the right common iliac artery (1) is confirmed and the partial occlusion of the left common iliac vein by thrombus (4) is also demonstrated, as are collateral vessels (5).

(c) The velocity map encoded through the plane of the image. Caudal velocities are shown in shades of white and cranial velocities in shades of black. The velocity profiles in the two iliac arteries (a) reach an identical peak velocity but the diameters are different (b). The velocity profile in the normal right iliac vein with plug flow is arrowed (c) and the much higher velocity in the partially occluded vein is arrowed (d).

will be extended to the right side of the heart, the pulmonary outflow tract and valve. As techniques improve, trans-septal catheterisation of the left heart will allow some simple procedures in the left atrium, the mitral region and the left ventricular outflow tract and the aortic valve. Magnetic resonance will be used to guide angioplasty catheters, certainly in the periphery and possibly also in the coronary arteries. Unlike intracardiac and intravascular procedures under X-ray vision which must be done in the limited available exposure time and require repeated injection of contrast medium, magnetic resonance screening can be continuous and the duration as long as necessary. The resolution of ultrasound is inadequate for the fine surgery which will be possible using cutting, sewing and dilating catheters.

15.5.8 Population screening and drug trials

Aortic compliance and pulse wave velocity have already been shown to be a likely method of detecting arteriopaths. The combination of one-shot imaging and automated analysis will increase the number of subjects who can be studied, thereby reducing costs and refining the data base. Aortic compliance has so far been studied in isolation and the contribution of peripheral vessel tone has not been established. It is likely that as magnetic resonance techniques improve and speed up, the contribution of measurements of compliance and velocity in the circulation to the early detection of vascular disease will improve. There have not been any serious attempts by the pharmaceutical industry to produce drugs which will reverse atheroma directly and there will not be any major investment in this area until the place of magnetic resonance in quantifying and analysing atheromatous plaques is recognised widely. When this does happen, it will be worth the manufacturers' research effort and investment to develop innovative drugs to control atheroma and magnetic resonance will be used to monitor their efficacy.

15.6 Constraints influencing the adoption of cardiovascular magnetic resonance

15.6.1 How much further has cardiovascular magnetic resonance to go?

The optimistic analysis of the future of magnetic resonance based on the current status of the technology assumes that this is an evolving field and there is still great potential for development. Is this assumption valid?

The hallmark of a young technology or science is that its activities begin by increasing exponentially, but later a physics barrier is reached when new developments become increasingly difficult and progress slows. On any objective count (numbers of workers in the field, numbers of papers published, number of conferences, number of sales representatives, etc.), activity in the cardiovascular magnetic resonance has at least doubled every year for the past 5 years, and it is still in the early phase of exponential growth. Unfortunately, the story is not as straightforward as that described by the simple growth curve. There is considerable inertia in the system. At first, the scientific advances are several years ahead of the awareness of the new technology but soon, if it shows promise, the true growth curve is overtaken by an associated excess of 'overheads' of staff, research units, publications, etc. The vital question in magnetic resonance relates to exactly where cardiovascular magnetic resonance is on the true growth curve. At first thought, there would be justification for believing the period of true exponential growth is drawing to a close because many of the obvious and easy advances and discoveries have been made. This is clearly not the case. How can we establish where magnetic resonance is placed on the curve? If we assume that it is at an early stage, we can speculate how the development from this prototechnology into a sound and solid discipline will take place. If there are no restraining influences, advances will leapfrog one another. As cardiology and vascular diagnosis place greater demands on the equipment, the major manufacturers will, if they remain true to form, respond by producing refinements on the existing equipment. Such incremental advances will be overtaken from time to time by the development of new generations of machine. Small specialist manufacturers working in association with science-based magnetic resonance units will make the quantum leaps in technology.

15.6.2 Will medicine embrace cardiovascular magnetic resonance?

The gap between fundamental discovery and everyday application in general science and technology has narrowed consistently in the last two centuries (figure 15.3). It took 112 years from fundamental discoveries in chemistry, to every-day photography, 56 years for the development of the telephone, 35 years for a wireless receiver to be available in many homes, 15 years to develop radar, 12 years for television, 6 years to produce the atom bomb and 5 years from the discovery of the gallium transistor to the ruination of every open space in the Western world. In contrast, there has not been a steady narrowing of the gap between fundamental discovery and medical application (figure 15.4). It took 185 years for the application of Fourier mathematics to image processing, a remarkably short 40 years for the application of anaesthetics (demonstrating a vested interest in the avoidance of pain), 40 years from tomography to CT, 46 years for blood transfusion, 10 years for the development of antibiotics (stimulated by World War II), 25 years for cardiac catheterisation, 30 years for clinical organ transplantation, and 40 years for cardiovascular magnetic resonance. The reasons for the disproportionately long acceptance time in medicine are complex. The traditional conservatism of the medical profession may be due partly to the fact that medicine is a vast subject taking a major proportion of a lifetime for the assimilation of the basic facts, making doctors unwilling to abandon these facts in favour of new ideas. In addition, the method of disseminating knowledge about new ideas is inefficient. There are too many publications for the busy doctor to follow. Pseudoscientific meetings are dominated by large numbers of repetitive papers while the proceedings of serious scientific specialist meetings are not seen by practising doctors. There is also the opportunity for clinicians to shelter behind clinical responsibility, claiming that their patients should be given the best of conventional medicine and not experimented upon, even though contemporary techniques are known to be flawed and do not offer the patient the best hope.

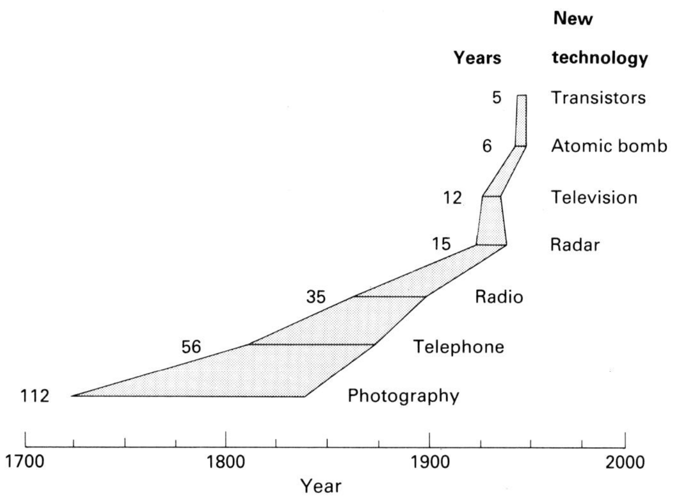

Figure 15.3. The time lapse between fundamental discovery which makes a new technology possible and its practical application has consistently narrowed in general science and technology.

Reluctance to change has been intensified by the ever-increasing publicity, sometimes anti-progress, sometimes overstated, and more often than not inaccurate reporting of pioneering medical procedures. Advanced treatment and experimental procedures on patients used to be a private matter between the patient, his relatives and the doctor. The world stage was changed by the publicity-seeking surgeons performing the first operations on Siamese twins. It became clear to other branches of medicine, particularly in countries where hospitals are dependent upon private referrals, that publicity-seeking might be used to advantage. Claims about breakthroughs were made without reference to reality. A prime example of this approach took place in the early 1960s when heart replacement became practical. There was rivalry between the artificial heart programme and heart transplantation. Large amounts of money could be got from a gullible venture capital market for the attractive but still unattainable artificial 'heart from the factory'. When Barnard transplanted a heart into Louis Waskanski in Cape Town in 1967, the world's press were pre-sensitised and what had been a private medical matter became the basis for poorly-informed public debate. No longer were the wishes or the hopes of the patient of paramount importance. Churchmen, politicians,

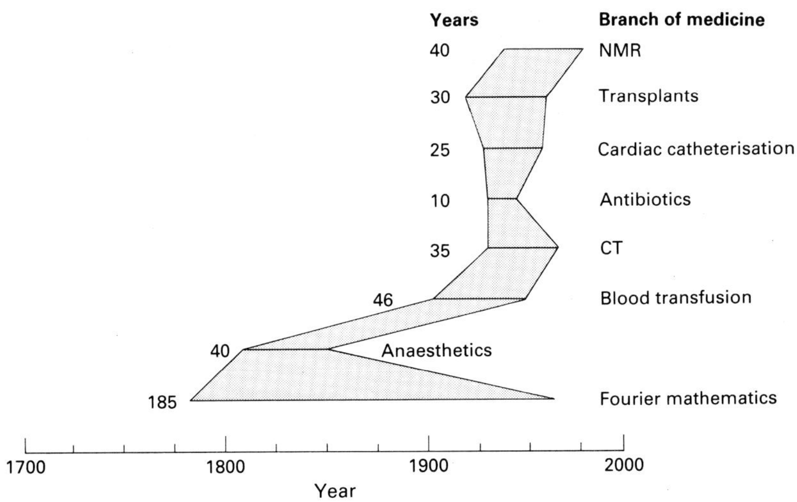

Figure 15.4. The time lapse between the fundamental discovery which makes a new branch of medicine possible has remained at about 20 years.

health-care administrators and financiers debated theoretical issues with more reference to theology and prejudice than to clinical need. From that era until the advent of cardiovascular magnetic resonance, the chances of a therapeutic revolution in medicine were diminished. Regulations, which are rarely based on measured consideration but usually on political expediency and pragmatism were introduced to supplement the control of doctors which hitherto had been the responsibility of their own ethical bodies. In 1990, political decisions about the use of precious biological material will be made without adequate medical input following debates about the use of foetal material. The creation of opportunity to regulate medicine from without is politically convenient because therapeutic life-saving procedures threaten to cost an ever greater proportion of the gross domestic product. For example, if the present rate of increasing costs of medical care continue, the USA will be spending over 20% of its GDP on medicine by the end of the century.

With all these constraints, it is likely that acceptance of cardiovascular magnetic resonance, the very vehicle which will reverse the trend of rising costs, will be unacceptably delayed. The main hurdle to overcome at the moment is finding sufficient money to buy magnetic resonance machines exclusively for cardiovascular magnetic resonance.

15.6.3 Cost

Magnetic resonance machines are still expensive and the prime cost difficult to justify to hospital authorities and grant-giving bodies. Thus manufacturers attempt to make a general purpose machine which can be sold to all potential users rather than units optimised for special applications. The cardiovascular magnetic resonance machine of the future will be very different from today's head camera. The present generation of machines are still expensive and are comparable in capital cost with PET cameras or a cardiac catheter laboratory. The machines of the 21st century will be comparable in price with Doppler ultrasound today. The running costs of a magnetic resonance unit are already lower than a catheter laboratory or a PET unit. The magnetic resonance unit can be run by a small specialised staff. The other two types of examination are multidisciplinary; the catheter laboratory needing surgical, anaesthetic, technical and radiographic skills and the PET laboratory needs staff to run the associated cyclotron.

The development costs of the present generation of magnetic resonance machines have been enormous and many have been duplicated unnecessarily. The total investment by the major manufacturers is measured in billions, and millions have been spent in replicating the technology of superconducting magnets pioneered by Oxford. The investment has not been amortised from profits from sales but by profitable maintenance contracts. Expensive maintenance will not be needed for new simpler modular machines using distributed microprocessor hardware. These will become like personal computers today, both reliable and throw-away items. Once software and hardware support are unnecessary, the stranglehold of the big manufacturers will be lost.

Since the founding of the secular and independent Royal Society in 1666 by King James, the business of science has been regulated by a strict code of conduct. Science has developed virtually unfettered by outside influences such as the Church and the Court which before that time inhibited the dissemination of unwelcome or heterodox ideas and results of experimentation. The way the system worked became the cornerstone of science. A discovery was made and publicised in a book, monograph or as a paper to be circulated amongst the scientifically literate and kept away from the masses who were not aware of what was going on. Other workers repeated the experiments or probed the hypotheses to see if they were valid (often rivalries and jealousies led to very rigorous testing). If the work was noticed, was sound and was in the mainstream, it was used as a basis for further development. This scientific discipline was 'policed' by the learned journals. Old copies of Nature contain descriptions of remarkable discoveries made by country vicars and amateur scientists as well as the professionals, all meticulously reported once only. Magnetic resonance has become the exception to the rules of science. Outside commercial influences prevail and the plethora of journals which exist to generate profit and fame pay only lip service to their role as arbiters.

The greatest driver to high cost has been the unnecessary quest for machines with a high field strength. The cost of a magnet varies as the cube of the bore and the square of the field strength, but the improvment in signal to noise increases linearly with field strength. For moving organs the position is complicated by chemical shift and motion artefact. Before most users became knowledgeable, some manufacturers succeeded in marketing the myth that a 1.5 T is ten times as good as a 0.15 T machine and that it would be possible to locate a lesion and to study its metabolism using magnetic resonance spectroscopy. This has not yet been shown to be possible, and as low-cost, low and mid-field machines become available, spectroscopy will be relegated to specialist machines in university departments. Acceptance of lower fields will allow cheaper open-access magnets.

15.6.4 Nuclear Overhauser effect

As stated above, the cost of a magnet varies as the cube of the bore and the square of the field strength. There is little that can be done about the size of the bore because the chest and the abdomen have to be fitted comfortably between the poles. The field strength however is potentially reducible. The magnetic resonance experiment depends upon getting energy in minute quantities into the nuclei of atoms and detecting the returned energy. The electrons present a barrier to these transferences of energy and theoretically if the electrons can be induced to spin in a way which enhances energy transference, the signal strength could be increased by a factor of 382. Unfortunately, the radio-frequencies required to influence electrons at the magnet field strength we are accustomed to are well into the microwave band with considerable potential for tissue damage. Field strengths low enough to exploit the nuclear Overhauser produce a very poor signal to noise ratio and it is unlikely that the beneficial effect will be more than a factor of 3 but the very low field magnets required will be a fraction of the cost of the present generation of magnets. Eventually, the magnet will consist of iron poles focusing the earth's field combined with more powerful gradients.

15.6.5 Interpretation

The radiologist is accustomed to interpreting X-ray films. Interpretation of magnetic resonance images differs in several ways. Unlike X-ray imaging, appearance in a magnetic resonance study does not depend on just two variables (dose and attenuation) to influence contrast, but many. A structure can be highlighted selectively by skilful choice of sequence, whereas an inappropriate magnetic resonance study can result in obscurity of pathology and even the suppression of important structures. There is a mass of anatomical information contained in possibly hundreds of slices in many unfamiliar planes. The appearance of the images varies widely with the choice of sequence. Each image can contain additional information about blood velocity, acceleration and chemical composition, all presented in new ways. There is no doubt that reporting an magnetic resonance scan can be daunting.

There will be changes in practice. Radiologists and cardiologists will need to be familiar with the capabilities of the different sequences and the best results will be obtained when they perform the examination themselves.

The mechanism or reporting on a magnetic resonance scan can be extremely difficult because there is so much information in a magnetic resonance study of the cardiovascular system. If a conventional, written report is to be comprehensive, it becomes too long and involved to be practical. A video moving film with annotation and a voice commentary made during the examination is easier and a more effective use of time and skill.

Cardiovascular machines will eventually be marketed as a complete diagnostic system with integral voice to hard copy as well as being equipped with a multi-standard video output which will have the capability of accepting a spoken commentary as well as annotation.

15.7 Who will use cardiovascular magnetic resonance?

It is obvious that the discipline must be run by the competent and dedicated, but will this be so? It is not obvious from which medical ranks the magnetic resonance specialists will be drawn.

When the Luftwaffe burned down part of the Parliament buildings in World War II it found surprising allies down below—the night staff of the Houses of Parliament, who refused to let the fire crews into the building, because only members and servants of Parliament had authority to enter there. On the very same night an incendiary bomb fell into a bonded warehouse, but customs officers would not let firemen into the premises without the necessary permit. The resulting fire wrecked a sorely needed wharf.

Every age and every country has its own crop of such stories, which make us heave with weary exasperation. We can be tolerant of computers that send out bills for £0.00. We do not expect fellow humans to be quite so punctilliously reflexive. Why, then are our expectations so frequently dashed? At the root of all such stories are systems that require humans to behave like computers:

Q: Has the bearer permit to enter?
A1: Yes—bearer may enter.
A2: No—bearer may not enter.

When such a binary function defines more than 80 percent of a person's job, and when that job is done for half a lifetime, it is not surprising that the person behaves with the mulish logic of a computer. Naturally no medical job is defined in such simple terms. Its basic algorithm is dressed up in the traditional finery of some service or 'in' group, and the in-group mentality is fostered by setting up insider-outsider demarcations. Outsiders who want to visit Insiderland must apply for permits, state their purposes, and show appropriate gratitude. Those who do not are spies or poachers.

At this point scientific or medical readers may recognise a vague unease. Imperceptibly the argument has moved away from a humble gatekeepers job to one that fits almost every branch of science—and every branch of medicine including radiology and cardiology. In creative science and industrial application, success justifies almost any amount of spying and poaching: but in normative science, which is what most scientists practice, either activity is a breach of accepted standards. Of course all draw lines around their various areas of work: this is thoracic, that cardiac; this is biochemical, that biophysical; those are neurotic signs, those psychotic; and so on. Such demarcations are useful only as long as we treat them like contour lines—abstract marks on our conceptual map of a given area. They help us to understand how parts of a field are related, but do not prevent us from wandering freely over it. The dangers of the other extreme are obvious, when what should be simple contours sprout barbed pickets and all the marks of a private preserve. It is in the in-between state, where the fences are genteelly unobtrusive and each specialist's right to 'his' or 'her' preserve is tacitly accepted, that insidious damage can be done.

Nowhere does this argument apply more clearly than in medicine. Our field of study, the human animal, collective and individual, is carved up among several hundred specialisations. The divisions are scored ever deeper by the career structure where remuneration and prestige depend in part on protectionism. The methods of funding research, the attitude of administrative bodies and the success and even the survival of each given area of specialisation depend on its keeping to itself a given area.

Because most advances in magnetic resonance (even the discipline itself) come from without the medical profession it is not obvious which speciality should be entrusted with its care and development or even whether a new discipline is needed. Concentrating cardiovascular magnetic resonance in one particular area, say, radiology or cardiology, without regard to the overall needs of society, the prevention of the most common diseases, is quickly subject to the law of diminishing returns. It will be important to unite the relevant fragments of medicine if magnetic resonance is to fulfil its potential, indeed if we fail to work towards medical unity the goal of a healthy cardiovascular system will, like the rainbow's end, recede before us as fast as we pursue it. A broad, wide base is needed. Epidemiologists and those interested in preventive medicine may eventually give cardiovascular magnetic resonance it best chance.

Peter Ustinov tells a story that reveals the close affinity between specialisation and lunacy. A golfer early in his round drove a ball clean off the links. When later he got back to the clubhouse he found it in uproar. 'Whats the matter?' he asked the professional coach. 'Have you not heard?' said the pro. 'Someone drove off the links and hit a cyclist who fell in front of a school bus. The bus swerved to avoid him and overturned down an embankment. Forty children dead'. 'I drove that ball,' said the golfer, 'What can I do?' 'You should try holding the club a little more like this,' said the pro, demonstrating.

There are few specialist doctors with any insight who can laugh at this particular story with a completely easy conscience. For most of us who really care about patients our specialities are as important and all consuming as golf was to that pro. The dunce's cap with which we should have crowned the parliamentary watchman and customs officers begins to look and feel uncomfortably like the ceremonial headgear we ourselves wear on formal academic occasions.

This line of thought has been forced on me by the commitment to decide who would give magnetic resonance cardiology its best chance of turning promise into performance. Its future is not only as a safe and patient acceptable non-invasive comprehensive diagnostic technique giving more accurate information than we are used to, but also as a vehicle for change from the management of end-stage cardiovascular disease to prevention.

The problem is deeper than just the unification of doctors with different training and knowledge bases.

Magnetic resonance is a physics based technology, it was conceived by physicists, developed by physicists but is used, often in an empirical way, by doctors. Should physicists be in charge? The medical users may not understand a nuclear spin quantum number of 3/2, how spatial resolution is achieved using phase encoded gradients and how the image, which can be made to contain information about velocity and chemical composition, is produced, but they do know what they are looking for and can guide the physicists, diverting them from fascinating esoteric problems the solution of which leads into a by-way.

Some reasonably successful magnetic resonance units are 'physics driven', others are based on diagnostic radiology departments, and a few are run by cardiologists. All of these have their unique shortcomings. The most successful cardiac magnetic resonance research units are idiosyncratic depending on leadership which owes no allegiance to any of the traditional areas. They have a structure based on equality between physicists and clinicians. Even this symbiosis is insufficient for progress. A third group of clinical scientists, mostly medically qualified with additional scientific training, who know what the magnetic resonance physics can do and the requirements of clinical application, are needed to translate physicists' basic discoveries into practical clinical techniques.

People envisaged a time when two scientists in closely related fields would hardly understand each other. Experience is precisely the reverse. No matter how obscure and remote-seeming the science in apparently unrelated aspects of cardiovascular magnetic resonance, there is often something to be found which is seen to be relevant by a receptive mind.

Far from allowing physicists and clinicians to compete for power or grow apart there should be the strongest incentive for them to unite; we desperately need a community of action that depends on something more substantial than coincidence.

The classic example of a community of that kind was the Manhattan Project, which led to the first fission bombs. It united just about every known physical and chemical science in one joint effort. If the atom bomb had depended on the haphazard serendipidity we rely on to develop and use magnetic resonance, the world would still be wondering if Rutherford hadn't been right when he said that the atom would never provide man with a source of power.

What was it that brought together, on the one hand physicists so abstract that they were practically philosophers and, on the other, high-voltage engineers who tended to scoff at equations that included the square root of -1? It was more than administrative decision, or organisation, or money. The nature of the project soon convinced such radically different workers that they belonged to the same team. Above all though, they were able to relate to one another because of the work of men like Einstein, Bohr, Planck, Rutherford, Cockcroft and Heisenberg who had provided a uniform conceptual framework for their operation. A remarkably similar framework forms the basis of magnetic resonance physics, we need only to add the names of Fourier, Bloch, Purcell, and Hounsfield for completeness. The complexity of magnetic resonance itself and its application to cardiology is daunting and there is no hope that some unified equations of medicine and physics will pop into some thinker's mind and that the whole field of combining physics and preventive cardiology will suddenly be lit with a single light of crystalline clarity and undreamed of intensity. Realising this we might be forgiven for concluding that our field has no conceptual unity. As a result, for example, designers of magnets, computer programmers, paediatric cardiologists, epidemiologists and radio-frequency, electrical and mechanical engineers may feel little in common with one another. Such resignation is shortsighted and harmful. A concept does not have to be universal (like $E = mc^2$) in order to provide a form of unity in our field. But it must be fundamental enough to relate to the prime purpose of understanding human physiology and departures from the normal.

It is not clear in 1990 which discipline will win the irrelevant (and trivial) 'turf battle' which is already waging between radiologists and cardiologists to the near exclusion of the essential physicists. What is clear however is that unified teams will continue to dominate real scientific advance. The scientific advance is so important that grant-giving bodies must act responsibly and support original fundamental magnetic resonance work. Many millions are spent on magnetic resonance research. How cost effective is this vast expenditure? For commercial reasons, industrial expenditure is subject to market perceived forces and misguided planning results from misjudgment.

Unfortunately, efficiency does not always enter the picture in awarding grants. Research funds handled by government, universities and the older charities are scrutinised by accountants looking for irregularities—

not by investment manager types looking for return. Cost effectiveness is often low and the mechanism stochastic. Department A gets money out of charity X with the voting support of faculty B. Faculty B of course will rely on the support of department A next time round.

15.8 The place of magnetic resonance in the grand design

Magnetic resonance is the most powerful diagnostic technique so far developed. (It is important to recognise that magnet-related diagnosis is in no way therapeutic. The use of lodestone to cure headache was finally debunked in the early part of the 16th century.) The very words 'diagnosis' and 'therapy' symbolise the nominal and unreal divisions that history has forced upon us and that continue to trap us until this day. In the 18th century, doctors had thousands of remedies for diseases they could not accurately recognise. The 19th century went into praiseworthy reaction—which as in so many other fields it overdid: no remedy should be attempted, was the rule until accurate diagnosis had been made. The pendulum swung too far and diagnosis became an end in itself. The great men of medicine had but one function: to pin down disease with the same superior mastery that Sherlock Holmes and his many lookalikes displayed in pinning down criminals. Once the great diagnosticians had spoken, the management of the patient could be left to lesser men—surgeons, junior doctors and general practitioners, just as Holmes left his criminals to the slower-witted police. In many fields, this unhealthy division between diagnosis and therapy (even between primary treatment and after care) persists today.

What is diagnosis? It is a process for extracting information from a complex, interdependent, intercommunicating set of physical and chemical events (the reason for resorting to this cumbersome definition will soon become clear). And therapy? It is a process for changing those same events so that they either revert to a normal pattern or assume a new state of equilibrium. In short, these two elements correspond to the two processes we can discern in any complex control circuit: feedback and control. Both are fundamentally involved in the handling of information—inward and outward bound. To ensure that we are not now pursuing a mere analogy, we need only look at the power levels involved in each element.

In any cybernetic system it is of the essence that the energy consumed by the sensing elements (thermostats, voltmeters, rev counters, etc.) should be minute compared with the energy consumed to maintain or change the system. Thermostats do actually cool the rooms that house them, but pity the man who sets out to measure the loss to the room. Similarly, in diagnosis, those methods that rely on physiological energy consume a minute proportion of it. An electrocardiogram, for instance, consumes energy in the microjoule range to record a single heartbeat. This is the electrical energy that, tapped from the body and amplified, moves the pen. Similarly, the receiver aerial of a magnetic resonance machine removes some energy from the patient. The heartbeat itself consumes between 40 and 400 joules, and the therapeutic restarting of the heart consumes 300 joules of energy in one powerful shock. These relationships between the energy demands of the feedback and command circuits are characteristic of all efficient self-regulating systems. Cardiovascular magnetic resonance is a little different from the electrocardiogram in that energy is added to perturb the system and to measuring the return of the system to equilibrium. It is essential, therefore, that the magnetic resonance experiment should be confined to energies which are small in proportion to the natural processes of the body.

In short, therefore, the entity that unites both diagnosis and therapy is information, and this same entity provides that fundamental unifying concept mentioned earlier in this chapter. Life is a system obsessed with information. The genes that control our growth, our defences, our susceptibilities—and often, too, our manner of death—are no more than four chemicals of a particular architecture arranged in particular sequences that constitute a code. They operate, in turn, through molecules (enzymes) of a precise architecture that determine both mode and speed of interaction. Thus the network of chemical pathways we call metabolism is the information network of a homeostat. Even in sickness it remains an efficient network; to be sure, it is then processing wrong information or using wrong channels, but it is nonetheless a functioning network. Only in terminal states, when the volume of informational traffic falls below the critical volume that makes for a self-adjusting therefore self-sustaining, living organism, do the strands of the network begin to fall apart.

Medical machines are adjuncts to this information network. They work either by extending existing channels (as in biochemical analysis) or by providing

Table 15.1. Diagnostic and therapeutic procedures from many areas of medicine in relation to the arenas in which they operate. Such a classification emphasises the wide-ranging abilities of magnetic resonance

Interaction between:	Macrosystems (direct)	Macrosystems (indirect)	Microsystems	Molecular systems
Medium:	Physical manipulation	Sound, magnetic resonance	Vision, magnetic resonance	Chemical activity, magnetic resonance
Subject:	Large systems	Large and microsopic	Cells	Molecules
Examples:	Physical examination Sphygmomanometer Thermometer Surgery Physiotherapy Cardio-pulmonary bypass Renal dialysis	Magnetic resonance (imaging) Radiology Electrocardiogram Ultrasound Nuclear medicine Pacemakers Psychotherapy Radiotherapy	Magnetic resonance (chemical shift imaging) Histology Haematology Immunisation	Magnetic resonance (spectroscopy) Biochemistry Chemotherapy

new channels, unknown in nature (as in magnetic resonance). By classifying these channels—or, more strictly, the arenas within which these channels are linked—we arrive at a kind of spectrum, somewhere along which any given diagnostic machine (including of course the magnetic resonance machine) can be placed. It is therefore important to determine where the magnetic resonance machine fits into this spectrum. This will indicate whether magnetic resonance is another trivial diagnostic instrument or whether it has a fundamental place in the management of disease. Later, we shall argue that it has a specific place in allowing harmless population screening so that the transition to the era of post-Hippocratic (preventive) medicine can be achieved.

Such a spectrum is shown in table 15.1. Obviously many more subdivisions could be made, but, because the idea of classifying diagnosis in this way will be novel to many, it is limited to four simple arenas. The first two relate to the familiar macroscopic world, the world which can be manipulated in real time and the resultant activity observed. The second two cover the microscopic and quantum arenas, where the real biological action is but where our approach before magnetic resonance was clumsy and circuitous. The contrast between the two could hardly be greater. There are a vast range of machines that operate in real time at the macroscopic level—a level at which it is really quite impossible to manipulate the bionetwork in any but the grossest ways; and until magnetic resonance there were only slow, cumbersome, off-line machines (none therapeutic) that let us probe the mysteries of that network, but not yet in real time.

The nature of biological activity places fundamental limits on the improvements that can be made at the macrosystem level. We are close to a state of diminishing returns already. That is to say, we can make machines handier, more stable and more reliable but, great though these advances may be, they will not yield fundamentally new kinds of information about the human organism. For instance, we shall probably soon be able to record the electrocardiogram by radiotelemetry using devices that will slip into a vest pocket and yet be sophisticated enough to monitor the heartbeat of at-risk patients and give them, and the hospital looking after them, 2 or 3 hours warning of an impending attack (at least, of those attacks that signal their onset in electrocardiographic abnormalities). Such an advance would be of benefit to many sufferers. It would be wrong to suggest that this and similar developments should not be pursued vigorously and nothing in this chapter should be construed as an attempt to denigrate improvements in instrumentation. But we delude ourselves if we think that ultimate progress lies along a path strewn with piecemeal advances in physics and engineering. Real hopes must surely be pinned on the new insights into living chemistry, which until recently was the Cinderella of bio-engineering. It is this chemistry that magnetic resonance promises to analyse at first indirectly by functional measurements then by direct analysis.

All the activities called 'living' are under chemical control. It has been shown that many conditions not previously thought to have a significant genetic component, such as dental caries, coronary thrombosis and diabetes, have at least in part a genetic basis. Indeed, it is probable that growth, disease, and natural aging without the ravages of acquired occlusive vascular disease are all aspects of the same genetic process. If so, the prospects for medical progress aided by magnetic resonance are bright indeed. For it is no longer necessary to think of the genes as being locked away in some unattainable Mendelian fastness; we know plenty of chemicals that can get at them—all, alas, harmful—but nevertheless it shows that the genes are not beyond our reach. We know, too, that natural pathways exist for turning the genes on and off, as it were. The most stupendous example of this is in the creation of a complete animal, a frog,[6] not by the conventional processes that have evolved over millions of years but by removing the nucleus from an egg and replacing it with the nucleus of a cell taken from the intestine of an already advanced tadpole. The characteristics of the resulting frog are thus determined entirely by a nucleus taken from a specialised cell. The fact that the frog is in every way indistinguishable from others of its species shows that all the information needed for the development of an entire organism is contained in the nucleus of every cell in that organism's body. And from this it follows that during specialisation, cells do not lose genetic information, but merely switch off the genes they do not need (in practice, most of the genes are thus switched off). This experiment shows that, in at least one set of circumstances (nuclear transplantation), all those genes can be reactivated. From other studies we know that genes can be diverted from their purpose (this is how viruses persuade our cells to stop making normal protein and to replicate viruses instead) and that they can change during life (the genetic abnormalities of cancer being an example). More recently, the techniques for producing recombinant DNA—genetic engineering—have been used.

To sum up: all biological activity is under genetic control, and genes can be diverted, modified, and switched on and off. Here is the basis for fundamental advance in medicine which has been recognised by the major government-sponsored funding bodies in the USA and the UK, the National Institute of Health and the Medical Research Council. Only from such premises can we develop the magnetic resonance machines that will eventually fill out the two threadbare columns of our spectrum, and enable us to delete 'off-line' and substitute 'on-line and real-time.'

15.9 Population screening

Magnetic resonance population screening has already been touched on. Magnetic resonance offers for the first time a non-invasive and accurate method of establishing normal performance in the cardiovascular system. It will not be enough merely to know the normal ranges of, say, right atrial contribution to cardiac output, normal velocity in the left renal artery, right ventricular mass in smokers and non-smokers, invaluable those these might be. On their own they are not nearly enough. It will be necessary to correlate these ranges with one another and full information profiles. By the time the young readers of this chapter are approaching middle age, it will be considered inferior practice to diagnose or treat a patient (except in emergencies which with proper health maintenance will be less common) without a full knowledge of his or her cardiovascular performance over a period of time. The profiles will also include personality, aptitudes, preference, habits and disease patterns, in fact any factor which shows some significant relationship. Even today, those who doubt the value of such a philosophy should remember that we could improve the efficiency of medicine by any chosen yardstick by improved diagnosis, even if there were no matching advance in therapy. Attempts to correlate risk factors for cardiovascular disease are the norm. However the correlations are always limited and the proponents of the risk factor philosophy are reluctant to admit that they may not even be aware of the major factors. Careful correlation of normal ranges established by magnetic resonance will offer much more powerful studies of the factors influencing disease. As an example, everybody knows that lung cancer correlates with smoking. How many however remember that lung cancer also correlates significantly with coffee drinking, with sugar intake, eating of spicy food, a high rate of sexual intercourse, with body type, with personality and with emotional type. There must be many other factors as yet unknown, notably the genes which are at the heart of the correlation. The genes are the predisposing factors and some of the other correlations are multipliers—including smoking, one of the most powerful multipliers of all. As doctors in our present state of ignorance, we are justified in a blanket condemnation of smoking. We are right to advise every patient to give it up, but as biologists we must be fascinated by the fact that some are more susceptible than others, with the possibility that occasional people could chain smoke all their lives and live a full life without developing lung cancer, bronchitis, emphysema, occlusive vascular disease, bladder cancer or any of the other ailments that correlate with smoking. In the same way, there appear to be people who can gorge on cholesterol-rich foods, grow obese and never suffer a hint of vascular occlusions just as there are patients who do all the right things yet fall victim to disease after disease. The classical response to this seeming injustice, the effects of fate, is now no longer acceptable. It is known that the onset of a disease or disorder is not the result of some cosmic dice rattle but the result of multiple aetiological factors in our environment. If we can use magnetic resonance to study the normal and to pin down these factors for each disease, we could use magnetic resonance to turn medicine into a truly predictive science. No longer will we need to tell patients that they have a number of risk factors which may cause blockage of vital arteries but we may be able to tell each individual, for example, that he must change his lifestyle or he will inevitably succumb or, on the other hand, his chances if he continues in his lifestyle of major cardiovascular disease are so remote that he can disregard them.

The mechanism of the major killing diseases will not be understood until there is a new insight into every field of medicine. We still say, for instance, that colds are caused by viruses. In fact, colds merely correlate highly with virus invasion but not vice versa, that is not all virus invasions lead to colds even amongst people who have no antibodies against the viruses in question. Why, therefore, do such people not catch cold despite their lack of orthodox defence? If we really understood disease processes, there should be no difficulty in framing an answer to this question. The fact that it cannot be answered is just another aspect of the lamentably backward state of modern medicine which has been based on high-tech curative procedures. At least it is possible to pinpoint the deficiencies in our thinking with some accuracy and it is possible to map a path along which improvements must lie. When magnetic resonance has been used intelligently to show what correlates positively or negatively with the established normal, it will be possible to ask 'why' questions with some certainty that answers exist. Why, for instance, do extroverts with strong libidos, excitable tempers, a taste for rich foods and cigarettes, suffer more from lung cancer than unemotional, undersexed introverts who like plain food and do not smoke. This simple question can be asked because a great amount of research has been done into this one disease. When similar studies of cardiovascular disease have been made using the opportunities given by the new instrument, as yet unsuspected patterns will emerge. The patterns will suggest mechanisms, the mechanisms will generate theories, the theories will demand testing. To test these theories, it will be necessary to refine magnetic resonance machines and eventually the empty columns in the spectrum of disease will be filled.

If magnetic resonance is to achieve its promise as a comprehensive cardiovascular diagnostic instrument and a screening tool, original thinking and not rehashed applications of present-day measurements and concepts will need to be applied. Rather than debating whether magnetic resonance can be used to mimic existing tests and whether X-ray based procedures can be replaced by quantitative magnetic resonance studies, the following questions should be addressed:

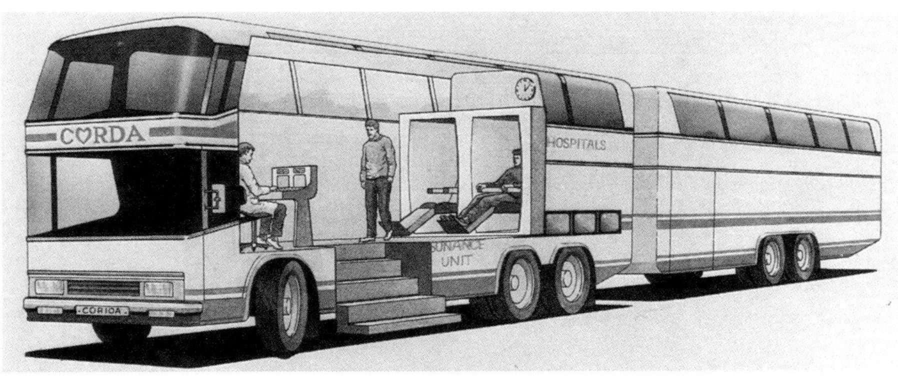

Figure 15.5. An artist's impression of a new generation machine with one common back-end combined with a new type of open-access magnet using both poles of a superconducting coil combined with iron reflector plates. The unit is designed to incorporate educational video equipment as part of the contribution of magnetic resonance to a better understanding by the general public of the natural history and the causative factors of acquired cardiovascular disease in response to the public demand for better care discussed at the beginning of this chapter. The trailer could house a similar unit.

- Is occlusive vascular disease an inescapable part of the ageing process or is it preventable?
- What is the natural history of the disease process before it produces symptoms?
- Are preventive and therapeutic measures likely to arrest or even reverse the formation of lethal plaques?
- Can magnetic resonance imaging answer these questions?

The answer to the first of these questions has already been shown to be in the affirmative. There is no doubt that the remainder of these fundamental questions will not be answered affirmatively as soon as they should unless the medical profession uses magnetic resonance wisely and that equipment manufacturers produce appropriate machines.

The answer to the last of these questions could and should also be in the affirmative. It is likely that by the end of the forecast period, new generation 'back-end' systems capable of serving two one-shot images using a simple central microprocessor and distributed dedicated boards with many megaflops of memory will be generally available. These will be combined with innovative magnets which will use both poles of the magnet projecting 'balls' of magnetism into space and these will be incorporated in mobile units for population screening. Such a unit of the future is depicted in figure 15.5.

15.10 Power equals responsibility

The magnetic resonance cardiovascular machine promises to become the Promethean machine which will displace most other cardiovascular diagnosis. It will fall to the unpusillanimous doctors (whoever they may be) and physicists to take the great opportunity offered by magnetic resonance and to use it to benefit both patients and potential patients from the normal population as quickly as possible cutting across the traditional medical obstacles to progress.

Certainly, like all advances of great potential benefit, I can only end by saying how I should hope to use them if I lived that long. And, like everyone who delivers an ethical opinion, I like to feel that my morality springs from something more than the local needs and customs of my own time. It is possibly a delusion, but I should like to foster it by going back three centuries for one of its most perfect expressions, in Dryden's Oedipus, the play he wrote with Nathaniel Lee:

Of no distemper, of no blast he died,
But fell like autumn-fruit that mellowed long,
Ev'n wondered at because he dropp'd no sooner.
Fate seemed to wind him up for fourscore years
Yet freely ran he on ten winters more;
'Till, like a clock worn out with eating time,
The weary wheels of life at last stood still.

Any medical worker would surely be proud to have helped offer such a life and such a way of going to anyone who wanted it.

References

1 Editorial. *Med Sci Res* 1989; **17**: 536.
2 Marmot MG, Davey Smith G. Why are the Japanese living longer? *Br Med J* 1989; **299**: 1547–51.
3 *Medicine in the 1990s: a Technological Forecast*. London: Office of Health Economics, 1969.
4 Bogren HG, Mohiaddin RH, Klipstein RH, *et al*. The function of the aorta in ischaemic heart disease: a magnetic resonance and angiographic study of aortic compliance and flow patterns. *Am Heart J* 1989; **118**: 234–47.
5 Bogren HG, Klipstein RH, Firmin DN, *et al*. Quantitation of antegrade and retrograde blood flow in the human aorta by magnetic resonance velocity mapping. *Am Heart J* 1989; **117**: 1214–22.
6 Burch P. *An Inquiry Concerning Growth, Disease and Ageing*. London: Oliver and Boyd, 1968.

Index

Page references in italic indicate figures